Evidence-Based Orthodontics

Evidence-Based Orthodontics

Second Edition

Edited by

Greg J. Huang

School of Dentistry
University of Washington
Seattle
Washington, USA

Stephen Richmond

School of Dentistry
Cardiff University
Cardiff
Wales, UK

Katherine W. L. Vig

Harvard School of Dental Medicine
Boston
Massachusetts, USA

WILEY Blackwell

Registered Office(s)
John Wiley & Sons, Inc., 111 River Street, Hoboken, NJ 07030, USA

Editorial Office
111 River Street, Hoboken, NJ 07030, USA

Library of Congress Cataloging-in-Publication Data

Names: Huang, Greg J., editor. | Richmond, Stephen, editor. | Vig, Katherine W. L., editor.
Title: Evidence-based orthodontics / edited by Greg J. Huang, Stephen Richmond, Katherine W.L. Vig.
Description: 2nd edition. | Hoboken, NJ : Wiley, 2018. | Includes bibliographical references and index. |
Identifiers: LCCN 2018010564 (print) | LCCN 2018011366 (ebook) | ISBN 9781119289920 (pdf) |
    ISBN 9781119289951 (epub) | ISBN 9781119289913 (paperback)
Subjects: | MESH: Orthodontics | Malocclusion | Evidence-Based Dentistry
Classification: LCC RK521 (ebook) | LCC RK521 (print) | NLM WU 400 | DDC 617.6/43–dc23
LC record available at https://lccn.loc.gov/2018010564

Cover Design: Wiley
Cover Images: (Dental images) Courtesy of Greg J. Huang; (Pyramid) Courtesy of Wiley

Set in 10/12pt Warnock by SPi Global, Pondicherry, India
Printed and bound in Singapore by Markono Print Media Pte Ltd

10 9 8 7 6 5 4 3 2 1

Contents

List of Contributors

Azrul Safuan Mohd Ali, BDS
Applied Clinical Research and Public Health
School of Dentistry
College of Biomedical and Life Sciences
Cardiff University
Cardiff, UK

Matina V. Angelopoulou, DDS, MS
Department of Developmental Sciences
Marquette University School of Dentistry
Milwaukee, WI, USA

Philip Benson, BDS, PhD, FDS(Orth)
Academic Unit of Oral Health, Dentistry and Society
School of Clinical Dentistry
University of Sheffield
Sheffield, UK

Niko Bock, DMD
Department of Orthodontics
University of Giessen
Giessen, Germany

Anne-Marie Bollen, DDS, MS, PhD
Department of Orthodontics
University of Washington
Seattle, WA, USA

Macario Camacho, MD
Otolaryngology-Head and Neck Surgery
Division of Sleep Surgery and Medicine
Tripler Army Medical Center
Honolulu, HI, USA

Stephanie Shih-Hsuan Chen, DDS, MSD
Taipei City
Taiwan

Domenico Dalessandri, DDS, MS, PhD
Department of Orthodontics
School of Dentistry
University of Brescia
Brescia, Italy

Scott Deacon, BDS, MSc, MFDS, MOrth, FDS(Orth)
South West Cleft Service
University Hospitals Bristol NHS Foundation Trust
and University of Bristol
Bristol, UK

Damian Farnell, BSc, PhD
Applied Clinical Research and Public Health School
of Dentistry
College of Biomedical and Life Sciences
Cardiff University
Cardiff, UK

Camilo Fernandez-Salvador, MD
Otolaryngology-Head and Neck Surgery
Tripler Army Medical Center
Honolulu, HI, USA

**Padhraig Fleming, BDent Sc (Hons),
MSc, PhD, FDS RCS, MFDS RCS, FDS RCS,
MOrth RCS, FDS (Orth) RCS, FHEA**
Barts and The London School of Medicine and
Dentistry
Queen Mary University of London
London, UK

Carlos Flores Mir, DDS, DSc, FRCD
Department of Dentistry
University of Alberta
Edmonton, Alberta, Canada

James Fricton, DDS, MS
School of Dentistry
University of Minnesota
Minneapolis, MN, USA

Jennifer Galloway, BDS, BMSc, MDSc, MFDS RCPS
Applied Clinical Research and Public
Health School of Dentistry
College of Biomedical and Life Sciences
Cardiff University
Cardiff, UK

Geoff Greenlee, DDS, MSD, MPH
Department of Orthodontics
University of Washington
Seattle, WA, USA

Gordon Guyatt, MD, MSc, FRCP, OC
Department of Medicine
McMaster University
Hamilton, Ontario, Canada

Jayne Harrison, BDS, MDentSci, PhD, MOrth RCSEd, FDS(Orth)RCPS, FDTFEd
Orthodontic Department
Liverpool University Dental Hospital
Liverpool, UK

Hong He, MDS, PhD
Department of Orthodontics
School and Hospital of Stomatology
Wuhan University
Wuhan, Hubel,China

Fang Hua, BDS, MSc, PhD
Department of Orthodontics and Center for
Evidence-Based Stomatology
School and Hospital of Stomatology
Wuhan University
Wuhan, Hubei, China

Greg J. Huang, DMD, MSD, MPH
Department of Orthodontics
University of Washington
Seattle, WA, USA

Guilherme Janson, DDS, MSc, PhD, MRCDC
Department of Orthodontics
Bauru Dental School
University of São Paulo
Bauru, São Paulo, Brazil

Eleftherios G. Kaklamanos, DDS, Cert, MSc, MA, Dr Med
Hamdan Bin Mohammed College of Dental
Medicine
Mohammed Bin Rashid University of
Medicine and Health Sciences
Dubai, United Arab Emirates

Visnja Katic, PhD, DMD
Research Assistant
Department of Orthodontics
Faculty of Medicine
University of Rijeka
Rijeka, Croatia

O. P. Kharbanda, BDS, MDS, M Orth RCS, M MEd, FDS RCS, Hon, FAMS
Division of Orthodontics and Dentofacial
Deformities
Centre for Dental Education and Research
All India Institute of Medical Sciences
New Delhi, India

Malcolm Kohler, MD
Department of Pulmonology
University Hospital Zurich
Zurich, Switzerland

Vasiliki Koretsi, DDS, Dr Med Dent
Department of Orthodontics
University Hospital Regensburg Regensburg
Germany

Eleni Koumpridou, DDS, DOrth
Department of Orthodontics
Center for Dental and Maxillofacial Health
Medical Faculty
University of Wuerzburg
Wuerzburg, Germany

Wenli Lai, DDS, PhD
State Key Laboratory of Oral Diseases and
Department of Orthodontics
West China Hospital of Stomatology
Sichuan University
Chengdu, China

Débora A. Lentini-Oliveira, DDS, MSc
Neuro-Sono Sleep Center
Department of Neurology
Federal University of São Paulo
São Paulo, Brazil

Anne Littlewood, BA(Hons), MA, MPhil
Cochrane Oral Health
University of Manchester
Manchester, UK

Simon J. Littlewood, BDS, FDS(Orth)RCPS,
MDSc, MOrth RCS
Orthodontic Department
St Luke's Hospital
Bradford, UK

Claudia Trindade Mattos, DDS, MSD, PhD
Department of Orthodontics
School of Dentistry
Universidade Federal Fluminense
Niterói, Brazil

Marcello Melis, DMD, PharmD
Private Practice
Cagliari, Italy

Reint Meursinge Reynders, DDS, MS, MSc, PhD
Milan
Italy

Declan Millett, BDSc, DDS, FDSRCPS, FDSRCS,
DOrthRCSEng, MOrthRCSEng, FHEA
Oral Health and Development
Cork University Dental School and Hospital
University College
Cork, Ireland

Peter Ngan, DMD
Department of Orthodontics
West Virginia University
Morgantown, WV, USA

Riccardo Nucera, DDS, PhD, MSc
Department of Biomedical and Dental Sciences
and Morphofunctional Imaging
Section of Orthodontics
School of Dentistry
University of Messina
Messina, Italy

Kevin O'Brien, BDS, FDS, DOrth RCS, PhD
School of Dentistry
University of Manchester
Manchester, UK

S. H. Ong, DDS
Department of Orthodontics
University Medical Center Groningen
University of Groningen
Groningen, The Netherlands

Nikolaos Pandis, DDS, MS dr. Med Dent MSc,
DLSHTM, PhD
Department of Orthodontics and Dentofacial
Orthopedics
Dental School/Medical Faculty
University of Bern
Bern, Switzerland

Moschos Papadopoulos, DDS, Dr Med Dent
Department of Orthodontics
School of Dentistry
Aristotle University of Thessaloniki
Thessaloniki, Greece

Spyridon N. Papageorgiou, DDS,
Dr Med Dent
Clinic of Orthodontics and Pediatric Dentistry
Center of Dental Medicine
University of Zurich
Zurich, Switzerland

Pertti Pirttiniemi, DDS, PhD
Professor and Chair
Oral Development and Orthodontics
Institute of Dentistry
University of Oulu
Oulu University Hospital
Medical Research Center
Finland

Lauren K. Reckley, MD
Otolaryngology-Head and Neck Surgery
Tripler Army Medical Center
Honolulu, HI, USA

Yijin Ren, DDS, MSc, PhD
Department of Orthodontics
University Medical Center Groningen
University of Groningen
Groningen, The Netherlands

Stephen Richmond, BDS, D'Orth, RCS, MScD, FDS, RCS (Ed & Eng), PhD FHEA
Applied Clinical Research and Public Health
School of Dentistry
College of Biomedical and Life Sciences
Cardiff University
Cardiff, Wales, UK

Anibal M. Silveira, DDS
Department of Orthodontics, Pediatric Dentistry
and Special Care
School of Dentistry
University of Louisville
Louisville, KY, USA

Badri Thiruvenkatachari, BDS, MFDS RCS, MDS, MOrth RCS, FDS RCS, PhD
School of Dentistry
University of Manchester
Manchester, UK

Alessandro Ugolini, DDS, PhD, Spec. Orthodontics
Orthodontics Department
University of Genoa
Genoa, Italy

Aslıhan Uzel, DDS, PhD
Department of Orthodontics
Faculty of Dentistry
Çukurova University
Balcalı, Turkey

Alexandre R. Vieira, DDS, MS, PhD
University of Pittsburgh
School of Dental Medicine
Pittsburgh, PA, USA

Katherine W. L. Vig, BDS, MS, D.Orth, FDS RCS
Department of Developmental Biology
Harvard School of Dental Medicine
Boston, MA, USA

Yan Wang, DDS, PhD
Department of Orthodontics
Laboratory of Oral Diseases
West China Hospital of Stomatology
Sichuan University
Chengdu, Sichuan, China

Belinda Weltman, HBSc, MSc, DMD, MS, FRCD(C)
University of British Columbia
Vancouver, British Columbia, Canada

Robert J. Weyant, MS, DMD, DrPH
Department of Dental Public Health
School of Dental Medicine
University of Pittsburgh
Pittsburgh, PA, USA

Caryl Wilson-Nagrani, BDS, MFDS(RCSEng), MOrth(RCSEd), FDSOrth(RCSEd), PhD, FHEA
Applied Clinical Research and Public
Health School of Dentistry
College of Biomedical and Life Sciences
Cardiff University
Cardiff, UK

Anastasios Zafeiriadis, DDS, MSc, DrDent
Department of Orthodontics
School of Dentistry, Faculty of Health Sciences
Aristotle University of Thessaloniki
Thessaloniki, Greece

Khalid H. Zawawi, BDS, DSc
Department of Orthodontics
Faculty of Dentistry
King Abdulaziz University
Jeddah, Saudi Arabia

Alexei Zhurov, BSc, MSc, PhD
Applied Clinical Research and Public Health
School of Dentistry
College of Biomedical and Life Sciences
Cardiff University
Cardiff, UK

Vasileios F. Zymperdikas, DDS
Department of Orthodontics
Faculty of Dentistry
Aristotle University of Thessaloniki
Thessaloniki, Greece

Foreword

Evidenced based orthodontics (EBO) provides tools for using the relevant literature to determine the benefits and risks of alternative patient management strategies in the context of the individual patient's presenting condition.

The term evidence-based medicine (EBM) first appeared in the medical literature in 1991; it rapidly became something of a mantra. EBM is sometimes perceived as a blinkered adherence to randomized trials, or a health-care manager's tool for controlling and constraining recalcitrant physicians. In fact, EBM and EBO involve informed and effective use of all types of evidence, but particularly evidence from the medical literature, in patient care.

EBM's evolution has included outward expansion – we now realize that optimal health care delivery must include evidence-based nursing, physiotherapy, occupational therapy, and podiatry – and specialization. We need evidence-based obstetrics, gynaecology, internal medicine, and surgery – and, indeed, orthopedics and neurosurgery. And, of course, we need evidence-based orthodontics.

Applying EBO to management decisions in individual patients involves use of a hierarchy of study design, with high-quality randomized trials showing definitive results directly applicable to an individual patient at the apex, to relying on physiological rationale or previous experience with a small number of similar patients near the bottom rung. Ideally, systematic reviews and meta-analyses summarize the highest quality available evidence. The hallmark of evidence-based practitioners is that, for particular clinical decisions, they know the quality of the evidence, and therefore the degree of uncertainty.

What is required to practice EBO? Practitioners must know how to frame a clinical quandary to facilitate use of the literature in its resolution. Evidence-based orthodontic practitioners must know how to search the literature efficiently to obtain the best available evidence bearing on their question, to evaluate the strength of the methods of the studies they find, extract the clinical message, apply it back to the patient, and store it for retrieval when faced with similar patients in the future.

Traditionally, neither dental schools nor medical schools or postgraduate programs have taught these skills. Although this situation is changing, the biggest influence on how trainees will practice is their clinical role models, few of whom are currently accomplished EBO practitioners. The situation is even more challenging for those looking to acquire the requisite skills after completing their clinical training.

This text primarily addresses the needs of both trainees and of this last group, orthodontic practitioners. Appearing over 25 years after the term EBM was coined, the text represents a landmark in a number of ways. The book represents a successful effort to comprehensively address the EBO-related learning needs of the orthodontic community, and summarize the key areas of orthodontic practice.

To achieve its goals of facilitating evidence-based orthodontic practice, the text begins with chapters that introduce the tools for evaluating the original orthodontic literature, including research designs, searching for relevant trials, and making sense of randomized trials and systematic reviews. Those interested in delving deeper into issues of how to evaluate the literature, and apply it to patient care, can consult a definitive text, the *Users' Guides to the Medical Literature* (Guyatt G et al. 3rd edition, McGraw-Hill Education, 2015).

The current text goes on to provide evidence summaries to guide each of the key common problems of orthodontic practice. Thorough and up to date at the time of writing, they provide a definitive guide to evidence-based orthodontic practice today – with over 50 brief summaries of relevant evidence including self-ligating versus conventional brackets, the impact of orthodontic treatment on apical root resorption, and the success rates for temporary anchorage devices.

That evidence will, of course, change – and in some areas change quickly. Clinicians must therefore use this book not only as a text for the present, but as a guide for updating their knowledge in the future. That future will hopefully hold the advent of an evidence-based secondary journal for orthodontics, similar to those that have been developed in other areas, including evidence-based mental health, evidence-based nursing, and the ACP Journal Club, which does the job for internal medicine. These publications survey a large number of journals relevant to their area and choose individual studies and systematic reviews that meet both relevance and validity screening criteria. The results of these studies are presented in structured abstracts that provide clinicians with the key information they need to judge their applicability to their own practices, similar to the summaries that comprise the second section of this text. Fame and fortune await the enterprising group who applies this methodology to produce evidence-based orthodontics.

Whatever the future holds for the increasing efficiency of evidence-based practice, the current text provides an introduction to a system of clinical problem-solving that is becoming a prerequisite for modern orthodontic practice.

Dr. Gordon Guyatt

1

Evidence-Based Orthodontics – Its Evolution and Clinical Application
Katherine W. L. Vig

Introduction

Health-care information escalated towards the end of the twentieth century. This created a serious challenge for clinicians trying to make informed decisions for their patients concerning the relative effectiveness of alternative treatment interventions. The lack of systematic reviews from prospective well-designed clinical trials led to delays in incorporating and testing new information while fostering the continuation of less-effective, less-efficient, and even harmful interventions; the proponents believing clinical experience, as the gold standard, for supporting and recommending treatment procedures and interventions.

Medicine pioneered an evidence-based approach to clinical practice in the eighteenth century at a time when navigation was important for overseas trading in Britain. Long voyages to Australia and the Far East were undertaken with sailors deprived of fresh fruit and vegetables, resulting in scurvy and other medical problems. James Lind MD, surgeon to the British Navy, wrote a *Treatise of the Scurvy* which was ignored for many years but considered the first controlled clinical trial to be translated into clinical practice by equipping long-distance trade ships with lemons and limes to avoid the ship's crew succumbing to scurvy.

In 1971, the British epidemiologist, Archie Cochrane (Figure 1.1), in his influential monograph entitled *Effectiveness and Efficiency* (Cochrane 1971) introduced this "new" concept in clinical medicine that all treatment interventions must be proven to be effective. This was supported by an early example in which data were combined from multiple clinical trials investigating premature births and infant mortality. By 1974, all controlled trials in perinatal medicine had been systematically identified and entered into a clinical trials register. By 1987, the year before Archie Cochrane died, 600 systematic reviews on health-care topics had been conducted. How one man, whose ideas were initially unacceptable to the medical community, had such a profound impact on medicine is recounted in the autobiographical monograph *One Man's Medicine* (Cochrane and Blythe 1989). His revolutionary observations and convictions were fashioned by his experiences of growing up in Britain during the tumultuous years surrounding the two World Wars, and the death of his father in the First World War. The loss of his father had a profound effect on the young Archie Cochrane, with the responsibilities expected from the eldest son to take over as head of the family to care for his mother and siblings.

Archie Cochrane and the development of evidence-based medicine

The early years

Archie Cochrane was born in a small town in Scotland in 1909 to a privileged and wealthy family. His successful grandfather and great-grandfather pioneered the textile industry and benefited from the textile manufacture of the popular Scottish tweeds. As a young boy with an elder sister, two younger brothers, and devoted

Evidence-Based Orthodontics, Second Edition. Edited by Greg J. Huang, Stephen Richmond and Katherine W. L. Vig.
© 2018 John Wiley & Sons, Inc. Published 2018 by John Wiley & Sons, Inc.

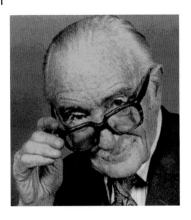

Figure 1.1 Professor Archibald Leman Cochrane CBE, FRCP, FFCM (1909–1988). The Cochrane Collaboration is named in honor of Archie Cochrane, a British medical researcher who contributed greatly to the development of epidemiology as a science. *Source:* courtesy of the Cochrane Collaboration.

parents, he lived an affluent but disciplined life in a large house with multiple servants. His youthful world was disrupted in 1914 when the First World War was declared. His father joined a Scottish regiment and was killed in 1917 while attempting to rescue a wounded brother officer. Archie Cochrane was 8 years old and now carried the responsibilities of being the eldest son with three siblings and a grieving mother. The desolation accompanying the loss of his father was followed by the death of his younger brother to tuberculosis during the severe wartime restrictions.

Archie Cochrane was educated in the traditional upper-class prerogative of "building character" by sending young boys to preparatory boarding school, followed by a prestigious and expensive "public" school, before entering University. Archie Cochrane excelled in athletics and mathematics, and his aptitude for literature resulted in his successful admittance to King's College, Cambridge. A rugby football accident curtailed the time he devoted to acting, riding, tennis, and golf but made him focus on his studies. He graduated with a double first-class honors degree. His grandfather's death, while he was at Cambridge, resulted in his becoming independently wealthy early in his adult life, which he believed contributed to his later success. However, this was also the time of another family tragedy when his remaining younger brother died in a motorcycle accident. Archie was now the eldest and only son of his family, and he undertook responsibility for his widowed mother and elder sister.

The influences in developing an evidence-based approach

Archie Cochrane was a man of the turbulent 1930s who witnessed the events leading to the Second World War. His emotional and intellectual independence and conviction of moral values caused him to often reject political solutions. When he was a medical student at University College Hospital, in London, the Spanish civil war broke out, and Archie Cochrane risked his life and career by volunteering to join the Spanish Medical Aid Unit following Franco's invasion. A year later he returned to England to complete his medical training while believing fascism a menace to Western civilization.

His experience of seeing the consequences of war prepared him for joining the British Army during the Second World War and serving overseas. His fluency and aptitude for languages, including German, French, and Spanish, resulted in his joining a commando regiment that included 70 Spanish refugees from the civil war who had enlisted in the British Army. The regiment was deployed to Crete where Archie was captured by the invading Germans. He spent the next 4 years as a prisoner of war (POW), serving as the medical officer to a camp of 20 000 POWs from diverse cultures and countries, whom he cared for with compassion and fortitude (Doll 1997).

This ordeal resulted in his abiding beliefs in patient care and that medical interventions should be available for all individuals whatever their circumstance. As the medical officer in the POW camp he shared the same diet and conditions as his fellow prisoners. His courage and endurance as a compassionate medical officer resulted in his first clinical trial. He was emaciated and jaundiced himself, with pitting edema above the knees, but he set up a trial with yeast he had acquired from the German prison guards. He describes this as "my first, worst, and most successful clinical trial" (Cochrane 1984).

Having survived the Second World War, he subsequently spent time in the United States before returning to England with a mission and commitment to change the imperfect British medical system. His firm belief in finding evidence for the effectiveness of medical interventions resulted in the development of randomized clinical trials (RCTs) and systematic reviews of the scientific literature. This initiated a new era in medicine – one that would ultimately influence dentistry. A new evidence-based approach to patient care was destined to revolutionize clinical practice, and the methodology had its roots in his experiences as a POW medical officer with limited medical supplies, never knowing what might or might not work. This uncertainty proved to be fertile ground for Archie to test his theories, as it allowed him to ethically randomize patients to alternative treatments. This randomization usually resulted in well-matched groups that received different interventions, thus allowing the investigation to determine the most effective treatment.

The Cochrane legacy

The Cochrane Collaboration was established a year after Archie Cochrane's death and is recognized in the twenty-first century as an international organization that prepares, maintains, and promotes accessible systematic reviews of the effectiveness of health-care interventions from which well-informed decisions emerge (Antes and Oxman 2001).

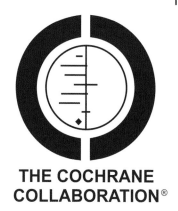

THE COCHRANE COLLABORATION®

Figure 1.2 The Cochrane Collaboration logo. The outer blue semicircles represent the Cochrane Collaboration and the inner circle the globe to represent international collaborations. The forest plot of clinical trials represents the effectiveness of administering corticosteroids to pregnant women delivering prematurely; the diamond to the left of the "no effect" line indicates the meta-analysis favored the intervention.

The familiar logo of the Cochrane Collaboration (Figure 1.2) exemplifies and recognizes the impact of Archie Cochrane's life. The circle, representing the global and international collaboration, encircles the forest plot, which depicts the results of a quantitative meta-analysis. This forest plot represents one of the earliest systematic reviews and meta-analyses of the literature on the therapeutic intervention of corticosteroids in women who were to deliver their babies prematurely. By a statistical combination of data from the clinical trials, the highest evidence, and ultimately the gold standard for clinical practice in caring for pregnant women delivering prematurely, was established. The benefits of the effectiveness of administering perinatal corticosteroids were undeniably correlated with the outcome of perinatal and neonatal survival with a consequent reduction in mortality and morbidity.

The Cochrane Collaboration

The Cochrane Collaboration (Cochrane Collaboration 2017) has influenced and driven the science and methodology of systematic reviews and has been compared to the revolutionary Human Genome Project in its potential implications for contemporary health care (Naylor 1995). Nevertheless, changing the standard of care in clinical practice does not move quickly, and information gained from research experience has a long gestation period and time lag before it becomes incorporated into clinical practice.

Historically, medical and dental regimens have remained unchanged even when well-designed clinical trials have provided counterevidence. Treatment decisions based on clinical experience and beliefs are difficult to change, and it has been shown to take an average of 17 years for the findings from clinical trials to be implemented into clinical practice. For example, there were clinical trials in 1960 of thrombolytic therapy and the administration of streptokinase. By 1975, 40 RCTs had been conducted, and by 1985 there were 50 000 patients enrolled, with evidence that thrombolytic therapy was effective. When a systematic review and meta-analysis conclusively showed the effectiveness of thrombolytic agents, it was finally accepted as a standard of care in 1990. If the contemporary methodological approach to evidence-based practice had been established 30 years previously, many lives could have been saved. Unfortunately, even in the twenty-first century, when evidence is convincing, clinicians may still find it difficult to relinquish their beliefs based on their clinical experience.

The influence of an evidenced-based approach

The establishment of the evidence-based approach resulted in rapid changes in the health-care system and in the education of students and residents in the health-care professions. A paradigm shift had occurred from the paternalistic choice of a treatment intervention by doctors for their trusting patients to a partnership in which the doctor and patient make choices together to determine the "best" treatment. It was therefore incumbent on the health-care provider to have knowledge of the best available evidence pertaining to the risks, costs, benefits, burden of care, and probability of success for alternative treatment interventions. The caveat was that if evidence exists to support the effectiveness and efficiency of treatment interventions, an integration of the best research evidence with clinical expertise and patient values and preferences should occur (Sackett *et al.* 1991, 2000). Although the new movement of Evidence Based Medicine and Clinical Trialists was flourishing in Britain with the leadership of the Cochrane Collaboration, other influences were playing their part on the other side of the Atlantic. Alvan Feinstein MD, Professor of Medicine and Epidemiology at Yale, promoted "clinical care as science," and advanced knowledge with clinimetrics. The term clinimetrics, as its name suggests, embraced science, technology, and clinical care with reproducible consistency as the basic science underlying clinical decision making. During his formative years, in 1963 David Sackett read a paper by Alvan Feinstein on Boolean algebra and taxonomy and wrote Feinstein a fan letter, following which Alvan Feinstein became a mentor to Sackett (Smith 2015). Clinicians and academics interested in evidence-based medicine consider Cochrane, Feinstein, and Sackett as the "fathers" of a new and currently flourishing movement of evidence-based medicine. Dentistry has embraced an evidence-based approach and has ridden on the coattails of medicine in teaching and practicing an evidence-based approach, and conducting systematic reviews and meta-analysis of treatment interventions with well-defined, reliable, and valid outcomes.

The impact of David Sackett and clinical epidemiology resonated with the orthodontic attendees when Bob Moyers invited David Sackett to participate in the Moyers Symposium on three occasions over a 30-year period, starting in 1985. By 2015, when Sackett attended his third Moyers Symposium, he cited his comments from 1985 when he excoriated orthodontics, suggesting the trials in orthodontics was lagging behind "such treatment modalities as acupuncture, hypnosis, homeopathy and orthomolecular therapy and on a par with scientology, dianetics and podiatry" (Sackett 1995). There were no RCTs in orthodontics prior to 1967 and there was a rate of one trial every 2 years during the next decade. By 1994, when Sackett next participated in the Moyers Symposium, orthodontic trials had increased 18-fold, and by 2005 had risen to 129 per year (Sackett 1995, 2014). David Sackett's unique perspective and encouragement in the world of orthodontics had a major influence on the now classic orthodontic Class II RTCs funded by National Institutes of Health/ National Institute of Dental and Craniofacial Research. So who was the late David Sackett and what influenced his interest in an evidence-based approach in medicine (Figure 1.3)?

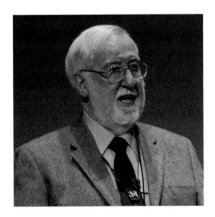

Figure 1.3 David Lawrence Sackett, OC, MD, MMSc, FRSC, FRCP (Canada, England, and Scotland). *Source:* Per Kjeldsen with permission of Dr. James McNamara.

The influence of David Sackett and medical clinical trials

David L. Sackett (1934–2015) was born in Chicago, the third son of "a bibliophile mother and artist-designer father" (Smith 2015). His childhood was not without adversity as he was bedridden for months with polio, from which he recovered as a 12 year old. He became a voracious reader and as he recovered from polio he became an accomplished runner. He started his medical training at the University of Illinois in 1956 and in 1962 was drafted into the US Public Health service as a result of the Cuban missile crisis. He also had a Master of Science degree from the Harvard School of Public Health. He was diverted from a career in bench science by his love for clinical medicine, and was influenced by Walter Holland, Professor of Clinical Epidemiology at St Thomas's Hospital Medical School in London, to have an enduring interest and career in clinical epidemiology. He was only 32 years old when he was recruited to the new Canadian Medical School at McMasters University, in Hamilton, Canada. This was a difficult decision as Sackett did not want to leave the United States. Nevertheless, the opportunity to develop a different way to educate medical students by finding evidence from systematic reviews rather than conventional teaching "in my clinical experience" was irresistible. This proved a new and exciting challenge, embraced by a new generation of medical students who flourished in the innovative educational methods, although these were not popular with the senior experienced clinicians. Sackett was not a man with a big ego and once considered an expert it was time to move on and let new talent emerge. This trait was exemplified by his decision, when he was 49 years old, to repeat his Medical Residency. He considered clinical practice had changed so much that he was no longer a "good enough doctor anymore". It took courage to return to medical school but he believed he would become a better doctor if he adopted contemporary methods and became updated. Sackett believed that evidence-based medicine went beyond critical appraisal by combining evidence from research with clinical skills and the values and preferences of patients (Sackett 2015). In 1994, Sackett became a clinician at the John Radcliffe Hospital in Oxford where he was the Director of the Center of Evidence-based Medicine. Five years later, in 1999, he gave his last lecture on evidence-based medicine in Krakow and retired from clinical practice. He returned to Canada to live with his wife and family in a wood cabin beside a lake and set up the Trout Research and Education Center (Smith 2015).

The application of evidence-based dentistry to orthodontics

One method of achieving an evidence-based approach in dentistry and its advanced specialty programs is to carry out a systematic review of all RCTs from which a quantitative analysis of the available data can be statistically included into a meta-analysis. This approach was developed in medicine, with the benefit of patients and doctors making informed decisions on the most effective treatment intervention. The basis of a systematic review is that it provides a method of identifying all the available literature on a topic and synthesizing it into an easily accessible knowledge base. The clinician practicing in the twenty-first century has the computer literacy to access electronic data bases to make informative choices and decisions. As this approach became accepted in dentistry, leaders in the field developed a Cochrane Oral Health Group.

The Cochrane Oral Health Group/ Collaboration

The Cochrane Collaboration is made up of over 50 review groups, of which the Cochrane Oral Health Group (COHG) is one (Shaw 2011). Originally, the COHG was established in 1994 in the United States by Alexia Antczak Bouckoms, based at Harvard University in Boston Massachusetts. In 1996, the editorial base of the COHG (COHG 2017) was relocated to the School of Dentistry, University of Manchester, in England, with Professors Bill Shaw and Helen Worthington as the coordinating editors (Shaw 2011). The COHG is part of the Cochrane Collaboration based in Oxford, England and the University of Dundee in Scotland, directed by Professor Jan Clarkson, and comprises an international network of researchers involved in producing and disseminating systematic reviews of controlled RCTs in the field of oral health. Searching for trials to include in a systematic reviews is a complex process; in order to avoid bias in the results of the review, it is important to include as many relevant trials as possible (see Chapter 3 of this text). The search process relies on initially defining the question, and this has been described in detail in Chapter 2. Finding the best available evidence from sources of published and unpublished studies requires a standardized systematic approach to avoid the different types of recognized bias (Eggar *et al.* 2001). The quality of data retrieved from a careful, systematic, and standardized review of the scientific literature may be quantitative and/or qualitative in nature (Glasziou *et al.* 2001). Therefore, discrete steps to find the relevant studies are required in searching computer databases to retrieve a body of literature that then requires careful selection and appraisal.

Evidence-based dentistry in education: Commission on Dental Accreditation guidelines

Dentistry did not adopt this revolutionary concept in guiding clinical practice and the education of dental students and residents in the advanced specialty programs until the mid-1990s. To a certain extent, it was forced on the profession by several events that occurred in 1995 owing to the publication of *Dental Practice Parameters for Oral Health* (McNeil *et al.* 1995). The American Dental Association practice parameters stressed the need to develop and implement aids to assist in clinical decision making, which stated the need for:

- condition-based parameters, not procedure-based;
- integrated oral health care in an interdisciplinary approach;
- parameters to aid clinical decision making;
- process of care to be emphasized as well as the outcome;
- balancing patient needs with scientific soundness.

In the same year, the Institute of Medicine report (Field 1995) was published on the future of dental education. This had 22 recommendations, which among others emphasized the need to implement:

- evidence-based care;
- patient-centered treatment;
- elimination of unnecessary/ineffective treatment interventions;
- scientific evidence, outcome research, and formal consensus processes in clinical practice guidelines;
- research to evaluate outcomes of alternative treatments.

With the need to make major changes in the practice and education of oral health-care professionals, at the end of the twentieth century the Pew Trust also identified the critical challenges necessary for health-care professions (Pew Health Professions Commission 1995).

Making rational decisions in orthodontic practice

In orthodontics, clinical experience suggests that some conditions are best treated early for biological, social, or practical reasons, whereas others should be deferred. So how do we reconcile these conflicting issues? When anterior crossbites exist in the early mixed dentition due to a Class I crowded dentition or with a mild developing Class III skeletal pattern, should we wait until the permanent successors have erupted in the late mixed dentition or correct earlier to avoid perpetuating the malocclusion with possible labial gingival recession on the mandibular incisor from the traumatic incisor relationship (Vig *et al.* 2007)? When using a protraction face mask in an attempt to move the nasomaxillary complex forward, our knowledge of craniofacial growth and development indicates early intervention when the circum-maxillary suture system should be responsive. Correcting the anterior crossbite early supports the concept of effective and efficient early treatment intervention. However, with further growth the Class III skeletal pattern may result in the anterior crossbite being re-established. Problems exist when using an evidence-based approach to clinical decision making in orthodontics, as the scientific literature in our specialty has relatively few prospective RCTs, and this study design is considered to provide the highest level of evidence.

So how are clinical judgments made when they cannot be based solely on evidence at the highest level but rather rely on lesser-quality studies and/or clinical experience? One of the most common early orthodontic treatment interventions is the correction of posterior crossbites in the mixed dentition, which may be considered a well-accepted clinical practice. But what evidence exists in the scientific literature? A systematic review published by Harrison and Ashby (2001), *Orthodontic treatment for posterior crossbites,* resides in the Cochrane database of systematic reviews. This is a very comprehensive review of randomized and controlled clinical trials in the scientific literature that reported data on the outcomes of crossbite correction. An extensive number of publications on this topic exist, but until a systematic approach was made to review the literature and identify the quality of studies that should be included, stronger inferences could not be made. The result of the search strategy to identify studies of orthodontic treatment for posterior crossbites, limited by a priori inclusion criteria, resulted in only seven RCTs and five controlled clinical trials. Cochrane reviews have the advantage of being regularly updated as new information becomes available. The updated abstract included studies since 2001, and for this update 113 abstracts were assessed for potential inclusion. Of these, 38 papers were obtained and assessed for eligibility. An additional five reports for three RCTs and one controlled clinical trial (CCT), together with another report to a previously included CCT, satisfied the inclusion criteria.

It becomes clear when trying to quantify the evidence using systematic reviews and meta-analyses that a definition of evidence-based clinical practice requires the careful and considered use of statistics and may be defined as "the enhancement of a clinician's traditional skills in diagnosis, treatment, prevention and the related areas through the systematic framing of relevant and answerable questions and the use of mathematical estimates of probability and risk" (Donald and Greenhalgh 2001). The advantage of a systematic review is that it will limit bias by a methodological approach to strict inclusion criteria of articles, and the conclusions are more reliable and accurate (Greenhalgh 2001). This is covered in Chapter 2 of this text.

Even when evidence is available, clinicians may still be unable to relinquish their beliefs based on their clinical experience. In orthodontic clinical practice, treatment decisions are made based on early intervention for Class II patients being beneficial, even when evidentiary data does not appear to support the effectiveness, efficiency, and benefits of this approach. (O'Brien and Sandler 2011).

Orthodontics, while the oldest specialty in dentistry, recognizes that strong scientific evidence is an important goal for the future of the profession. However, patients are waiting to be treated even though we cannot provide good estimates for the outcomes of alternative treatments at the time of the consultation. In the face of this uncertainty, it becomes even more important for patients to have their preferences considered during the treatment planning stage (Vig and O'Brien 2017).

Advances are often first brought to our attention by anecdotal case reports and observation, as was the discovery of penicillin. Although low on the strength of evidence, these initial reports still have value, as do case series, retrospective studies, and clinical experience. Although there is a paucity of clinical trials in orthodontics from which systematic reviews may be conducted, the methodology is still relatively new. In medicine there was also considerable opposition to Archie Cochrane's insistence that clinical trials needed to be done to establish evidence for the effectiveness of clinical interventions. The lack of RCTs in orthodontics does not mean we should accept the present state of orthodontics as a science but rather that we should demand more rigor in designing clinical trials to determine what works, what doesn't work, and what is just inspired rhetoric with little scientific support or substance. If the very expensive RCT cannot answer the question/hypothesis we would like to test, then perhaps well-designed cohort studies should be a starting place.

The American Dental Association website

The initiative by the American Dental Association (ADA 2017) to develop a website for both clinicians and the public to access current information has provided a rich resource to search for the best information we have concerning alternative treatment interventions. By identifying authors who are publishing in a field of interest, it is possible to easily contact, communicate, and collaborate with researchers all over the world.

Research cannot be set up overnight, but undertaking a systematic review on a chosen topic will allow areas of strength and weakness to be identified. This will reveal further fertile research opportunities and stimulate the development of hypothesis-driven research.

The future of an evidence-based approach in orthodontics

Attacks on an evidence-based approach and severe criticism of clinical epidemiology and the evaluative clinical sciences was in response to the impact and change in clinical practice standards. Doctors were urged to defend clinical reasoning based on the clinician's experience and their understanding of pathology and physiological mechanisms. If we cannot accept applying the highest level of evidence, we will be doomed to muddle along with our best guess. A choice needs to be made based on the alternative outcomes of a clinical intervention combined with the patient's preferences and the clinician's expertise. In the interest of providing the best available care to our patients, the current best evidence must be incorporated into the treatment recommendations that each clinician makes.

References

American Dental Association (ADA), 2017. *Center for Evidence-based Dentistry*. Available at: http://www.ebd.ada.org. Accessed November, 2017.

Antes G, Oxman AD, 2001. The Cochrane Collaboration in the 20th century. In: M Egger, GD Smith, DG Altman, eds. *Systematic Reviews in Health Care: Meta Analysis in Context*, 2nd ed. New York: BMJ Books.

Cochrane AL, 1971. *Effectiveness and Efficiency: Random Reflections on Health Services*. New York: BMJ.

Cochrane AL, 1984. Sickness in Salonica: my first, worst and most successful clinical trial. *BMJ*, 289, 1726–1727.

Cochrane AL, Blythe M, 1989. *One Man's Medicine. an Autobiography of Professor Archie Cochrane*. London: Cambridge University Press.

Cochrane Collaboration, 2017. Available at: www.cochrane.org. Accessed November, 2017.

Cochrane Oral Health Group (COHG), 2017. Available at: http://www.ohg.cochrane.org. Accessed November, 2017.

Doll R, 1997. A reminiscence of Archie Cochrane. In: A Maynard, I Chalmers, eds. *Non-Random Reflections on Health Services Research*. New York: BMJ Books, 7–10.

Donald A, Greenhalgh T, 2001. *A Hands-on Guide to Evidence-Based Health Care: Practice and Implementation*. Oxford: Blackwell Science.

Eggar M, Smith JD, Altman DG, 2001. *Systematic Reviews in Health Care: Meta-Analysis in Context*, 2nd ed, New York: BMJ Books.

Field MJ, 1995. *Dental Education at the Crossroads: Challenges and Change*. Washington DC: National Academy Press.

Glasziou P, Irwig L, Bain C, *et al.*, 2001. *Systematic Reviews in Health Care*. London: Cambridge University Press.

Greenhalgh T, 2001. Papers that summarize other papers (systematic reviews and meta-analysis). In: *How to Read a Paper. The Basics of Evidence Based Medicine*. New York: BMJ Books, 120–138.

Harrison JE, Ashby D, 2001. Orthodontic treatment for posterior crossbites. *Cochrane Database Syst Rev*, 18 (3) CD000979.

McNeil KJ, Aurbach FE, Brotman DN, *et al.*, 1995. Dental practice parameters; parameters for 12 oral health conditions. *J Am Dent Assoc* (Suppl.) 126, S1–S37.

Naylor CD, 1995. Grey zones of clinical practice: some limitations to evidence-based medicine. *Lancet* 345, 840–843.

O'Brien K, Sandler J, 2011. The treatment of Class II malocclusion – have we evidence to make decisions? In: Huang GH, Richmond S, Vig KWL, eds. *Evidence-based Orthodontics*. Blackwell Publishing Ltd.

Pew Health Professions Commission, 1995. *Critical Challenges: Revitalizing the Health Professions for the Twenty First Century*, 3rd report of the Pew Health Professions Commission. San Francisco, CA.

Sackett DL, Haynes RB, Guyatt GH, *et al.*, 1991. *Clinical Epidemiology: a Basic Science for Clinical Medicine*, 2nd ed. Boston: Little, Brown.

Sackett DL, 1995. Nine years later: A commentary on revisiting the Moyers Symposium. In: Trotman CA, McNamara JA Jr, eds. *Orthodontic Treatment: Outcome and Effectiveness*, Volume 30, Craniofacial Growth Series, Center for Human Growth and Development. Ann Arbor, University of Michigan, 1–5.

Sackett DL, Strauss SE, Richardson WS, *et al.*, 2000. *Evidence-based Medicine: How to Practice and Teach EBM*. Edinburgh: Churchill Livingston.

Sackett DL, 2014. On the vanishing need for MD randomized trialists at Moyers Symposia. In: *The 40th Moyers Symposium: Looking Back...Looking Forward*. McNamara JA Jr, ed. Volume 50, Craniofacial Growth Series, Center for Human Growth and Development. Ann Arbor, University of Michigan, 145–165.

Sackett DL, 2015. Why did the randomised clinical trial become the primary focus of my career? *Value Health* 18, 550–552.

Shaw WC, 2011. Evidence-based care in context. In: Huang GJ, Richmond S, Vig KWL, eds. *Evidence-based Orthodontics*. Blackwell Publishing Ltd., 283–291.

Smith R, 2015. Obituary: David Sackett – physician, trialist and teacher. *BMJ* 350, h2639

Vig KWL, O'Brien K, Harrison J, 2007. Early orthodontic and orthopedic treatment. The search for evidence: will it influence clinical practice? In: McNamara JA, ed. *Early Orthodontic Treatment; is the Benefit Worth the Burden*, Craniofacial Growth Series Vol. 44. Ann Arbor, MI: Center for Human Growth and Development, University of Michigan, 13–38.

Vig KWL, O'Brien K, 2017. Making rational decisions in an era of evidence-based orthodontics. In: Kapila SD, Vig KWL, Huang GJ, eds. *Anecdote, Expertise and Evidence: Applying New Knowledge to Everyday Orthodontics*. Craniofacial Growth Series Vol. 53. Ann Arbor, MI: Center for Human Growth and Development, University of Michigan, 1–16.

2

Clinical Research Design

Robert J. Weyant

Introduction

Dr. Jones is an orthodontist who recently graduated from training and is now in private practice, having purchased her practice from a retiring orthodontist. After several months, Dr. Jones noted that she was receiving a large number of referrals from community general practice dentists of young children aged 7–9 who have prominent front teeth (i.e., Class II malocclusion). The referrals were implying that the young patients would benefit from early treatment, and most of these patients were told by their referring general dentists that if they received "early" treatment (by age 9), they could avoid more extensive treatment when they were older (in adolescence, after age 12). Dr. Jones was happy to have the referrals but was not sure she could tell the patients with confidence that they would be less likely to need orthodontic treatment as adolescents if they received "early" treatment now. Moreover, Dr. Jones was taught that both headgear and functional appliances were appropriate approaches for treatment of children with prominent upper front teeth but was not sure which approach would be best. Dr. Jones felt that she needed more information so that she could discuss treatment in an informed manner with her patients and make scientifically sound clinical decisions about recommending treatment.

The above vignette provides the reader with a common situation encountered frequently by clinicians, that is the need for additional, high-quality evidence from the scientific literature to assist them in their clinical decision making. In this mode, clinicians are consumers of the scientific literature as opposed to producers of science; consequently, they need a broad understanding of research methods and designs so that they can properly interpret the scientific basis for clinical practice. Whether orthodontics or any area of medicine is a science is debatable because the nature of the problems addressed by medical and dental care draws on ethics, culture, and economics in a way not commonly found in chemistry, physics, and biology. Nevertheless, as with all of biomedicine, orthodontics can thank empirical research for helping to refine and optimize contemporary approaches to patient care. The research underlying clinical practice ranges from basic sciences, such as genetics and physiology, to social sciences, such as psychology and sociology. All of these clinical evaluative sciences inform clinical practice, and all are fundamentally derived from the same overarching scientific process or method. At its best, research helps to improve the quality of care and patient outcomes, but when the science is poor or misunderstood, its misapplication can lead to just the opposite result. Hence, understanding the elements of good research and what makes science important to clinical practice is needed as a basis for clinical care. This chapter is designed to aid in this understanding.

Evidence-Based Orthodontics, Second Edition. Edited by Greg J. Huang, Stephen Richmond and Katherine W. L. Vig.
© 2018 John Wiley & Sons, Inc. Published 2018 by John Wiley & Sons, Inc.

The scientific method

The scientific method is, in fact, part of a broader area of philosophy known as *epistemology*. Epistemology is the branch of philosophy that deals with the nature of and limits to human knowledge (Salmon *et al.* 1992). A proper discussion of epistemology and the philosophy of science are well beyond the scope of this chapter. Suffice is to say that our concern in clinical practice is to have the best "knowledge" available to help our patients. There are many ways of humans "knowing" something, including intuition, faith, reason, authority, testimony, personal experience, and science. The distinction of importance here is between belief (I think something is true) and knowledge (something is actually true). Arguably, then, of all the ways we have of knowing something, the scientific method provides us with the best approach if our goal is obtaining objective, valid, and useful information.

Science pursues knowledge by essentially asking and then answering questions. Simple enough. But the devil is in the details. The veracity of the information generated by this process is entirely dependent on the rigor and objectivity employed in how one seeks out the information to answer the question. Moreover, the specific approach to answering the question, that is, the research design, places inherent limits on the conclusions (answers) that can be made. This chapter provides a brief overview of basic research development, the common clinical research designs, their uses, strengths, and limitations, and a discussion of best practices that apply broadly to any research endeavor. The intent is to provide a broad overview framed in terms related to clinical orthodontics.

Developing a hypothesis

Although it is seemingly straightforward, asking the right question is key to moving science forward. The questions of science are derived from many sources, including intuition, clinical experience, and reading the scientific literature.

Any question that is focused on naturalistic answers (as opposed to metaphysical answers) is fair game for science. Some questions only serve to satisfy the questioner's curiosity, whereas other questions are the motivators that advance a scientific discipline. The degree to which a question is framed to address a gap in our general knowledge of a subject is the degree to which a question serves to motivate research and move science forward. These are questions that focus us on those areas that lie just beyond our current understanding of how things work. Consequently, science tends to move forward incrementally by constantly working at the frontier of our current understanding and carefully taking the next logical step forward. Scientists (and clinicians) working in a field generally know where that boundary is between current knowledge and our need for new information, and it is this knowledge that allows them to create new questions that lead to the research that advances the field.

Dr. Jones in the vignette has implicitly asked a question that derives from her clinical experience with her new patient population: Can early orthodontic treatment reduce or prevent the need for additional treatment later in adolescence?

Based on one's experience in an area, it is possible to offer a prediction of what the answer to a question might be. In science this provisional answer is referred to as a hypothesis. From the above example, Dr. Jones might hypothesize that early treatment will, in fact, reduce the need for later treatment for a substantial number of her patients. Any orthodontist understands this question, and most would have an opinion about the answer. In contrast, for naive individuals (i.e., nondentists), not only would they not have an answer to this question, they also would be very unlikely to think of the question.

When asking a question about treatment outcomes, one is essentially asking about causality. Does treatment A cause outcome B? One of the fundamental goals of clinical research is to establish causality. In so doing we improve our understanding of underlying mechanisms and we provide an opportunity to design clinical interventions aimed at improving the quality of clinical care. In our example, Dr. Jones wishes to know if early treatment is causally related to subsequent occlusal status (and hence the need for additional treatment).

An important concept that underlies the notion of causality in clinical research is that most associations in biomedicine are probabilistic (stochastic) rather than deterministic. This means that at the level of clinically

Table 2.1 Hill's viewpoints on the aspects of an association to be considered when deciding on causality.

Hill's Viewpoint	Interpretation
Strength of association	The stronger the associations (larger effect size) between the hypothesized causal agent and the effect, the less likely the association has occurred by chance or is due to an extraneous variable (i.e., confounding).
Consistency	A relationship when observed repeatedly in different people or under different circumstances increases the likelihood of it being causal.
Specificity	An effect is the result of only one cause. In Hill's day this was considered more important than today.
Temporality	It is logically necessary for a cause to precede an effect in time.
Biological gradient	This is also known as a dose–response relationship and implies that as the exposure to the causal agent increases, the likelihood of the effect occurring increases.
Plausibility	The causation we suspect is biologically plausible. However, Hill acknowledged that what is biologically plausible depends upon the biological knowledge of the day.
Coherence	Data should not seriously conflict with the generally known facts of the natural history and biology of the disease.
Experiment	Experimental evidence provides the strongest support for a causal hypothesis.
Analogy	At times, commonly accepted phenomenon in one area can inform us of similar relationships in another.

Source: Hill 1965.

measured outcomes, the likelihood that some outcome will occur as the result of some exposure is not a certainty. For example, if someone is a life-long smoker, they are more likely to experience some sort of lung or heart problem than a nonsmoker. Not all smokers experience lung or heart problems, and some nonsmokers indeed develop these conditions, but smoking certainly increases one's chances of developing these problems. Consequently, assessing causality in probabilistic systems is challenging and requires an understanding of statistics and research methods. Moreover, this implies that the research must occur in populations (groups) of individuals (patients) as we are often attempting to detect only slight changes in the marginal likelihood of an outcome.

There is a rich philosophy underlying the notion of establishing causality that goes beyond the scope of this chapter. However, the philosophical discussion of causality can often be immobilizing when there is a pragmatic need to move forward with clinical decision making. Fortunately, there are well-regarded heuristic criteria that are considered, when present, to strongly suggest a causal association. Some of the criteria most widely used are guidelines, first put forward in 1965 by Sir Austin Bradford Hill (1897–1991), a British medical statistician, as a way of evaluating the existence of a causal link between specific factors (Hill 1965). He wished to avoid the philosophical and semantic problems often encountered in discussions of causality and rather move to the pragmatic situation in which those aspects of an association that, if present, would most likely lead to the interpretation of causation (Hill 1965). His "viewpoints" (Table 2.1) are put forward as suggestions and specifically were not called criteria for estimating causality. With the exception of the temporal association (i.e., the cause must precede the outcome), all of these are conditions that suggest, but are not required when making the case for, a causal association. It should be noted that Hill is not the only person to suggest such factors, but his are the most widely recognized.

Testing a hypothesis

Testability is the hallmark of a well-structured hypothesis and the foundation for high-quality scientific investigation. Although the philosophy underlying the testing of hypotheses is beyond the scope of this text, the common approach is based on deduction and extends from the work of philosopher Karl Popper. This approach is known as *refutation or falsifiability*. Falsifiability means that a hypothesis can be shown to be false through observation or experimentation.

To make a hypothesis fully testable, it must go through a process of operationalization. This means that all of the elements of the hypothesis must be specified in such a way that will allow them to be measured. Moreover, it also implies the need for some a priori determination of what constitutes the standard by which the hypothesis will be declared, "falsified."

Once the hypothesis if fully operationalized, the investigator can then move forward with the empirical investigation, the aim of which is to attempt to falsify his or her hypothesis. If successful in demonstrating that the hypothesis is false, then that hypothesis should be discarded and, ideally, a new hypothesis, benefiting from this new information, created and the process repeated. Failing, through rigorous effort, to demonstrate that a hypothesis is false does not necessarily demonstrate that it is true, but it provides the initial evidence that it may be true.

It is rarely the case that a single study is considered definitive proof of the veracity of a hypothesis. Rather, each experiment (or observational study) done to test a hypothesis provides evidence that supports or refutes the hypothesis. Over time, this so-called weight of evidence accumulated through multiple investigations, often by different investigators, provides a sense of the veracity of the hypothesis. Consequently, most knowledge created through the scientific process is considered provisional. Some say that hypotheses should not be defined as true or false but rather as useful or not useful in accurately predicting outcomes.

In the example above, Dr. Jones as an orthodontist in full-time private practice would not likely address her desire to know more about the association between early treatment and its effect on later treatment need through her own research efforts. Rather she would likely search for publications where this issue has been studied. Her ability to understand the elements that go into creating high-quality clinical research and what types of research designs are used to test various types of hypotheses will give her the knowledge necessary to select and critically evaluate appropriate publications for consideration.

Research quality issues

Even the casual student of science appreciates that science demands carefully constructed and objective processes be used in generating information (data) to test (falsify) hypotheses. All well-designed clinical research shares common features that serve to reduce bias and ensure valid findings. These features are mentioned in brief here, and interested readers can find more detailed information in the References at the end of the chapter.

Measurement issues

Accurate measurement is a hallmark of good science. Poorly selected or designed measures lead inevitably to the inability to properly test a hypothesis and ultimately to spurious results. Thus, great care is required when operationalizing a hypothesis to ensure that all of the important elements of the hypothesis can be measured in a valid and reliable manner. In the example, the notion of malocclusion needs to be defined – a case definition. This should include a detailed definition of what elements (e.g., overjet, overbite, ANB, etc.) will be included and exactly how they will be measured. Similarly, "early treatment" will need to be defined in terms of age, duration, forces, and appliances to be used.

Population (study subjects)

The subjects or participants in a study (including any control or comparison group) need to be defined with respect to all relevant demographic and biomedical characteristics. In the example, age and orthodontic status would be important to consider, whereas gender and race would perhaps be less so. Inclusion and exclusion criteria need to be clearly specified and based on a sound rationale. Descriptions of the population serve to provide important information on study relevance to readers.

A related issue is the use of a control or comparison group. This is of extreme importance if we are to conclude that an intervention has had an effect. If the treatment and control groups are not similar, then it can be difficult to conclude that the treatment was the causative agent for any outcome. In experimental studies this is often accomplished through randomization.

Data acquisition needs to be carefully considered to assess feasibility. Failure to be able to accurately collect relevant data has been the downfall of many clinical studies. If the forces applied by headgear cannot be measured in the study in a valid manner, it will be impossible to determine the association between the treatment and outcome. In cases of rare conditions, the inability to accumulate enough subjects can lead to underpowered studies.

Statistical analysis and sample size

Choosing the right approach to statistically analyze study results is crucial for obtaining a valid test of the hypothesis. Given the complexity of making an appropriate choice for statistical analysis in most modern clinical studies, successful analysis will hinge to a great degree on the inclusion of a well-trained research methodologist from the beginning to the end of the study.

A related issue that also hinges on the advice of a research methodologist is the sample size, or number of subjects to be included. There needs to be a sound rationale provided for the sample size selected. Moreover, in negative studies (studies that fail to show support for the hypothesis) a post hoc power estimate is important. The reader should be informed if the study's failure to find a significant result was based on the validity of the hypothesis or the inadequacy of the study design. The appropriate number of subjects to be included in a study cannot be determined in the abstract as it is dependent on features of the study design, actual effect size of interest (clinically important), expected variability in the data, and approach to analysis.

Placebo

A placebo is a material, formulation, or intervention that is similar to the test product or procedure, but without the use of an active ingredient or efficacious process. The "placebo effect" is the degree to which a benefit (or harm) is experienced by a study subject when a placebo, rather than an active ingredient or process, is used in an experimental study. The degree of benefit experienced as the result of the use of a placebo can be substantial and hence must be considered when evaluating the efficacy of a therapeutic intervention. Placebo effects are greatest for outcomes that are highly subjective or psychogenic in nature (e.g., mood changes, pain sensation) and are negligible for things that are not under psychological control (e.g., reduction of overjet after nonapplication of orthodontic forces). It is considered good practice to employ a placebo when practical and ethical. When a placebo effect occurs, it serves to reduce the effect size and consequently requires a larger sample size to evaluate the efficacy of an intervention.

Duration

The need to conduct a prospective study for a sufficient length of time to observe the anticipated outcome is another issue related to feasibility and study cost. The study must run for long enough to observe the development of the outcome of interest. In caries studies, perhaps 2 years would be needed. For orthodontic relapse, perhaps much longer follow-up is needed.

Research designs

In addition to establishing a hypothesis, ensuring that all variables therein can be accurately measured, and having access to an appropriate population of subjects, the best research design to use to test the hypothesis is a major decision for an investigator. The strengths and weaknesses inherent in every design will determine how well the hypothesis can be tested and what conclusions can be made at the end of the study. The selection of design is based on factors related to the hypothesis being tested as well as feasibility, ethical concerns,

Table 2.2 Research designs ordered from least potential for bias (top) to greatest potential for bias (bottom).

Meta analyses
Systematic reviews
Experimental trials (randomized controlled trials)
Cohort studies
Case–control studies
Human trials without controls (quasiexperiments)
Cross-sectional studies
Simple descriptive studies
Case reports
Personal opinion

budget, and often other factors. Some questions readily suggest an appropriate design. For example, evaluating the efficacy of a new treatment is generally done using a randomized controlled trial (RCT), whereas disease prevalence studies are done using a cross-sectional design. The initial investigation of etiology is often done using a case–control design. The section below briefly introduces the most common designs used in clinical research and lists their uses, strengths, and weaknesses (see also Table 2.2). This list is not comprehensive, as hybrid and quasiexperimental designs are not included. But a general understanding of the four designs listed will illustrate important concepts and give the reader a good introduction for understanding the majority of what is encountered when reading the orthodontic literature.

Research designs can be divided into two groups, experimental and observational, based on the degree of control the investigators exert over the conditions of the study. Experimental studies are those for which the investigators actively manipulate the conditions under study, for example, when the investigator gives some of the study subjects a therapeutic intervention. Observational studies are those for which there is effectively no manipulation of study conditions by the investigators. Rather, investigators simply observe and measure conditions that occur within the subjects.

The ability to assign study subjects, especially through use of randomization (e.g., RCT) and the ability to closely measure important aspects of the exposures and outcomes (e.g., RCT and cohort) of a study can greatly reduce bias and, when possible, are the preferred designs for testing hypotheses about causality.

Space allows here only the most basic description of each of the research designs. Each design on its own has been the topic of full texts, and interested readers can find references at the end of the chapter. The vignette above can be used to show how various clinical questions can relate to research designs.

Imagine that Dr. Jones has the following questions relating to the uncertainty over early treatment:

1) How many children in the community are affected by early malocclusion of this type (Class II)?
2) Is thumb sucking a risk factor that could increase the likelihood of Class II malocclusion?
3) What proportion of children with early Class II malocclusion would grow out of a need for orthodontic intervention if they did not receive early treatment?
4) Is headgear more efficacious than functional appliances for early treatment of Class II malocclusion?

Observational research designs

Cross-sectional design

Question 1 above is a question of disease prevalence and would best be addressed through a cross-sectional study. Cross-sectional studies are the most common observational research design used in clinical and epidemiological research and are used to estimate disease prevalence and to explore relationships between variables through correlational analysis.

The cross-sectional design can be either descriptive, such as a prevalence study, or analytic, such as a study correlating risk factors and disease status. DeAngelis (1990) notes that the name *cross-sectional*, "comes from the image of taking a slice across a stream of activity that is flowing from some point of onset toward some outcome." This all-at-once approach to gathering data provides the design's greatest strengths and weaknesses.

The strength of the design includes its relative low cost, as there is no need to follow up with subjects. It is also possible to screen large numbers of variables, especially when a questionnaire or record review approach is used to collect data. The study duration is also often quite short in cross-sectional designs, with all data immediately available for analysis after the one phase of data collection.

The major weakness of the design also comes from the all-at-once nature of the data collection because the temporal relationships between variables can be confused. Hence, this design is not considered optimal for assessing causal associations. Additionally, the external validity of the study, the ability of the investigators to draw conclusions about a larger group of interest beyond just the study subjects, is based on the quality of the sampling process used to select study subjects. If the selection of study subjects is done well, cross-sectional studies can have high external validity.

Other uses of the cross-sectional design include opinion (survey) research and normative values studies (e.g., Bolton 1958).

Given the weakness in establishing causal associations, these studies are often used as a means for creating new questions or for hypothesis generation rather than for testing hypotheses. Correlations found in cross-sectional studies in general should be followed up in subsequent research using other designs that allow for better characterization of the hypothesized association with regard to the conditions indicating causality, as noted by Hill (1965).

Case–control

The case–control design is a versatile one that is often used as an initial exploration of etiology, hence appropriate for Question 2 above. A case–control design should begin with a statement about the source population giving rise to the so-called cases (Rothman and Greenland 1998). In the example, cases would be defined as children with Class II malocclusion, and the source population could be something such as all children living in Dr. Jones's community between the ages of 7 and 9. The control group would also be selected from this source population and would be children without the condition (no Class II malocclusion).

The design is considered retrospective in that the exposures of interest (potential etiological factors) will all have occurred prior to the initiation of the study and are collected through historical assessment (e.g., record review, questionnaire, subject interview). In this example, it could be hypothesized that thumb sucking could be a risk factor, and parents could be asked questions about their child's past habits in an interview or with a questionnaire.

The advantage of this design is the fact that you start the study by enrolling subjects who already have the condition or outcome of interest (e.g., Class II malocclusion). Hence, diseases that are rare or have long latency periods (e.g., certain cancers) can be efficiently studied without the need to recruit large numbers of subjects (when diseases are rare) or waiting for decades for an outcome to develop (when diseases have long latency periods). However, this design is not limited to rare disease or those with long latency.

Because the exposures that potentially could have resulted in the outcome have already occurred, this design also sidesteps any ethical concerns about exposing study subjects to potential harm or not providing needed care in the quest for information on etiology. Thus, this is a commonly used design in the study of toxic exposures leading to diseases such as cancer.

There are two main concerns with the case–control study design. One is information bias based on poor recall or documentation of past exposures. It may be difficult to accurately recall past exposure for many subjects, particularly when they occurred far in the past or when they are not readily quantifiable. In the example, some measure of the concept of "thumb sucking" would need to be developed and used to evaluate the exposure level for each child.

The second, and often the greater concern, is the bias introduced by poor selection of the control group. Selecting an appropriate control group is far from a trivial task and can be the downfall of a case–control study through the introduction of uncontrolled selection bias. Rothman and Greenland (1998) and Sackett (1979) address these biases at length and provide insight into strategies to overcome them.

Cohort

This prospective design consists of assembling a group of subjects who, at the time of study initiation, are free of the outcome (disease) of interest but vary in their exposure to the potential etiological agents of interest. The individuals are then followed over time by periodically reassessing the subject to determine if and when the outcome develops. The study must run until sufficient numbers of individuals develop the outcome to be able to statistically analyze the results or until some critical phase has passed. These designs are the preferred observational design when examining causal associations and can also be used to study the natural history of a disease. Thus, this is the design of choice when determining Question 3 above: how many children will grow out of a need for orthodontic treatment if they remain untreated?

Cohort studies often create a rich and complex dataset that allows for numerous hypotheses to be tested. Because much of the measurement of the exposures of interest are done by the investigators (rather than through record reviews or subject recall), the design is considered to be the observational design with the lowest potential for bias. Moreover, conclusions related to causality are strengthened by the ability to establish the temporal association between exposure and outcome. Given that the investigators do not control exposures among the study subjects, the ethics of studying harmful exposures (e.g., smoking) are avoided.

The main weaknesses of this design are its cost to assemble and follow a cohort, often for years, with subjects lost to follow-up as the study unfolds, and the potential for other causal factors confounding the results, because exposures are not randomized or controlled.

Experimental

Randomized controlled trial

The randomized clinical trial (RCT) is the sine qua non for establishing efficacy and safety of therapeutic interventions and would be the design of choice for Question 4 above. Since its development in the 1950s (Randal 1998), the methods have undergone refinement, with current best practices for RCTs formalized in the *Consolidated Standards of Reporting Trials* (CONSORT) statement (Altman *et al.* 2001). Details of this potentially complex design can be found in Meinert (1986).

In its simplest form, the RCT is a means to compare two approaches to treating a given condition or disease. The first step requires recruiting a population of individuals, all of whom have the condition or disease of interest. This group is then divided into two groups through a formal randomization process, the purpose of which is to make the groups as similar are possible with respect to all potential factors that could be related to their response to the treatment(s) under study. Randomization involves assigning individuals to one of the study groups through a random process to maximize the probability that study groups are similar as to disease status, as well as medical, demographic, social, or other relevant conditions, and independent of the investigators' knowledge of subjects. Once the two groups have been assembled through randomization, it can be assumed that any difference in response to the two therapies under study is related to the efficacy of the therapies and not to some underlying difference in the two groups (e.g., age, disease severity, or comorbidities).

Each study group is provided with a different therapy. Generally, RCTs are used to compare a "new" therapy to a traditional therapy, but in some cases it is ethical to compare a new therapy with no treatment or placebo. The decision on what is the proper comparison therapy with a new therapy is based on ethical considerations and the current standard of care. When a new therapy is introduced, its assignment to patients in an RCT is considered ethical only when there is a state of equipoise. *Equipoise* is a state of presumed equality between the new therapy and the old, where it is truly unknown if the new therapy offers any benefit (or harm) compared to the old. It is only when the condition of equipoise exists that it is considered ethical to randomly assign patients into the new or traditional treatment groups. When a current efficacious therapy exists, new therapies must be compared with current therapies. Only when no current efficacious therapies are available can a "no treatment" or "placebo" group be used.

Once the groups are assigned and the therapies initiated, the study subjects are followed over time to determine how well the therapies did in treating the condition of interest. At the same time, unwanted outcomes (adverse events) are monitored to ensure subject safety and determine the hazards of the new therapy. For any research funded by the National Institutes of Health, a Data Safety and Monitoring Board (DSMB) needs to be in place to ensure that any harm arising from the therapies under study is noted and, if necessary, the study can be stopped to prevent further subject harm.

The advantage of the RCT is its ability to minimize bias. Bias is minimized through the construction of two equal groups for study assembled through randomization. Additionally, the investigators can exert careful control over the delivery of the therapeutic intervention and can carefully monitor the changes in subject health status. Thus, it is unlikely that any outcomes that are observed are the result of uncontrolled bias. Consequently, RCTs are said to have high internal validity (internal validity is defined as the degree to which a study provides truth about a cause-and-effect relationship within the study sample).

The major disadvantages of the RCT are its cost and, at times, low external validity (external validity is defined as the ability to generalize the findings from the study to a larger population of interest). The cost of providing care and following a large number of subjects can be substantial. For many medical therapies, for example, new drugs or new devices, the Food and Drug Administration (FDA) requires RCTs to document safety and efficacy prior to FDA approval for use and sale in the United States. In dentistry, this is somewhat less common due to the nature of many dental therapies. For example, over-the-counter products such as toothpaste and oral rinses do not need to go through an FDA-approved RCT process. Many surgical interventions, dental implants, and orthodontic devices are all exempt from FDA oversight. Manufacturers are often reluctant to incur the cost of establishing efficacy using a large RCT if they can market their products without such trials. Consequently, many of the approaches to treatment and many of the devices used in dentistry are lacking established efficacy as determined by an RCT.

The reasons for low external validity in RCTs are related to the nature of the subjects who can be successfully recruited into an RCT design. Oftentimes an individual who volunteers for a research study is substantially different (e.g., sicker or more compliant with therapy) than an individual in the community with the same condition who does not volunteer. Hence, it is often unclear if the findings from the RCT will be broadly applicable to individuals with the condition who were not included in the study.

As a result of the concerns over low external validity and safety, many RCTs represent only the initial assessment of therapeutic efficacy. Many drugs and devices continue to be followed once they are approved for the market through postmarket surveillance programs. These programs provide for reporting of unexpected outcomes and serve to identify rare side effects after the therapy is in broader use.

It should be noted that although RCTs are well suited for identifying the efficacy of a new therapy, they may not be a good estimate of effectiveness. Efficacy is the potential of a therapy to provide a benefit under "ideal" conditions. *Ideal* refers to the optimal selection of subjects and delivery of the therapy, conditions which are optimized in RCTs. Most RCTs have stringent inclusion and exclusion criteria that select for subjects most likely to benefit from the therapy. Additionally, the delivery of the therapy in regards to compliance or provider skill is also monitored to ensure optimal delivery. The low risk of bias and careful control of operational procedures contribute to the RCTs' high internal validity.

Effectiveness is the ability of the therapy to provide a benefit under more "real world" conditions, as found in routine clinical practice. Once efficacy is established within the RCT, most therapies are then made widely available and enter routine practice. It is here where the delivery of the therapy may differ in substantial ways from those encountered in the RCT. For example, the stringent exclusion criteria found in the RCT may now be ignored, hence sicker patients or patients with comorbid conditions that alter the efficacy of the therapy may begin to receive it. Additionally, especially with surgical interventions (e.g., dental implants), provider skill may vary from that of the providers trained for the RCT. Consequently, benefits to patients may not approach the level found in the RCT. This difference can be substantial and should be understood by the clinician when considering therapeutic options and providing informed consent.

Quasiexperiments

The other common experimental designs are known collectively as quasiexperimental designs. The main difference between these designs and RCTs is that the quasiexperimental designs lack a randomized control group. In fact, they often lack a separate control group altogether and rely on before and after designs with the same group. These designs are popular in the social and behavioral sciences but would not be adequate for new drug- or device-approval studies. A complete description of these designs is provided by Campbell and Stanley (1963).

Systematic reviews and meta-analysis

Systematic reviews and meta-analytic studies represent the latest wave of innovations that are changing the way in which information is gathered, summarized, and distributed for use by clinicians. In the early days of evidence-based medicine (and dentistry), which is to say the 1990s, clinicians were taught how to review and evaluate individual studies so that they could conduct personal reviews of the literature and arrive at an informed approach to care. The skills needed to master the scientific literature were not trivial and required a considerable amount of effort to master. However, once mastered, they provided the clinician with the ability to sort through the mass of clinical literature, tease out those papers worth reading, and determine what information was valid and relevant enough to inform their clinical practice.

A major shortcoming of this approach was that the amount of clinical literature being produced, tens of thousands of articles each year, was so vast that any busy clinician could only hope to read a small portion of it. Consequently, much information inevitably would be missed, leading to a partial understanding of the status of current research on a given topic. Even worse, it could potentially create an information bias or confirmation bias if a clinician limited his or her reading only to research that conforms to the clinician's existing beliefs or practices.

Problems with the published literature are highlighted by this quote from the Cochrane Collaboration website (2017):

> It is a difficult task for practitioners to keep up-to-date with the relevant evidence in their field of interest: the major bibliographic databases cover less than half the world's literature and are biased towards English-language publications; textbooks, editorials and reviews that have not been prepared systematically may be unreliable; much evidence is unpublished, but unpublished evidence may be important; and more easily accessible research reports tend to exaggerate the benefits of interventions.

The fact that there was useful information not being used by clinicians, either due to time constraints limiting their ability to search and read the literature or lack of knowledge about how to interpret studies, was brought to light by Archie Cochrane as far back as the 1970s (Cochrane 1972). Cochrane noted that there was useful information being ignored by clinicians as well as the persistent use of therapies that were documented as being ineffective. Cochrane thought that this could be remedied by making high-quality information more easily available in a form that properly summarized the current knowledge on a topic in an unbiased and easily understood manner. He received funding from the British National Health Service to set up a program to develop and disseminate information to medical practitioners. The approach they used evolved into what is now known as systematic reviews and led to the establishment of the now well-known Cochrane Collaboration, the foremost creator and distributor of systematic reviews for medicine and dentistry in the world.

Features of a systematic review

A systematic review summarizes the results of available carefully designed health-care studies (usually controlled trials) and provides a high level of evidence on the effectiveness of health-care interventions.

The reviewers set about their task very methodically, following step by step an advance plan. The steps typically followed in conducting a systematic review are as follows:

- Create a rationale or statement of purpose based on a question about clinical practice.
- Conduct a search for evidence. This almost always includes computerized databases (e.g., Medline), but can also include hand searches of relevant journals, non-English-language journals, and the gray literature (e.g., nonpublished reports, theses, dissertations).
- Identify studies that meet basic inclusion criteria (Cochrane reviews often limit included studies to RCTs.)
- Review these studies in detail for relevance.
- If the studies are not relevant, reject them.
- If the studies are relevant, evaluate their methodological quality.
- If quality is sufficient, extract data.
- Analyze the data in context with other studies.
- Summarize and draw conclusions.

When the underlying measurements used in RCTs are similar enough, it may be possible to mathematically combine the results of several studies to conduct a new analysis of the combined data. This is called a meta-analysis and is a means to improve the overall sample size and hence statistical power of the analysis. It also allows for an estimate of an overall effect that may better capture the real effect of a treatment or intervention.

For most clinicians, reading systematic reviews and meta-analyses is the preferred approach for answering a clinical question regarding patient care. Systematic reviews, when done using well-established and valid search criteria such as those employed by the Cochrane Collaboration, provide, in general, a much more exhaustive examination of the state of the current research. They also provide an objective selection of studies and data extraction processes. Consequently, they can quickly provide the reader with, arguably, the highest quality, least-biased evidence available on the efficacy, safety, and value of any given therapy and allow us to resist the influence of Glacow's law, which states "one half-baked observation I made personally is equal in validity to 12 randomized, double-blind trials." (Kunin 1979). Thus, systematic reviews are highly recommended as the first choice for evidence in support of clinical decision making. Dr. Jones would be well served in her quest to understand the benefits of early treatment by referring to the Cochrane Review that addresses this topic (Harrison *et al.* 2007).

Translational research

In its examination of health-care delivery in the United States, the National Academy of Sciences, Institute of Medicine (IOM 2001) found there were three main problems characterizing health-care delivery. These problems were: (1) an *underuse* of therapies that are known to benefit patients; (2) an *overuse* of therapies known to not benefit patients; and (3) the *misuse* of therapies leading to avoidable errors in delivery that fail to provide full benefit or result in unnecessary harm to patients. Collectively, they called this the "know–do gap".

Translational research is the interdisciplinary field of biomedical research that aims to reduce this gap by advancing methods that are shown to be effective in moving high-quality scientific evidence into routine patient care, thus improving prevention, diagnosis, and therapies (Cohrs 2015). Two important subareas within translational research of direct relevance to clinical orthodontics are the study of strategies for the dissemination of new evidence and for its implementation into routine clinical practice.

Dissemination research aims to optimize how information is delivered to busy clinicians to maximize its utility in clinical practice. Optimizing information transfer faces several barriers in dental practice. Research suggests that dentists rely heavily on peers for clinical information and validation of new approaches to care (Spallek *et al.* 2010; O'Donnell *et al.* 2013), causing concern that this process can be arbitrary and subject to unknown biases. Even when high-quality scientific information is sought, access to the relevant scientific literature presents barriers for dentists when they lack access to academic medical libraries. Moreover, much of the scientific literature on a topic consists of numerous individual studies that vary in quality, are spread across numerous journals, and are often published over many years. Thus, grasping the full extent of the current understanding about a particular clinical topic can be challenging.

Several dissemination strategies have been developed to address this challenge of summarizing the evidence around a clinical topic. Of particular relevance here is the development of secondary sources of evidence. Secondary sources include systematic reviews (as discussed in Section Systematic reviews and meta-analysis) and clinical practice guidelines (discussed in Section Clinical practice guidelines). Both of these approaches aim to transparently and without bias summarize the evidence around a given topic of clinical relevance and present it in a manner that is easily understood and, with guidelines, applicable to patient care. Grimshaw *et al.* (2012) refers to these secondary sources or evidence summaries as the basic unit of knowledge translation.

Clinical practice guidelines

Turning scientific evidence into clinically actionable information that can be routinely applied to improve patient care is the ultimate goal of clinical research. As important as systematic reviews are in accurately summarizing current knowledge around prevention, diagnoses, and therapies, they are not designed to provide clinicians with actionable recommendations on how best to use that knowledge in patient care. Translating research findings into recommendations around patient care is the role of clinical practice guidelines.

The US Institute of Medicine (IOM 2011) defines clinical practice guidelines as "statements that include recommendations intended to optimize patient care that are informed by a systematic review of evidence and an assessment of the benefits and harms of alternative care options". As can be seen from this definition, the need for a systematic review as a point of departure for guideline development means that high-quality guidelines attempt to base recommendations upon the best (i.e., least biased) information available on a topic. Guideline development typically follows a process whereby current evidence from a systematic review is evaluated by an expert panel. Based upon this evidence review, the panel ideally makes unambiguous and actionable recommendations as to the indications, benefits, and harms of various treatment options.

As there are no rules as to who can undertake guideline development, their quality varies. The Guideline International Network provides standards as an aid in assessing guideline quality (Qaseem *et al.* 2012). Briefly, these standards emphasize the need for a guideline development panel that includes diverse stakeholders and research methodologists. Also emphasized is the need for transparency in the decision-making process, assessment of evidence quality, periodic updates as new evidence becomes available, and identification of conflicts of interest.

The overarching goal of guideline developers is to broadly influence the quality of patient care. Thus, guidelines tend to be widely disseminated and easily accessible for clinicians. Some important guideline databases are the following:

National Guideline Clearinghouse (NGC) (www.guideline.gov/)
Scottish Intercollegiate Guideline Network (SIGN) (www.sign.ac.uk/)
Translating Research into Practice (TRIP) (www.tripdatabase.com/)
UpToDate (www.uptodate.com/home)
American Dental Association Center for Evidence Based Dentistry (http://ebd.ada.org/en)
Guideline International Network (www.g-i-n.net)

Mindful that patients cannot benefit from treatment they do not receive, implementation science was developed to facilitate bridging the final gap required to bring evidence into routine practice. Implementation science is thus concerned empirically with examining how the contextual factors in the clinical care environment facilitate or impede adoption of high-quality evidence into care delivery. Implementation efforts typically focus on strategies that ensure high-quality clinical practice guidelines are appropriately and routinely applied in care delivery. In so doing, the aim is to ensure that all patients who would benefit from a specific treatment are given that treatment, thus improving patient and population health outcomes. It thus becomes the role of the attending clinician to apply their clinical skills in determining which individuals would benefit from the guideline recommendations and which patients would benefit from a different approach.

Implementation science is an acknowledgement that dissemination alone of high-quality evidence rarely results in the desired outcome, that is clinicians incorporating new evidence as part of their routine patient care. It has been shown repeatedly that knowledge of appropriate care alone is insufficient in most cases to produce modifications in clinicians' behavior (Francke *et al.* 2008). In fact, Bonetti *et al.* (2009) found no association between dentists' knowledge and behavior. Several other studies of dentists' behavior report similar findings, where knowledge of the effectiveness of particular intervention was unrelated to a willingness to provide those therapies to patients (O'Donnell *et al.* 2013; Tellez *et al.* 2011).

This failure to translate knowledge into action has been found to be the result of a complex interplay of numerous individual and contextual factors. These factors include psychological resistance to change as well as structural, financial, and policy barriers that generally accompany any substantial change in the type of treatments provided. Implementation science studies the nature of these barriers and then suggests approaches aimed at overcoming the identified barriers, with the goal of making the delivery of appropriate evidence-based care routine.

One should anticipate expanded production of clinical practice guidelines and their adoption into dental care delivery. Factors that will drive this include the growing emphasis on value-based payment, which emphasizes both patient and population health outcomes, and economic factors resulting in consolidation of dental practices and rapid growth of multiprovider care delivery groups. The result of these changes will be an emphasis on evidence-based practice and accountability for care delivered. This is a welcome change and both patients and dentists will benefit.

References

Altman DG, Schulz KF, Moher M, *et al.*, 2001. The revised CONSORT statement for reporting randomized trials: explanation and elaboration. *Ann Intern Med* 134, 663–694.

Bolton WA, 1958. Disharmony in tooth size and its relation to the analysis and treatment of malocclusion. *Angle Orthod* 28, 113–130.

Bonetti D, Johnston M, Pitts NB, *et al.*, 2009. Knowledge may not be the best target for strategies to influence evidence based practice: using psychological models to understand RCT effects. *Int J Behav Med* 16, 287–293.

Campbell DT, Stanly JC, 1963. *Experimental and Quasi-experimental Designs for Research*. Boston: Houghton Mifflin.

Cochrane Collaboration, 2017. *Cochrane Collaboration*. Available at: www.cochrane.org/ (accessed Nov. 2017).

Cochrane AL, 1972. *Effectiveness and Efficiency: Random Reflections on Health Services*. London: Nuffield Provincial Hospitals Trust.

Cohrs RJ, Martin T, Ghahramani P, *et al.*, 2015. Translational medicine definition by the European Society for Translational Medicine. *New Horiz Transl Med* 2, 86–88.

DeAngelis C, 1990. *An Introduction to Clinical Research*. New York: Oxford University Press.

Francke AL, Smit MC, de Veer AJE, *et al.*, 2008. Factors influencing the implementation of clinical guidelines for health care professionals: A systematic meta-review. *BMC Med Inform Decis Mak* 8, 38.

Grimshaw JM, Eccles MP, Lavis JN, *et al.*, 2012. Knowledge translation of research findings. *Implement Sci* 7, 50.

Harrison JE, O'Brien KD, Worthington HV, 2007. Orthodontic treatment for prominent upper front teeth in children. *Cochrane Database Syst Rev* (3), CD003452.

Hill AB, 1965. The environment and disease: association or causation? *Proc R Soc Med* 58, 295–300.

Institute of Medicine (IOM), 2001. *Crossing the Quality Chasm: A New Health System for the 21st Century.* Washington, DC: National Academies Press.

Institute of Medicine (IOM), 2011. *Clinical Practice Guidelines We Can Trust.* Washington, DC: National Academies Press.

Kunin CM, 1979. *Practical Aspects of Antibiotic Review.* Atlanta: American Health Consultants.

Meinert CL, 1990. *Clinical Trials: Design, Conduct, and Analysis.* New York: Oxford University Press.

O'Donnell JA, Modesto A, Oakley M, *et al.*, 2013. Sealants and dental caries. Insight into dentists' behaviors regarding implementation of clinical practice recommendations. *J Am Dent Assoc* 144, e24–e30.

Qaseem A, Forland F, Macbeth F, *et al.*, 2012. Guidelines International Network: toward international standards for clinical practice guidelines. *Ann Intern Med* 156, 525–531.

Randal J, 1998. How randomized clinical trials came into their own. *J Natl Cancer Inst* 90, 1257–1258.

Rothman KJ, Greenland S, 1998. *Modern Epidemiology*, 2nd ed. Philadelphia: Lippincott Raven.

Sackett DL, 1979. Bias in analytic research. *J Chronic Dis* 32, 51–63.

Salmon MH, Earman J, Glymour C, *et al.*, 1992. *Introduction to the Philosophy of Science.* Indianapolis: Hackett Publishing Co.

Spallek H, Song M, Polk DE, *et al.*, 2010. Barriers to Implementing evidence-based clinical guidelines: a survey of early adopters. *J Evid Based Dent Pract* 10, 195–206.

Tellez M, Gray SL, Gray S, *et al.*, 2011. Sealants and dental caries: Dentists' perspectives on evidence-based recommendations. *J Am Dent Assoc.* 142, 1033–1040.

3

Electronic Searching for Clinical Trials Information

Anne Littlewood

Introduction

While systematic reviews may include studies utilizing any research designs, it is obviously best to restrict the content of systematic reviews to randomized trials, as they will provide the most valid and least biased findings. This is the strategy that Cochrane has adopted, and this chapter is largely based on the methods utilized by Cochrane review teams.

Searching for trials information to include in systematic reviews is a complex process; in order to avoid bias in the results of the review, as many relevant trials as possible must be found. There are many sources that can be searched, including MEDLINE and Embase (Excerpta Medica Database). These databases are growing month by month and advanced searching techniques are required to ensure that all relevant studies are found, but not at the cost of being overloaded by too many citations.

Searching electronic databases for systematic reviews requires a balance between sensitivity (number of relevant articles found as a proportion of all the relevant articles) and precision (the number of relevant articles found as a proportion of *all* articles). Searches for Cochrane systematic reviews attempt to aim for maximum sensitivity, so that no relevant articles are missed. This chapter will cover which databases to search, and how to construct a sensitive search strategy. It should be noted that this type of search is not suitable for all requirements. If a searcher needs a quick answer to a clinical question, this approach would not be needed. This kind of rigorous systematic process is only expected when a searcher wishes to avoid publication bias and retrieve as many articles as possible on a given topic.

Where to search: choosing databases

No one single resource covers all the information that is needed for a systematic review. A range of databases should be searched in order to make sure that all eligible trials are found and included. A search will normally cover the more mainstream medical databases, MEDLINE and Embase, and trials and systematic review information within the Cochrane Library as a minimum. Non-English language literature, gray literature, and trials registers are further sources of reports of clinical trials. Researchers should always check what is available to them via their institution or medical library.

MEDLINE

MEDLINE is a resource from the United States, based at the National Library of Medicine. Records date back to 1946, and 4600 journals have been added to the resource. It currently contains over 23 million citations in 40 languages (US National Library of Medicine 2017), and has a well-deserved reputation as the most

Evidence-Based Orthodontics, Second Edition. Edited by Greg J. Huang, Stephen Richmond and Katherine W. L. Vig.
© 2018 John Wiley & Sons, Inc. Published 2018 by John Wiley & Sons, Inc.

comprehensive medical science database (Collins 2007). MEDLINE is available through several database providers, including Ovid and EBSCO, via a subscription. MEDLINE is also available for free online via the PubMed service: http://www.ncbi.nlm.nih.gov/sites/entrez

Embase

Embase is the European equivalent of MEDLINE, based in the Netherlands and produced by the publisher Elsevier. It has coverage of over 8500 journals since 1947, and has 31 million citations (Elsevier 2017). It has a particular focus on pharmacological sciences, and also provides access to non-English language references and conference proceedings.Like MEDLINE, it is available via Ovid, but Embase also provide the service directly via Embase.com. Both of these services are subscription based, and require users to pay a premium to search and download citations. However, much of Embase's content is available via Scopus (https://www.scopus.com/), although its search interface is not as sophisticated as Ovid or Embase.com.

The Cochrane Library

The Cochrane Library is published by John Wiley and Sons and is produced by Cochrane. The Cochrane Database of Systematic Reviews contains all the published Cochrane reviews and protocols, at the time of writing there are over 9000 records, covering all the subject areas of the Cochrane Review Groups (Cochrane Collaboration 2017). Almost 200 of these are in the field of oral health. The Cochrane Central Register of Controlled Clinical Trials (CENTRAL) comprises the trials registers collated and maintained by the Cochrane Review Groups, along with records of randomized and controlled clinical trials from PubMed and Embase. It currently contains over 900 000 clinical trials (Cochrane Collaboration 2017). Access to The Cochrane Library varies from country to country, but all of the content is available free to residents of many countries including: the UK, Australia, Denmark, Finland, Ireland, some Latin American countries and the Caribbean, New Zealand, Norway, Poland, Spain, and Sweden (see http://www.cochranelibrary.com/help/access-options-for-cochrane-library.html for information). The Cochrane Library operates a green and gold open access model; reviews published from 1 February 2013 are available to all for free after 1 year of publication (green access) or immediately if the authors have funded the review through the gold open access option.

The Cochrane Library can be accessed via www.cochranelibrary.com/.

Non-English language literature

MEDLINE, Embase, and CENTRAL within the Cochrane Library all provide access to non-English language citations of clinical trials, but there are alternative sources of information. One of the largest non-English language databases is the Latin American and Caribbean Health Sciences Literature Resource (LILACS), which provides access to references from journals published in South and Central America. It can be searched in English, Spanish, or Portuguese. Access in the UK can be gained through the Virtual Health Library (http://lilacs.bvsalud.org/en/). There are country-specific databases with some limited trials information, such as KoreaMED (www.koreamed.org). Other non-English language sources include: the Chinese National Knowledge Infrastructure (www.cnki.net/), and the various databases provided through the World Health Organization. These include resources for the Eastern Mediterranean (http://www.emro.who.int/his/vhsl) and Africa (http://indexmedicus.afro.who.int).

Trials registers

Information about clinical trials, both ongoing and completed, can be found on trials registers. Cochrane Review Groups all maintain a specialized register of trials in their subject area. Cochrane Oral Health's register currently contains approximately 32 000 references to published clinical trials information. Access to the Cochrane trials registers is normally arranged through the Review Group's Information Specialist (more information can be found at http://oralhealth.cochrane.org/trials).

Information on ongoing trials can be found on the ISRCTN Registry (www.controlled-trials.com/), a resource which is free to search and gives details including the study design, trial outcomes measured, and contact information. The US National Institutes of Health provide free access to http://clinicaltrials.gov, a database containing over 230 000 study records (US National Institutes of Health 2017). Its coverage aims to be global but there is an inevitable concentration on trials from the US. The information provided includes the trial's purpose, participants, and contact information. The World Health Organization provides a gateway to several trials registers at http://www.who.int/trialsearch. The registers covered include the Australia and New Zealand Clinical Trials Registry, the Chinese Clinical Trial Register, the German Clinical Trials Register, the Iranian Registry of Clinical Trials, and the Netherlands National Trials Register (World Health Organization 2017).

OpenTrials is an initiative that attempts to link all available information on every clinical trials ever conducted. It is a work in progress and is the result of a collaboration between Open Knowledge International and the University of Oxford's DataLab (Open Knowledge International and DataLab 2017). The Beta platform is available for searching: https://explorer.opentrials.net/.

Gray literature, dissertations and conference proceedings

Gray literature is the ephemera that is not formally published in books or journals. Along with dissertations and conference proceedings, it can be a useful source of trials information. Open Grey (www.opengrey.eu/) is the System for Information on Gray Literature in Europe, and is a database of references relating to reports, dissertations, and conference papers. Access is free of charge. Conference proceedings can be found via a number of resources including Zetoc (http://zetoc.mimas.ac.uk), and the Web of Science (http://isiwebofknowledge.com), accessible via subscription. Selected dissertation abstracts are also available online. EThOS (http://ethos.bl.uk) is a service provided by the British Library, and has 250 000 records of abstracts of dissertations from UK universities. Database provider ProQuest (www.proquest.com/) also provides a global dissertation and thesis service, although this is subscription only.

Clinical study reports

For research on drugs and medical devices, especially those developed in the last 5 years, searching clinical study reports (CSRs) for regulatory data is recommended (Schroll and Bero 2015). CSRs typically contain a lot more data than a clinical trials record from a database like ClinicalTrials.gov. The two databases most widely used for searching for CSRs are the European Medicines Agency (EMA) database (https://clinicaldata.ema.europa.eu/web/cdp/home), and the US Food and Drugs Administration (FDA) database (http://www.fda.gov/Drugs/InformationOnDrugs/default.htm).

Choosing the right platform

Many of the resources listed above are available via several different service providers: platforms that offer access to these electronic databases include Ovid, EBSCO, PubMed, EMBASE.com, and SilverPlatter. While most of these require a subscription to access, PubMed is free of charge. The subscription services are normally superior, in that they allow more sophisticated and advanced searching, and sometimes provide links to the full text of the citation. In most cases where there is access to both, the subscription service should be used in preference to the free version. Most university and medical libraries subscribe to at least one of the subscription services, and advice should be sought from a subject specialist or librarian as to which are available and how to access them. Search syntax and subject headings vary from platform to platform, so it is important to know how the database is being accessed so that the search can be tailored appropriately. A search designed for MEDLINE via Ovid will not work in MEDLINE via PubMed. All of the mainstream medical databases provide help on their websites to assist in developing a correct and structured search strategy.

How to search: constructing a search strategy

Electronic records

Most of the electronic databases mentioned above provide access to citations from journals, not the full text of the article. Some also contain access to citations from books, conference proceedings, and dissertations. Electronic records normally contain basic information about an article such as authors, title, journal, volume and issue, page numbers, language, and year of publication. In most cases, more detailed information can also be found, like an abstract and contact details for the authors, although some older articles may have been added without abstracts. Many of the databases above also index all the journal articles with keywords and controlled vocabulary to help in searching.

Controlled vocabulary

Most of the mainstream medical literature databases can be searched using a mixture of controlled vocabulary and free text. Controlled vocabulary is a list of words and phrases used to "tag" information in electronic databases, in order to group similar articles together. The most famous example in this context is MEDLINE's Medical Subject Headings (MeSH). MeSH terms are arranged in a hierarchy or tree. Broader concepts come near the top of the tree and more specific terms lower down.

These subject headings are assigned to the articles in MEDLINE by experienced indexers at the National Library of Medicine (NLM) in the United States. MeSH can be found for a topic by visiting the NLM's MeSH browser at: http://www.nlm.nih.gov/mesh/MBrowser.html.

Typing in a keyword will not only give the MeSH term for that topic, but will also show where the term comes in the MeSH tree. The MeSH term can be used in MEDLINE to search for any records that have been indexed with it. This means that you do not have to know the exact wording of the title or abstract in order to retrieve the article in a search. For example, if you were to search for the MeSH "Dental caries", any article indexed with this term would be retrieved, even if the article itself does not mention caries and talks about tooth decay instead.

MeSH can also be "exploded" to include all of the terms that are included in that subject heading on the tree. For example, exploding the term "Orthodontic Appliances, Removable" (Table 3.1), would also search the terms "Activator Appliances" and "Extraoral Traction Appliances", without you having to enter those

Table 3.1 Example of a MeSH tree: orthodontic appliances.

Orthodontic Appliances	
Occlusal Splints	
Orthodontic Appliances, Functional	
	Activator Appliances
Orthodontic Appliances, Removable	
	Activator Appliances
	Extraoral Traction Appliances
Orthodontic Brackets	
	Orthodontic Retainers
	Orthodontic Wires

additional terms into the search box. However, you can also focus your search by not exploding the term. An unexploded search for "Orthodontic Appliances, Removable" would only retrieve the records indexed with that term, and not the records indexed with "Activator Appliances" and "Extraoral Traction Appliances".

Controlled vocabulary is not only used in MEDLINE, but in other electronic databases also, including Embase and the Cochrane Library. However, the terms used do vary from database to database, so the subject headings may have to be translated to make the search work in electronic resources other than MEDLINE.

Free-text searching

Searching for MeSH terms or controlled vocabulary limits the search to only include those terms that appear in the keyword field of a record, whereas free-text searching can be applied in any field in the record: author, abstract, keywords, or even full-text. Most electronic databases support the searching of single words or phrases: such as "orthodontic appliances". Searchers should avoid, however, just using free text at the expense of controlled vocabulary. If free-text alone is used the search will be limited to just those words or phrases you have entered. For example, a search for "Jaw Abnormalities" as free text will search for only that phrase where it appears in the title, abstract or keyword fields. However, the same phrase exploded as a MeSH term will also pick up those records indexed with further terms: including cleft palate, retrognathism, and Pierre Robin syndrome, records that the free-text search for "Jaw Abnormalities" would miss. However, MeSH indexing is not always fully comprehensive either, especially for older or foreign language records.

Ideally a full search for a systematic review should contain a combination of controlled vocabulary and free text to ensure that all bases are covered.

Boolean operators

One or more terms can be combined in a search using Boolean operators: these are supported by most electronic databases. The most common operators are AND, OR, and NOT, with all letters capitalized. AND is used when the records retrieved from the search must contain all of the search terms. The OR command is used when the records retrieved in the search can contain either of the search terms whether or not they appear together in the record. The NOT command is for searches where one term can be retrieved but the other must not be, even if it appears alongside the included term.

To put this into context, if you were searching for a study on orthodontic treatment for crowded teeth, a search for "orthodontic appliances" AND "crowded teeth" would usefully combine both terms to only retrieve the articles which contain both phrases (Figure 3.1).

However, not all articles may include the term "crowded teeth", and this is where the OR command is used to join synonyms together. For example: "crowded teeth" OR "Class I malocclusion" OR "Class II malocclusion" would pick up all of the articles containing any of these phrases in a free-text search (Figure 3.2).

Figure 3.1 The AND command – "orthodontic appliances" AND "crowded teeth" will only retrieve articles containing both terms (the shaded area).

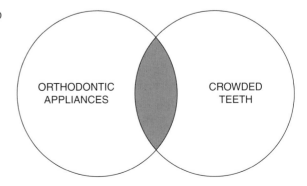

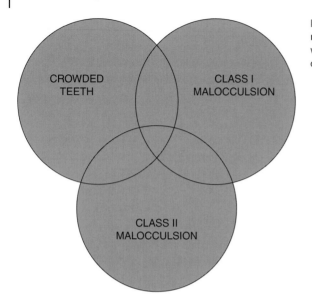

Figure 3.2 The OR command – "crowded teeth" OR "class I malocclusion" OR "class II malocclusion" will retrieve all articles with these terms, whether they appear together in the article or not. This is useful for finding synonyms.

The basic rule with Boolean operators is that AND will decrease the number of records retrieved in a search, where OR tends to increase the number of hits. Boolean operators can be combined together with parentheses. A search for ("crowded teeth" OR "Class II malocclusion") AND ("orthodontics") would search for all instances where the two phrases for the condition in question are discussed in the same article as orthodontics.

The Boolean NOT command should be used with caution, especially in the context of systematic reviews. Searches for systematic reviews should be designed to be as sensitive as possible, in order to make sure every clinical trial on a subject is retrieved. The NOT command is designed to exclude articles from a search so is rarely used in the construction of a search strategy for systematic reviewing. Use of the NOT command can also risk excluding articles that may be relevant. A search for "cancer NOT children" is designed to retrieve all articles about cancer but not cancer in children. However, if the abstract included the sentence "The participants in the trial were women with cervical cancer who had been pregnant and had children" then a search for "cancer NOT children" would not pick up this potentially relevant paper.

Truncation and wild cards

All of the mainstream databases discussed here support truncation, which enables searching on the "stem" of a word, which is useful when searching for words that could be pluralized. For example, a search for "child*" on PubMed would retrieve all articles containing the terms "child" or "child's" or "children", which saves time, as the search does not then have to include all variations on a word. Some databases will also support wild card searches, where a letter within a word can be replaced with a symbol so that the database search tool looks for all variations of a word. Within MEDLINE on the Ovid platform, the "?" symbol can be used as a wild card. For example, "wom?n" will retrieve articles containing the terms "women" and "woman" and "reminerali?ation" would retrieve the variant spellings "remineralisation" and "remineralization". Symbols for truncation and wild cards vary from database to database, so the Help or Frequently Asked Questions sections of websites should be checked to ensure the correct symbol is being used. *, $, % and ? are all commonly used for truncation or as wildcards.

Proximity operators

Some databases allow the searching of terms that are in close proximity to one another. This is a more precise method of searching than using "AND" but also more flexible than using a phrase search. A search for "dental anxiety" as a phrase would only search for those articles where the words appear next to each other. Searching "dental AND anxiety" would search for either term anywhere in the article. However, if a search for "dental near/6 anxiety" is conducted in The Cochrane Library, any references where the term "dental" is found within 6 words of the term "anxiety" will be retrieved. This can be a useful tool if you have many irrelevant results from an AND search and want to cut them down to a more relevant subset.

Not all database platforms support proximity searching. Most notably, PubMed does not, which is one of its limitations. As with truncation, the terminology for proximity searching varies from database to database. Ovid databases use "adj" for adjacent to, and EBSCO databases use the letter N. Again, the Help pages of each individual database should be checked to see if proximity searching is available and the correct terminology to use.

Building a search strategy

The first step in constructing an electronic search strategy is to identify relevant search terms or groups of terms that can be used as the basis of the strategy. It may be helpful at this stage to think in terms of participants or target population with the condition of interest, and the intervention of interest. For example, the systematic review entitled "Orthodontic treatment for prominent lower front teeth in children" can be broken down as:

Participants / population: Children
Intervention / treatment: Orthodontic treatment
Condition of interest: Class III malocclusion.

These kinds of section headings can help to provide a framework for the search. To date, bibliographic databases (unlike many search engines) are not especially intuitive, and will only search for the terms that are entered. It's therefore important to find as many synonyms as possible for each of these section headings.

If we take the example above, synonyms and related terms for orthodontic treatments or interventions could include:

- Fixed braces
- Facemasks
- Extraoral traction
- Reverse headgear.

Synonyms for the condition of interest in this case could include:

- Class III malocclusion
- Prominent lower front teeth
- Under-bite
- Reverse bite
- Prognathism.

Participants are more difficult to add to a search. For example, if the search was looking at adults, the term "adults" added to the search would not necessarily retrieve any more studies. The term "adult" may not be mentioned in all the studies on the topic. Participants could simply be called "patients" or "subjects", terms that may also include children! Participant information is better added to a search if you have a specific group of people or patients that are pertinent to the study, for example smokers or children, as in this case.

All of the synonyms identified for (in this example) the condition and the intervention should be listed. The NLM's MeSH browser should now be checked to see if any of the identified terms have a Medical Subject Heading: http://www.nlm.nih.gov/mesh/MBrowser.html. It is also worth checking where on the MeSH tree a term appears, to see whether any the subject headings above the identified term could be exploded to make the search more comprehensive. There may also be other synonyms in the MeSH tree that could be added to the search as free-text terms.

For the example above, the following MeSH terms were identified:

Condition
- Malocclusion, Angle Class III

Intervention
- Orthodontic appliances, Functional. This term can be exploded to include activator appliances
- Orthodontic appliances, Removable. This term can be exploded to include activator appliances and extraoral traction appliances.

Participants
- Child. This term can be exploded to include Child, Preschool.

Once the MeSH terms have been identified, the next stage is to start to build the free-text search. Taking the list of identified synonyms, the following questions need to be asked:

- Can any of the terms be truncated?
- Are there any alternative spellings?
- Are there any hyphens in any of the terms?
- Is it correct to explode the MeSH term? (in this case, does the population of interest include preschool children?)

Hyphens can be problematic, because the term could appear either with or without it in the literature. For example: "under-bite" could also appear as "under bite". Both versions should appear in the search strategy.

The search strategy for the condition can now be built. The example used here is for PubMed, and has been adapted from an Ovid search in a Cochrane Review (Watkinson *et al.* 2013). The first line is a MeSH term, the rest of the search is presented in free text. The square brackets after the terms are field tags, which indicate to PubMed which part of the record to search. [mh] represents the MeSH term, which can be exploded [mh:exp] or not exploded [mh:noexp]. A full list of field tags can be found on the NLM website: https://www.nlm.nih. gov/bsd/disted/pubmedtutorial/020_710.html. You can search just the author field, or the title, or keywords. Or you may want to combine two fields and search for words in the title and abstract. In PubMed, this would be achieved by typing [tiab] after your search term. In this example, we have searched all fields for the free-text terms (lines #2 to #6, there are no square brackets added to limit the search to particular fields), and the MeSH in line #1.

#1	Malocclusion, Angle Class III [mh:noexp]
#2	("Class III" AND malocclusion*)
#3	(Angle* AND "Class III")
#4	("Class III" AND bite*)
#5	(underbite* OR under-bite* OR "under bite*" OR "reverse bite*" OR reverse-bite* OR prognath*)
#6	"prominent lower front teeth"

These are the identified terms for the condition, and the identified MeSH term. Some have been truncated to pick up the plurals. Terms have been combined using AND / OR. Line #7 of the strategy should now combine all of these terms to tell PubMed that any or all of them could appear in the retrieved results.

#7	#1 OR #2 OR #3 OR #4 OR #5 OR #6

This completes the search for the condition. Terms for the interventions should now be added to the search:

#8	Orthodontic Appliances, Functional [mh:exp]
#9	Orthodontic Appliances, Removable [mh:exp]
#10	("growth modif*" AND jaw*)
#11	orthodontic*
#12	(extraoral AND traction)

#13   "chin cap*"
#14   ("face mask*" OR facemask* OR face-mask* OR "reverse head-gear" OR "reverse headgear")
#15   (orthopaedic OR orthopedic)
#16   #8 OR #9 OR #10 OR #11 OR #12 OR #13 OR #14 OR #15

The participants can then be added:

#17   Child [mh:exp]
#18   (child* OR adolescen* OR school-age* OR "school age*" OR teenage*)
#19   #17 OR 18

The final line of the strategy should bring together the condition, the intervention and the participants by using the AND command. This tells PubMed that you only want records about orthodontic interventions that are also about Class III malocclusion and children. The next line in this example should be:

#20   #7 AND #16 AND #19

Once the search strategy has been completed by combining the three sets of terms, the search should be tested in PubMed using the advanced search.
Questions to ask here are:

- Are the numbers of hits retrieved manageable for a systematic review? (generally less than 1000)
- Are any lines retrieving no hits? It may be that the wrong MeSH term has been used, or that one of the terms has been spelled or truncated incorrectly.
- Have any relevant keywords been missed?

Revisions should be made at this stage. If the number of hits is unmanageable, it may be possible to reduce the number by using proximity operators instead of "AND", depending on the platform. This is not possible in PubMed. Another way to cut down the number of hits is use of a search filter.

Search filters

Search filters are normally used to limit the search to particular study designs: for example, if the searcher is only interested in randomized trials or systematic reviews. They are designed to make the search more precise. There are standardized search filters available for use, and the InterTASC group have put together a web resource reviewing their efficacy. The website has filters for diagnostic tests, clinical trials, adverse events studies, economic evaluations, and qualitative research, among others: http://www.york.ac.uk/inst/crd/intertasc/.

Many of these have been peer reviewed by information specialists. An example would be the search filter that Cochrane has developed for finding randomized controlled trials in MEDLINE (Glanville *et al.* 2006). This filter has been tested against a "gold standard" of known records of randomized controlled trials within MEDLINE. The filter for PubMed has been published in *The Cochrane Handbook of Systematic Reviews for Interventions* (box 6.4a) (Lefebvre *et al.* 2009).

#1   randomized controlled trial [pt]
#2   controlled clinical trial [pt]
#3   randomized [tiab]
#4   placebo [tiab]
#5   drug therapy [sh]
#6   randomly [tiab]
#7   trial [tiab]
#8   groups [tiab]

#9	#1 OR #2 OR #3 OR #4 OR #5 OR #6 OR #7 OR #8
#10	animals [mh] NOT humans [mh]
#11	#9 NOT #10

Search filters can be added to a search by taking the last line of the subject search, and the last line of the search filter and adding an "AND" command, as in the example below:

#1	Malocclusion, Angle Class III [mh:noexp]
#2	("Class III" AND malocclusion*)
#3	(Angle* AND "Class III")
#4	("Class III" AND bite*)
#5	(underbite* OR under-bite* OR "under bite*" OR "reverse bite*" OR reverse-bite* OR prognath*)
#6	"prominent lower front teeth"
#7	#1 OR #2 OR #3 OR #4 OR #5 OR #6
#8	Orthodontic Appliances, Functional [mh:exp]
#9	Orthodontic Appliances, Removable [mh:exp]
#10	("growth modif*" AND jaw*)
#11	orthodontic*
#12	(extraoral AND traction)
#13	"chin cap*"
#14	("face mask*" OR facemask* OR face-mask* OR "reverse head-gear" OR "reverse headgear")
#15	(orthopaedic OR orthopedic)
#16	#8 OR #9 OR #10 OR #11 OR #12 OR #13 OR #14 OR #15
#17	Child [mh:exp]
#18	(child* OR adolescen* OR school-age* OR "school age*" OR teenage*)
#19	#17 OR 18
#20	#7 AND #16 AND #19
#21	randomized controlled trial [pt]
#22	controlled clinical trial [pt]
#23	randomized [tiab]
#24	placebo [tiab]
#25	drug therapy [sh]
#26	randomly [tiab]
#27	trial [tiab]
#28	groups [tiab]
#29	#21 OR #22 OR #23 OR #24 OR #25 OR #26 OR #27 OR #28
#30	animals [mh] NOT humans [mh]
#31	#29 NOT #30
#32	**#20 AND #31**

This will limit the search on orthodontic treatment for prominent lower front teeth in children to controlled clinical trials.

Translating the strategy

Once the MEDLINE strategy has been perfected, it needs to be translated for use in other databases. The golden rule is to check the help or frequently asked questions sections of the database website to ensure that the correct symbols are used to truncate, and that the correct terms are used in terms of controlled vocabulary. Controlled vocabulary varies from database to database, and MeSH terms are revised once a year, so these should be checked whenever the search is updated. The field tags and search terminology should also be checked, for example, is there another way of searching the title or abstract fields? If a line in your search retrieves less hits than expected, then it may need to be revised. Building a good search strategy is a process of trial and error, and all searches should be tested and revised accordingly.

Summary

- A range of sources should be searched to find eligible trials for a systematic review. These should include MEDLINE, Embase, and the Cochrane Library as a minimum.
- The method or platform for accessing the database is important, as a search designed for one platform will not necessarily work in another. PubMed is free to search, but the subscription services usually offer more advanced searching and should be used if available. Advice on access should be sought from a specialist medical librarian.
- A sensitive search strategy will be a mix of controlled vocabulary (such as MeSH terms) and free text or keywords.
- Free text can be truncated and many database platforms support wildcard and proximity searching.
- Search terms can be combined using Boolean operators: AND, OR, and NOT. AND will decrease the number of hits, OR will increase the number of hits. NOT should be used with caution.
- Search filters can be added to limit the search to particular study designs such as systematic reviews or randomized controlled trials.
- The creation of a search strategy is a trial and error process and all searches should be tested. The Help or Frequently Asked Questions pages of the electronic database should be checked for tips on how to structure the search.

Useful resources

MEDLINE via PubMED: http://www.ncbi.nlm.nih.gov/sites/entrez
Embase: http://www.embase.com (subscriber access only), Scopus makes most Embase content available for free: https://www.scopus.com/
The Cochrane Library: http://www.cochranelibrary.com/
Latin American and Caribbean Health Sciences Literature Resource (LILACS): http://www.bireme.br
KoreaMED: http://www.koreamed.org
Chinese National Knowledge Infrastructure http://www.cnki.net/
World Health Organization Gateway: http://www.who.int/
ISRCTN Registry (http://www.controlled-trials.com/
Clinical Trials.gov: http://clinicaltrials.gov
WHO International Trials Registry Platform: http://apps.who.int/trialsearch/
OpenTrials Beta search: https://explorer.opentrials.net/
OpenGrey: http://www.opengrey.eu/
ZETOC http://zetoc.mimas.ac.uk (subscribers only)
Web of Science: http://isiwebofknowledge.com (subscribers only)
EThOS: http://ethos.bl.uk
Proquest: http://www.proquest.com/ (subscribers only)
European Medicines Agency database: https://clinicaldata.ema.europa.eu/web/cdp/home
US Food and Drugs Administration database: http://www.fda.gov/Drugs/InformationOnDrugs/default.htm
National Library of Medicine MeSH Browser: http://www.nlm.nih.gov/mesh/MBrowser.html
InterTASC Search Filters Resource: http://www.york.ac.uk/inst/crd/intertasc/
The Cochrane Handbook (chapter 6): http://handbook.cochrane.org/
Cochrane Oral Health: http://oralhealth.cochrane.org/

References

Cochrane Collaboration, 2017. *About The Cochrane Library*. Available at: http://www.cochranelibrary.com/about/about-the-cochrane-library.html (accessed December 2017.

Collins J, 2007. Evidence-based medicine. *J Am Coll Radiol* 4, 551–554.

Elsvier BV, 2017. *Embase Fact Sheet*. Available at: https://www.elsevier.com/__data/assets/pdf_file/0016/59011/R_D_Solutions_Embase_Fact_Sheet-Web.pdf (accessed December 2017).

Glanville J, Lefebvre C, Miles JN, *et al.*, 2006. How to identify randomized controlled trials in MEDLINE: ten years on. *J Med Libr Assoc* 94, 130–136.

Lefebvre C, Manheimer E, Glanville J, 2009. Searching for studies. In: Higgins JPT, Green S, eds. *Cochrane Handbook for Systematic Reviews of Interventions*. Version 5.0.2 (updated September 2009). The Cochrane Collaboration. Available at: http://handbook.cochrane.org/ (accessed 9 December 2016).

Open Knowledge International and DataLab, 2017. *Open Trials*. Available at: http://opentrials.net/ (accessed December 2017).

Schroll J, Bero L, 2015. Regulatory agencies hold the key to improving Cochrane reviews of drugs. *Cochrane Database Syst Rev* (4), ED000098.

US National Institutes of Health, 2017. *ClinicalTrials.gov*. Available at: http://www.clinicaltrials.gov (accessed December 2017).

US National Library of Medicine, 2017. *MEDLINE Fact Sheet*. Available at: http://www.nlm.nih.gov/pubs/factsheets/medline.html (accessed December 2017).

Watkinson S, Harrison JE, Furness S, *et al.*, 2013. Orthodontic treatment for prominent lower front teeth (class III malocclusion) in children. *Cochrane Database Syst Rev*, (9), CD003451.

World Health Organization, 2017. *International Clinical Trials Registry Platform Search Portal*. Available at: http://apps.who.int/trialsearch/ (accessed 2 December 2017).

4

Making Sense of Randomized Clinical Trials and Systematic Reviews
Kevin O'Brien

One of the main reasons to carry out research is to reduce the uncertainty about any health-care intervention. When we consider that uncertainty pervades all aspects of our lives, we must remember that in clinical treatment there is rarely such a thing as 100% certainty. When we consider orthodontics, there is no doubt that there is a large amount of uncertainty in almost everything that we do. This is reinforced by the common experience that 10 orthodontists will come up with 10 different treatment plans for one patient!

It is well established that there is a hierarchy of research evidence that moves from the case report to the systematic review. Evidence from each level allows us to reduce clinical uncertainty. However, it is not always true that all clinical trials and systematic reviews provide us with information that we may feel is "certain". We still need to be able to interpret the results of these studies, in terms of reducing uncertainty in our personal clinical care.

In this chapter I intend to provide information that will help in reading and interpreting randomized trials and systematic reviews. You should consider that this is a broad guideline and I do not intend to cover all the detailed issues on trials and systematic reviews. Also, I would like to point out that none of the points are original, I have simply distilled several useful sources. Firstly, I will look at how I interpret a randomized trial and I will divide this into several broad sections that correspond to the main headings or sections of a paper.

How to interpret a randomized controlled trial

The abstract

In most journals the abstract should be structured. This should make interpretation of the paper easier and you can decide whether you want to read the paper in more detail. I read the abstract very carefully because I want to decide on two main facts about the paper. Firstly, I need to decide if it is a trial and this should be clearly stated in the methods section. Secondly, is the trial relevant to my interests? There is a large amount of research being published and we do not have sufficient time to read all the papers, so I tend to use the abstract as a broad filter to make the most use of my time. If the abstract outlines a study that I am interested in, I then make time to read it more carefully. I rarely just read the abstract of a paper that interests me, because the abstract does not always provide the important information that we need to use when we interpret the paper.

Evidence-Based Orthodontics, Second Edition. Edited by Greg J. Huang, Stephen Richmond and Katherine W. L. Vig.
© 2018 John Wiley & Sons, Inc. Published 2018 by John Wiley & Sons, Inc.

The introduction

I know it is tempting to skip past the introduction to a paper, but I always carefully read this so that I am clear on what the investigators are trying to discover. This may seem obvious but it is surprising how often the title or the abstract of the paper do not have a strong relationship to the study! The introduction also helps me update my knowledge on the subject of the study. At the end of the introduction I look very carefully at the hypothesis being tested. I then generally write this down and refer back to it as I read the paper.

The hypothesis

This is one of the most important parts of the paper. This is because the hypothesis provides the justification for the trial and the statistical analysis is based on testing the hypothesis. As a result, the hypothesis should be clear and understandable. If it is not, I start having doubts about the value of the paper.

As with a lot of statistical theory, there are discussions about the form of the hypothesis. Most orthodontic journals ask for the null hypothesis to be clearly stated. The null hypothesis refers to the situation in which the authors state that there is no relationship or difference between the interventions under test. If the null hypothesis is rejected, we may conclude that there is a difference between the interventions. Importantly, the null hypothesis is generally believed to be true, unless the study proves otherwise.

I also look to see if the hypothesis has generality. When the hypothesis is clear it should include information about the sample of participants to be studied in the trial. If this group has no resemblance to the patients I treat, I then start to consider whether this paper is going to have an effect on my practice.

Method

This is a most important section and it should be written carefully and clearly. I look for the following main points.

The patients and setting of the study

Is the sample of participants drawn from a population that is relevant to my clinical practice? This is important because if the findings of the study are going to influence practice, then the patients and treatment setting should be similar to our practice setting.

This then leads on the question of the generalizability of the study. This again means the relevance of the findings to our practice. If we consider various orthodontic studies, the levels of generalizability from high to low, for the average orthodontic office/ clinical practice, could be;

1) 10 to 16 year olds in a practice/office
2) 10 to 16 year olds being treated in a university/hospital setting
3) adults being treated in a practice/office
4) adults being treated in a university setting by residents.

In short, you need to identify whether the group of patients being treated are relevant to your clinical setting. If you feel that they are so far from the sphere in which you work, then you could argue that the findings of the study are not relevant to the care that you provide.

What was the control group?

It is very important that the control group is matched to the intervention group. You can decide this by carefully looking at the baseline data, which should be included in a table. It is also important that if an intervention involves a method of pain reduction that it is compared against either another pain control intervention or a placebo. It should not be compared against nothing. This is because it is unlikely that an operator would recommend no intervention to their patients. This will also take into account any placebo effect.

Did the authors carry out a sample size calculation?

This is very critical because this assures us that the study had sufficient power to detect a difference between the interventions. If the study does not have sufficient power there is a risk of incorrect acceptance of the null hypothesis. The power calculation should be based on previous literature and this reference stated. It is also good practice when you look at a power calculation to review the effect size that the authors are hoping to detect. Ideally, this should be based on the authors perception of what they feel is a clinically significant difference. You may not agree with this effect size and this helps your interpretation of the value of the study.

Was the intervention or treatment clearly described?

The authors should clearly state what their treatment involves and how it could potentially "work". I use this information to evaluate the studies relevance to the treatment that I am prepared to carry out.

Issues with randomization

The main reason to carry out a clinical trial is to find out about treatment using a form of research that minimizes bias. As a result, the following details of randomization are an essential requirement of reporting a trial. The most important concept is that the trial needs to have processes in place so that any bias caused by the preferences of the operators, or researchers, for certain treatment is minimized. As a result, the authors need to outline the following in some detail:

- How was the randomization done? For example, was it done by computer-generated randomization remotely from the site of the study (low risk of bias) or drawing lots for treatment out of a hat in the clinic (high risk of bias).
- How was concealment achieved? Concealment ensures that, when a person is being enrolled in a study, the operator has no idea what the treatment allocation for the patient is going to be. This is important because if they are aware of this treatment allocation, they may not enroll a patient into the study because of their potential bias about a particular type of treatment. The authors should also state who generated the allocation sequence and who enrolled the patients/subjects.

The ideal way to ensure adequate randomization, allocation, and concealment is to generate a random allocation of treatment using a computer, which is held at a site away from the clinic. The person who is enrolling the patient into the trial then contacts the center and provides details of the patient. Once this data is recorded the operator is then given details of the treatment allocation. There are many clinical trials units that will carry this out for people running studies.

Blinding

Blinding means that the participants, the operators and those recording the data do not know the treatment that the participant had received. This is very important because it ensures that any personal bias in providing the treatment, recording, and interpreting data is minimized. Ideally, a study should be triple blind so that the participant, the operator, and the person recording and analyzing the data does not know the treatment allocation. Unfortunately, this is not possible for any orthodontic study because it is impossible to conceal the treatment allocation from the patient and the operator. However, a realistic degree of blinding can be achieved by keeping the treatment allocation from the person who is recording the data, for example cephalometric analysis, study cast recording, etc.

Data

The authors should provide a flow diagram of the flow of participants through the study and this shows important features such as recruitment issues, total dropouts and any differences in dropouts between the intervention groups.

The data presentation should be clear and the means and 95% confidence intervals should be presented. This allows a reader to interpret any uncertainty in the data.

When I look at this data I consider two important features. Firstly, I look for clinical and statistical significance. I think that it is important to remember that these are related but have different meanings and are often confused. Statistical significance means that when the study results are analyzed the authors have found, for example, that the difference (effect size) between two interventions are statistically significant. That is, they may not have occurred by chance. Clinical significance means that the differences are so great that clinicians feel that they represent a difference that is clinically important. We need to remember that a difference may be "statistically significant," but so small that it is unlikely to make any difference to the treatment of the average patient. As a result, it is essential to interpret both the statistically significant difference and the effect size.

The other important issue is the interpretation of the 95% confidence interval. I have found the simplest way to explain this is an evaluation of how confident we can be with the findings of the study. For example, consider a study in which we want to identify the average overjet of 11-year-old children in the UK. We cannot make this measurement on all the children, so we select a sample and come up with a mean overjet measurement. Because this is a sample we are uncertain on the accuracy of this measurement and we calculate the 95% confidence interval. This will indicate the range of values that we would expect the overjet to fall within for 95 out of 100 repeats of the data collection. The narrower the confidence interval the less the uncertainty.

The results from a recent systematic review into methods of moving molars distally illustrate this point (Jambi *et al.* 2013). An analysis of the amount of distal movement achieved with different distalizing appliances is shown in Table 4.1.

If we evaluate this table, we can see that four studies were included in the meta-analysis. This shows that, for a total sample of 75 patients, the intraoral appliance is more effective than headgear in moving molars distally by 1.45 mm. It is clear that this difference is small and not very exciting. Nevertheless, we also need to look at the confidence intervals. These range from −2.74 to −0.15. This means that if we repeated this study 100 times then 95 times out of 100 the "true mean" will fall between −2.74 and −0.15. We can interpret this as representing a high degree of uncertainty in this area of our treatment. This is because the values represent a wide range, from nearly

Table 4.1 Forest plot of the amount of distal movement with intraoral appliances versus headgear.

Comparison 2 intraoral appliance versus headgear, outcome 1 movement of upper first molar

	Surgical anchorage		Conventional anchorage			Odds ratio IV, random, 95% CI		
A. Midpalatal implants								
Study	N	Mean (SD) (mm)	n	Mean (SD) (mm)	Weight (%)		Favors intraoral appliance	Favors headgear
Toy, 2011	15	−3.69 (3.45)	15	−0.77 (1.3)	21.2	−2.92 (−4.79, −1.05)		
Acar, 2010	15	−4.53 (1.46)	15	−2.23 (1.68)	29.5	−2.30 (−3.43, −1.17)		
De Oliviera, 2007	25	1.63 (5.49)	25	−0.14 (3.8)	14.9	1.77 (−0.85, 4.39)		
Bondemark, 2005	20	−2.2 (0.78)	20	−1 (1.32)	34.4	−1.20 (−1.87, −0.53)		
Subtotal (95% CI)	75		75		100	−1.45 (−1.87, −0.53)		

Heterogeneity: $Tau^2 = 1.15$; $Chi^2 = 10.91$ df = 3 ($P = 0.01$) $I^2 = 73\%$
Test for overall effect: Z = 219 ($P = 0.028$)
Test for subgroup differences not applicable.

(scale: −10 −5 0 5 10)

Abbreviations: CI, confidence interval; SD, standard deviation.
Source: Jambi *et al.* 2013. Reproduced with permission of The Cochrane Collaboration.

3.0, which is clinically significant, to 0.15 which is of no value. I can, therefore, conclude that the mean difference between treatments is not great and the finding has a high level of uncertainty. In reality, we do not know much about the comparative effectiveness of distalizing appliances and headgear. As a result, our decisions should be based on other factors such as our tolerance of risk in providing headgear with its inherent serious but rare risks.

The discussion and conclusions

Finally, when I read the discussion I look closely to see if the authors have justified their results, discussed the generalizability of their conclusions to clinical practice, and I look very closely to see if the conclusions are supported by the data! This is not always the case...

CONSORT guidelines

The evaluation of a trial is made much easier if the journal adopts a set of reporting guidelines called CONSORT (Consolidated Standards of Reporting Trials). If these are followed by both the authors of the paper and the editor of the journal, then most of the points that I have mentioned are covered. Most orthodontic journals have endorsed the CONSORT guidelines and this certainly makes the reading and interpreting of studies much easier.

How to read a systematic review

It seems that the number of published reviews is increasing and I feel that we are coming under pressure to keep up with the large amount of information that is coming our way. As a result, we need to be able to interpret systematic reviews in a time-efficient way. Again, these are my simple tips to rapid reading and interpretation.

The first step

This is to make an overall assessment of the quality of the review. My feeling is that Cochrane Systematic Reviews tend to provide the most useful information on clinical questions. This is because of the strict editorial and methodological steps that need to be taken to satisfy the Cochrane editors. I have now completed several Cochrane reviews and I think that they have the toughest editorial control of any publisher!

Another important criteria that sets Cochrane reviews apart from others is that the authors are committed to updating the review periodically. In theory, this results in the findings changing as new research is published. One example of this is the Cochrane review of Class II treatment that I helped produce. As additional evidence became available on the effect of early treatment on trauma, *the conclusions changed*.

I would like to point out that I am not suggesting that other reviews are not of value, but we need to bear in mind the overall quality of a review when we evaluate this form of literature.

Now that I have set out the context of the review, I will move to the main features that I look at when I read a review. This list is not exhaustive. It is simply a set of tips that I use and I hope are useful to you. I would like to use a Cochrane review on temporary anchorage devices (TAD) as an example.

Check the inclusion criteria

The review should clearly outline the inclusion criteria. The authors should state whether the studies that they included were randomized controlled trials (RCTs) and/or other types of study. In some reviews RCTs and controlled clinical trials are accepted. However, other reviews contain low-quality studies, for example retrospective designs with historic or convenience controls that are characterized by selection bias. When reading a review that includes retrospective studies you need to appreciate that the strength of any findings is diminished.

How were the papers selected?

Look closely at this section. In a good review the authors will provide a flow chart of how they obtained their papers. Ideally, they should provide information on each paper that they included and excluded.

The meta analysis and forest plot

The analysis of the data derived from the included papers is frequently presented as a forest plot. This is a clear way of presenting the data, but it can at first glance be confusing. I will go through an example forest plot from the TADS review (Table 4.2). This is the plot that illustrates the effectiveness of palatal implants and TADS compared to conventional forms of anchorage (Jambi *et al.* 2014). I have concentrated on the results for TADS and I have highlighted the relevant sections.

Table 4.3 shows that on the left hand side of the forest plot there is a summary of the data on sample size, etc. from each included study. You can look at this to build a picture of the number of studies and the subjects enrolled.

Table 4.2 An example forest plot from the temporary anchorage devices review.

Comparison 2 intraoral appliance versus headgear, outcome 1 movement of upper first molar

Study	N	Surgical anchorage Mean (SD)	n	Conventional anchorage Mean (SD)	Weight (%)	Odds ratio IV, Random, 95% CI	Favors surgical / Favors conventional
A. Midpalatal implants							
Boros, 2012	15	1.57 (1.06)	15	1.48 (1.56)	13.3	0.09 (−0.86, 1.04)	
Chesterfield, 2007	23	1.5 (2.6)	24	3 (3.34)	7.4	−1.50 (−3.32, 0.23)	
Feldman, 2007	54	−0.1 (0.67)	59	1.59 (1.74)	18.0	−1.69 (−2.17, −1.21)	
Subtotal (95% CI)	92		98		38.7	−1.02 (−2.31, 0.26)	

Heterogeneity: $Tau^2 = 0.99$; $Chi^2 = 10.71$ df = 2 ($P = 0.0005$), $I^2 = 81\%$
Test for overall effect: $Z = 1.56$ ($P = 0.12$)

Study	N	Surgical anchorage Mean (SD)	n	Conventional anchorage Mean (SD)	Weight (%)	Odds ratio IV, Random, 95% CI	Favors surgical / Favors conventional
B. Mini screw implants							
Liu, 2009	17	−0.06 (1.4)	17	1.47 (1.15)	14.2	−1.53 (−2.39, −0.67)	
Sharma, 2012	15	0 (0.021)	15	2.4 (0.712)	19.0	−2.40 (−2.76, −2.04)	
Shi, 2008	8	0.72 (1.23)	10	2.55 (0.69)	13.3	−1.83 (−2.78, −0.88)	
Upadhyay, 2008	18	0.78 (1.350)	18	3.22 (1.06)	14.9	−2.44 (−3.23, 1.65)	
Subtotal (95% CI)	58		60		61.3	−2.17 (−2.58, −1.77)	

Heterogeneity: $Tau^2 = 0.06$; $Chi^2 = 27.37$ df = 3 ($P = 0.23$), $I^2 = 30\%$
Test for overall effect: $Z = 10.48$ ($P < 0.00001$)

Total (95% CI)	150		158		100	−1.68 (−2.27, −1.09)	

Heterogeneity: $Tau^2 = 0.44$; $Chi^2 = 27.37$ df = 6 ($P = 0.00012$), $I^2 = 78\%$
Test for overall effect: $Z = 5.62$ ($P = 0.00001$)
Test for subgroup differences; $Chi^2 = 2.81$ df = 1 ($P = 0.09$), $I^2 = 64\%$

−4 −2 0 2 4

Abbreviations: CI, confidence interval; SD, standard deviation.
Source: Jambi *et al.* 2014. Reproduced with permission of The Cochrane Collaboration.

Table 4.3 An example forest plot from the temporary anchorage devices review with summary data from each study highlighted.

Comparison 2 intraoral appliance versus headgear, outcome 1 movement of upper first molar

	Surgical anchorage		Conventional anchorage			Odds ratio IV, Random, 95% CI		

A. Midpalatal implants

Study	N	Mean (SD)	n	Mean (SD)	Weight (%)		Favors surgical / Favors conventional	
Boros, 2012	15	1.57 (1.06)	15	1.48 (1.56)	13.3	0.09 (−0.86, 1.04)	
Chesterfield, 2007	23	1.5 (2.6)	24	3 (3.34)	7.4	−1.50 (−3.32, 0.23)	
Feldman, 2007	54	−0.1 (0.67)	59	1.59 (1.74)	18.0	−1.69 (−2.17, −1.21)	
Subtotal (95% CI)	92		98		38.7	−1.02 (−2.31, 0.26)	

Heterogeneity: $\text{Tau}^2 = 0.99$; $\text{Chi}^2 = 10.71$ df = 2 ($P = 0.0005$), $I^2 = 81\%$
Test for overall effect: Z = 1.56 ($P = 0.12$)

B. Mini screw implants

Study	N	Mean (SD)	n	Mean (SD)	Weight (%)			
Liu, 2009	17	−0.06 (1.4)	17	1.47 (1.15)	14.2	−1.53 (−2.39, −0.67)	
Sharma, 2012	15	0 (0.021)	15	2.4 (0.712)	19.0	−2.40 (−2.76, −2.04)	
Shi, 2008	8	0.72 (1.23)	10	2.55 (0.69)	13.3	−1.83 (−2.78, −0.88)	
Upadhyay, 2008	18	0.78 (1.350)	18	3.22 (1.06)	14.9	−2.44 (−3.23, 1.65)	
Subtotal (95% CI)	58		60		61.3	−2.17 (−2.58, −1.77)	

Heterogeneity: $\text{Tau}^2 = 0.06$; $\text{Chi}^2 = 27.37$ df = 3 ($P = 0.23$), $I^2 = 30\%$
Test for overall effect: Z = 10.48 ($P < 0.00001$)

Total (95% CI)	150		158		100	−1.68 (−2.27, −1.09)	

Heterogeneity: $\text{Tau}^2 = 0.44$; $\text{Chi}^2 = 27.37$ df = 6 ($P = 0.00012$), $I^2 = 78\%$
Test for overall effect: Z = 5.62 ($P = 0.00001$)
Test for subgroup differences; $\text{Chi}^2 = 2.81$ df = 1 ($P = 0.09$), $I^2 = 64\%$

−4　−2　0　2　4

Abbreviations: CI, confidence interval; SD, standard deviation.
Source: Jambi *et al*. 2014. Reproduced with permission of The Cochrane Collaboration.

Now look at the data for each study; this shows the effect size and 95% confidence intervals (Table 4.4).

In Table 4.5 I have highlighted the graphics around the vertical line. This is the line of "no effect". Now look at the graphics that are dispersed around the line. The upper ones are the means and confidence intervals for each study. If the CI line crosses the line of no effect, then there is no statistically significant effect of the intervention.

Now look at the diamond-shaped symbol at the bottom of the plot (Table 4.5). This represents the combined data. The horizontal width represents the confidence interval. If the diamond crosses the line, the difference is not statistically significant. You can see, in this example, that the diamond does not cross the line and reveals that TADS are more effective than other methods of anchorage.

Finally, look at the bottom right numbers (Table 4.6). This is the combined effect size and confidence intervals. Even if the result is statistically significant, you need to evaluate whether this is clinically significant.

Table 4.4 An example forest plot from the temporary anchorage devices review with effect size and 95% confidence intervals for each study highlighted.

Comparison 2 intraoral appliance versus headgear, outcome 1 movement of upper first molar

	Surgical anchorage		Conventional anchorage			Odds ratio IV, Random, 95% CI		
A. Midpalatal implants								
Study	**N**	**Mean (SD)**	**n**	**Mean (SD)**	**Weight (%)**		**Favors surgical**	**Favors conventional**
Boros, 2012	15	1.57 (1.06)	15	1.48 (1.56)	13.3	0.09 (−0.86, 1.04)		
Chesterfield, 2007	23	1.5 (2.6)	24	3 (3.34)	7.4	−1.50 (−3.32, 0.23)		
Feldman, 2007	54	−0.1 (0.67)	59	1.59 (1.74)	18.0	−1.69 (−2.17, −1.21)		
Subtotal (95% CI)	92		98		38.7	−1.02 (−2.31, 0.26)		

Heterogeneity: $Tau^2 = 0.99$; $Chi^2 = 10.71$ df = 2 ($P = 0.0005$), $I^2 = 81\%$
Test for overall effect: Z = 1.56 ($P = 0.12$)

B. Mini screw implants								
Liu, 2009	17	−0.06 (1.4)	17	1.47 (1.15)	14.2	−1.53 (−2.39, −0.67)		
Sharma, 2012	15	0 (0.021)	15	2.4 (0.712)	19.0	−2.40 (−2.76, −2.04)		
Shi, 2008	8	0.72 (1.23)	10	2.55 (0.69)	13.3	−1.83 (−2.78, −0.88)		
Upadhyay, 2008	18	0.78 (1.350)	18	3.22 (1.06)	14.9	−2.44 (−3.23, 1.65)		
Subtotal (95% CI)	58		60		61.3	−2.17 (−2.58, −1.77)		

Heterogeneity: $Tau^2 = 0.06$; $Chi^2 = 27.37$ df = 3 ($P = 0.23$), $I^2 = 30\%$
Test for overall effect: Z = 10.48 ($P < 0.00001$)

Total (95% CI)	150		158		100	−1.68 (−2.27, −1.09)		

Heterogeneity: $Tau^2 = 0.44$; $Chi^2 = 27.37$ df = 6 ($P = 0.00012$), $I^2 = 78\%$
Test for overall effect: Z = 5.62 ($P = 0.00001$)
Test for subgroup differences; $Chi^2 = 2.81$ df = 1 ($P = 0.09$), $I^2 = 64\%$

−4 −2 0 2 4

Abbreviations: CI, confidence interval; SD, standard deviation.
Source: Jambi *et al.* 2014. Reproduced with permission of The Cochrane Collaboration.

Strength of recommendations

Many reviews now include a statement on the strength of the recommendations that can be made from the review. Several now use the Grading of Recommendations Assessment, Development and Evaluation (GRADE) approach. I am not going to go through this in detail but those who are interested can read the original publication on GRADE (Guyatt *et al.* 2008).

You will see that they are concerned with looking at level of confidence in the effect size included in the review. In the TADS review the effect size was −2.17 mm with a fairly narrow confidence interval of (2.8–1.77). We concluded that we had moderate confidence in the findings.

Summary

I have tried to keep this as concise as possible. As a result, I have only outlined the features that I evaluate when I read a systematic review, I have not mentioned other features that are important and I appreciate that

Table 4.5 An example forest plot from the temporary anchorage devices review graphics dispersed around the line of no effect highlighted.

Comparison 2 Intraoral appliance versus headgear, outcome 1 movement of upper first molar

	Surgical anchorage			Conventional anchorage			Odds ratio IV, Random, 95% CI		
A. Midpalatal implants									
Study	**N**	**Mean (SD)**	**n**	**Mean (SD)**	**Weight (%)**			**Favors surgical**	**Favors conventional**
Boros, 2012	15	1.57 (1.06)	15	1.48 (1.56)	13.3	0.09 (−0.86, 1.04)			
Chesterfield, 2007	23	1.5 (2.6)	24	3 (3.34)	7.4	−1.50 (−3.32, 0.23)			
Feldman, 2007	54	−0.1 (0.67)	59	1.59 (1.74)	18.0	−1.69 (−2.17, −1.21)			
Subtotal (95% CI)	92		98		38.7	−1.02 (−2.31, 0.26)			

Heterogeneity: Tau^2 = 0.99; Chi^2 = 10.71 df = 2 (P = 0.0005), I^2 = 81%
Test for overall effect: Z = 1.56 (P = 0.12)

B. Mini screw implants									
Liu, 2009	17	−0.06 (1.4)	17	1.47 (1.15)	14.2	−1.53 (−2.39, −0.67)			
Sharma, 2012	15	0 (0.021)	15	2.4 (0.712)	19.0	−2.40 (−2.76, −2.04)			
Shi, 2008	8	0.72 (1.23)	10	2.55 (0.69)	13.3	−1.83 (−2.78, −0.88)			
Upadhyay, 2008	18	0.78 (1.350)	18	3.22 (1.06)	14.9	−2.44 (−3.23, 1.65)			
Subtotal (95% CI)	58		60		61.3	−2.17 (−2.58, −1.77)			

Heterogeneity: Tau^2 = 0.06; Chi^2 = 27.37 df = 3 (P = 0.23), I^2 = 30%
Test for overall effect: Z = 10.48 (P <0.00001)

| Total (95% CI) | 150 | | 158 | | 100 | −1.68 (−2.27, −1.09) | | | |

Heterogeneity: Tau^2 = 0.44; Chi^2 = 27.37 df = 6 (P = 0.00012), I^2 = 78%
Test for overall effect: Z = 5.62 (P = 0.00001)
Test for subgroup differences; Chi^2 = 2.81 df = 1 (P = 0.09), I^2 = 64%

Scale: −4 −2 0 2 4

Abbreviations: CI, confidence interval; SD, standard deviation.
Source: Jambi *et al.* 2014. Reproduced with permission of The Cochrane Collaboration.

some people may criticize this rather basic approach. However, understanding these key components will provide you with the information you need to read and interpret systematic reviews.

The interpretation of "negative" findings

I sometimes feel frustrated when I read a trial and the authors report that there is no difference between the treatments and further research is needed. But the interpretation of these negative findings is far from straightforward.

It is easy to interpret these "negative" findings by suggesting that the treatment did not have an effect. While this may be the case, this is not always correct. This has been discussed over many years and various researchers have stated that "absence of evidence does not mean evidence of absence." In other words, if we do not find difference in a study, then it is not correct to state that the treatment "does not work." The only thing that we can conclude is that the study did not detect any differences between the treatments.

Table 4.6 An example forest plot from the temporary anchorage devices review with effect size and confidence intervals highlighted.

Comparison 2 intraoral appliance versus headgear, outcome 1 movement of upper first molar

	Surgical anchorage		Conventional anchorage			Odds ratio IV, Random, 95% CI		
							Favors Surgical	Favors Conventional
Study	N	Mean (SD)	n	Mean (SD)	Weight (%)			

A. Midpalatal implants

Study	N	Mean (SD)	n	Mean (SD)	Weight (%)	Odds ratio IV, Random, 95% CI	
Boros, 2012	15	1.57 (1.06)	15	1.48 (1.56)	13.3	0.09 (−0.86, 1.04)	
Chesterfield, 2007	23	1.5 (2.6)	24	3 (3.34)	7.4	−1.50 (−3.32, 0.23)	
Feldman, 2007	54	−0.1 (0.67)	59	1.59 (1.74)	18.0	−1.69 (−2.17, −1.21)	
Subtotal (95% CI)	92		98		38.7	−1.02 (−2.31, 0.26)	

Heterogeneity: $\text{Tau}^2 = 0.99$; $\text{Chi}^2 = 10.71$ df = 2 ($P = 0.0005$), $I^2 = 81\%$
Test for overall effect: $Z = 1.56$ ($P = 0.12$)

B. Mini screw implants

Study	N	Mean (SD)	n	Mean (SD)	Weight (%)	Odds ratio IV, Random, 95% CI	
Liu, 2009	17	−0.06 (1.4)	17	1.47 (1.15)	14.2	−1.53 (−2.39, −0.67)	
Sharma, 2012	15	0 (0.021)	15	2.4 (0.712)	19.0	−2.40 (−2.76, −2.04)	
Shi, 2008	8	0.72 (1.23)	10	2.55 (0.69)	13.3	−1.83 (−2.78, −0.88)	
Upadhyay, 2008	18	0.78 (1.350)	18	3.22 (1.06)	14.9	−2.44 (−3.23, 1.65)	
Subtotal (95% CI)	58		60		61.3	−2.17 (−2.58, −1.77)	

Heterogeneity: $\text{Tau}^2 = 0.06$; $\text{Chi}^2 = 27.37$ df = 3 ($P = 0.23$), $I^2 = 30\%$
Test for overall effect: $Z = 10.48$ ($P < 0.00001$)

Total (95% CI)	150		158		100	−1.68 (−2.27, −1.09)	

Heterogeneity: $\text{Tau}^2 = 0.44$; $\text{Chi}^2 = 27.37$ df = 6 ($P = 0.00012$), $I^2 = 78\%$
Test for overall effect: $Z = 5.62$ ($P = 0.00001$)
Test for subgroup differences; $\text{Chi}^2 = 2.81$ df = 1 ($P = 0.09$), $I^2 = 64\%$

Axis scale: −4 −2 0 2 4

Abbreviations: CI, confidence interval; SD, standard deviation.
Source: Jambi *et al*. 2014. Reproduced with permission of The Cochrane Collaboration.

Why do "negative" findings occur?

I will now consider the possible reasons for "negative" findings. Firstly, the new treatment may indeed be no better than the other treatments under investigation. Alternatively, the study may not have sufficient power to detect a difference, even if it existed. This brings us back to the power calculation that I mentioned earlier. As a result, when you read a study with negative findings have a good look at the sample size calculation and look for these three main factors:

- Were the assumptions that they made in their calculation realistic and clinically significant?
- Did they clearly quote the source of the data that they used in their calculation?
- Was the sample size based upon the same outcome measure as the one that was tested in the study?

It is quite surprising to find that these three mistakes are commonly made in published trials. If these factors are not clear then you may conclude that the study could be underpowered and this may be a more compelling explanation for the finding of no difference between the treatments under investigation.

What if the "no difference" finding was true?

I will now consider the situation in which the finding of "no difference" may in fact be true.

We may come to this conclusion if the study is sufficiently powered. Nevertheless, we still need to be cautious in our conclusions. If I look back at some of my earlier work into Class II treatment, I concluded that:

> Early orthodontic treatment with the Twin-block appliance followed by further treatment in adolescence, at the appropriate time, does not result in any meaningful long-term differences when compared with one course of treatment started in the late mixed or early permanent dentition.

If we look at this carefully I feel that this conclusion is correct, because I stated that we did not detect a difference. It would have been very easy for me to conclude that early orthodontic treatment was not effective. Unfortunately, I know that I have said this in several presentations in the early days following our studies and I have fallen into the common mistake that I have described above.

How do we increase our certainty of "negative" findings

We need to remember that research aims to reduce uncertainty. In this respect, combining the results of several large, well carried out studies into a systematic review can increase the power of our study and enable us to be more certain. For example, when several studies provide data in a systematic review that shows "no difference" we can conclude with greater certainty that the treatment was not effective. This was the approach in a systematic review of early Class II treatment, when we concluded:

> There are no advantages for providing a two-phase treatment i.e. early from age seven to 11 years and again in adolescence compared to one phase in adolescence.

What are the clinical implications?

It is worth considering the clinical implications of this discussion. When the evidence of "no effect" is clear, we can explain to our patients that one treatment does not have an advantage over another. However, if there are no studies or the findings are not robust because of bias or lack of statistical power, then we should inform our patients that we do not know if one treatment is better than another. This information then helps them make an informed decision.

Final comments

I would like to emphasize that this is not an exhaustive list or set of instructions on how to interpret trials and systematic reviews. It is simply an outline of the method that I use when I am trying to assimilate the results from the many studies that are currently published. Some people may consider that this it not sufficiently precise. However, I have found it useful to help me reduce the uncertainty in my mind about some of the treatments that I have provided.

References

Guyatt GH, Oxman AD, Vist GE, *et al.*, 2008. GRADE: an emerging consensus on rating quality of evidence and strength of recommendations *BMJ* 336, 924.

Jambi S, Thiruvenkatachari B, O'Brien KD, *et al.*, 2013. Orthodontic treatment for distalising upper first molars in children and adolescents. *Cochrane Database Syst Rev* (10), CD008375.

Jambi S, Walsh T, Sandler J, *et al.*, 2014. Reinforcement of anchorage during orthodontic brace treatment with implants or other surgical methods. *Cochrane Database Syst Rev* (8), CD005098.

5

Understanding and Improving our Evidence
Padhraig Fleming, Greg J. Huang, and Nikolaos Pandis

Introduction

Orthodontists are regularly confronted with questions like, "Do self-ligating brackets increase treatment efficiency compared to conventional brackets?" or "Is it better to treat this patient using a one-stage or a two-stage approach?" To compound matters, commercial companies compete to capture the interest of clinicians by claiming their unique products will improve clinicians' practices. However, clinical decisions should be evidence-based, combining a regard for patient wishes, professional experience, and the best available evidence (Figure 5.1). This overarching approach to clinical decision making in health care is now accepted as the gold standard. While dentistry and orthodontics lagged behind pioneering medical specialties in recognizing the importance of evidence-based decisions, it has now become firmly established (Sackett *et al.* 1985).

Evidence-based practice has been criticized for trying to develop a "one size fits all" approach to clinical care; however, the fact that certain questions are not amenable to randomized designs for ethical or practical reasons is well accepted (Straus and McAlister 2000; Straus *et al.* 2007). Evidence-based science prioritizes evidence in terms of its importance, applying different weights during decision making, depending on the level of confidence associated with the study results. At the lower end of the quality hierarchy lies expert opinion, and at the upper end are high-quality meta-analyses and systematic reviews or randomized controlled trials (RCTs) with low risk of bias (Harbour and Miller 2001). Results from primary studies that are of high quality carry greater weight during the decision-making process and may be more influential in systematic reviews (Santoro and Gorrie 2005). Systematic reviews aim to synthesize high-quality evidence to determine the efficacy and safety of interventions more accurately, to resolve controversies and uncertainty surrounding treatment modalities, and to facilitate development of clinical practice guidelines. High-quality RCTs are an integral part of systematic reviews and allow us to be confident about the review results. Understanding and identifying quality features of RCTs and systematic reviews is of critical importance for adopting evidence-based orthodontics.

While the volume of orthodontic research (and indeed biomedical research) has increased exponentially, a greater appreciation of the importance of better execution and reporting of studies has also emerged. In particular, a range of reporting guidelines that apply to dentistry have been developed (Sarkis-Onofre *et al.* 2015). These are freely accessible on the Internet (www.equator-network.org) and include guidelines on the design and reporting of randomized and nonrandomized studies, as well as systematic reviews. Promoting better adherence to these established guidelines and enhancing the transparency and awareness of orthodontic research among clinicians and patients are among the challenges to the acceptance of evidence-based orthodontics. In this chapter, the current status of evidence-based orthodontics will be discussed, the design and appraisal of clinical trials will be addressed, and future research directions and challenges will be considered.

Evidence-Based Orthodontics, Second Edition. Edited by Greg J. Huang, Stephen Richmond and Katherine W. L. Vig.
© 2018 John Wiley & Sons, Inc. Published 2018 by John Wiley & Sons, Inc.

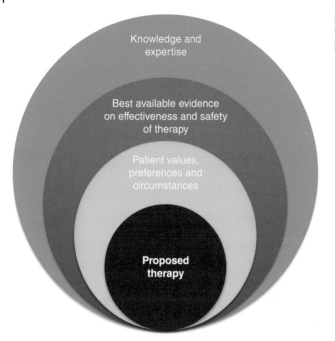

Knowledge and expertise

Best available evidence on effectiveness and safety of therapy

Patient values, preferences and circumstances

Proposed therapy

Figure 5.1 Evidence-based orthodontics amalgamating the best evidence with clinical expertise and individual patient values.

Maximizing value in clinical trials

A randomized controlled trial is a *preplanned experiment that aims to assess the effects or benefits of at least one treatment in humans.* An RCT employs randomization to assign participants to the arms of the study, with the aim of creating groups that are similar in all respects, other than the intervention or factor of interest (Moher *et al.* 2010). The use of a control group is important so that genuine treatment effects can be isolated from changes that might occur due to natural improvement, biased patient selection, and/or biased patient responses. The elimination or minimization of bias is important in order for an RCT to arrive at valid results. *Bias is systematic error that leads to distortion of the true treatment effect* and may arise at different stages of the trial, including design, conduct, analysis, and reporting. Bias calls into question the trial results, is difficult to quantify, and probably impossible to completely eliminate; however, there are methods to reduce it. Therefore, a key objective of every trial is to adopt procedures and processes that minimize bias (Higgins *et al.* 2011a,b).

A spotlight has been placed on deficient conduct and reporting of research in recent years (Glasziou *et al.* 2014). Specific aspects leading to wasted research and suboptimal yield from clinical trials include failure to ask the most important research questions, inappropriate research methods, regulatory issues, under-reporting, and inadequate reporting. Three of these factors (trial methodology, trial reporting, and research outcomes), as they relate to RCTs, will be considered in turn. These each have repercussions for the yield from systematic reviews and, in view of their potentially profound influence on public health policy, the configuration of services, and the delivery of care, should be carefully addressed during the planning and execution of clinical trials.

Orthodontic randomized controlled trials: methodology and reporting

Metaepidemiological research in orthodontics has indicated that clinical trials are not immune from methodological weaknesses, with problems such as inadequate randomization procedures, blinding, and handling of missing data pervasive (Lempesi *et al.* 2014). As such, in appraisals of orthodontic RCTs, the following questions are important (Moher *et al.* 2010):

1) What is the research question?
2) Can the results be trusted?
3) What are the results of the trial?
4) How can the results/ conclusions be applied?

Research question

A well-formulated question should clearly outline the participants, the intervention(s) and comparators, and the outcome measures (the PICO approach). The inclusion/ exclusion criteria applied to select the trial participants, as well as the settings and location where the trial was undertaken, help in understanding to whom the trial results are applicable (external validity or generalizability). The details of the intervention(s), such as the expected duration of wear of a functional appliance or the type of retention regimen, are important in understanding the wider applicability of the results. The use of control group(s) is an important element of an RCT, as it serves the purpose of helping to reveal the true treatment effect by discounting effects that might occur naturally. Close attention to the nature of controls is necessary, as use of historic controls or those exposed to nonstandard therapy may exaggerate the effects of the "new" intervention (Papageorgiou *et al.* 2016). Clinical trials may use one or several outcomes that may be further classified as primary and secondary. Clear descriptions and prespecification of outcomes is important, as this mitigates against selective reporting, in which interesting results or results aligned with a researcher's own bias may be preferentially reported.

Can the results be trusted?

Internal validity (quality of methodology) refers to whether all of the important steps were appropriately followed during the design of the trial, conduct of the study, and analysis of the results. Low methodological quality (usually accompanied by high risk for bias) should reduce the weight given to the evidence from an RCT during clinical decision making. The methodological components that are of interest when assessing internal validity are given in the following sections.

Design
Was proper randomization applied?
Randomization is the process of randomly generating and allocating interventions to trial arms such that neither the investigators nor the participants know or may predict what treatment the patients will receive. Random assignment of individuals to treatment, with proper *allocation concealment*, is of paramount importance in reducing *selection bias* and controlling *unobserved confounders* (factors that obscure the effect of therapy), thereby improving the internal validity of RCTs (Juni *et al.* 2001; Jadad *et al.* 1996). Proper randomization produces treatment groups that are similar in both known and unknown factors that may be associated with the outcome, meaning that any outcome differences between treatment groups can be attributed with confidence to the therapy. Proper randomization includes *generation of the random allocation sequence* and *allocation concealment*. Sequential treatment assignment, as well as allocation schemes that follow, for example, days of the week, or using participant initials are not considered random methods and have been characterized as "quasirandomized" methods (Pocock 1983). Appropriate randomization methods may include use of random tables and computer-based random number generators.

Allocation concealment is the process used to ensure that the produced randomization lists, and consequently the treatment to be assigned to the recruited participants, cannot be known or predicted by all involved parties. The objective of allocation concealment is to reduce selection bias, and its implementation is always possible (Wood *et al.* 2008; Pildal *et al.* 2007). Allocation concealment may be easily applied using opaque sealed envelopes; however, centralized assignment of treatment is considered more appropriate (Haag 1998). Allocation concealment and blinding describe two different procedures. Blinding refers to whether patients and investigators have knowledge of the intervention that has been allocated, and occurs after the intervention has been administered (Chalmers *et al.* 1987).

Was blinding of participants, investigators, and other trial staff undertaken?

Blinding (or masking) refers to the steps taken to ensure that all parties involved in a trial are unaware of the type of treatment each participant receives. Blinding is usually feasible when interventions are similar or can be made to appear similar (i.e., preparation of placebo for drugs trials); however, there are situations when blinding is not feasible and, depending on the intervention and the type of outcome, bias may be introduced (Boutron *et al.* 2008). Bias from lack of blinding may be generated at the patient level and at the investigator/staff level *(detection bias)*. In orthodontics, depending on the intervention, blinding may be difficult to implement, especially at the investigator level, particularly if he/she is the one delivering the treatment. However, it may be possible to blind the outcome assessor, the data analyst, and other relevant staff. The ideal situation is triple blinding, which indicates that the patients, the investigators/ providers, and the assessors/ statisticians are all blinded.

Were the treatment groups similar at baseline?

If randomization has been carried out properly, treatment groups should be similar with respect to baseline characteristics. *Baseline data* collected from all participants may include data on demographic variables (such as age, sex, and ethnicity) and clinical characteristics, including type of malocclusion, baseline crowding, overjet, and level of oral hygiene. A table delineating baseline data permits rapid assessment of similarities and differences between participants in the respective groups. Small differences between groups in terms of baseline characteristics are expected and usually occur due to chance. During critical appraisal, an effort should be made to detect large and important differences between group participants at baseline, as this may reflect improper randomization and associated selection bias.

RCT conduct

Were all participants followed up until the end of treatment?

Minimal losses of trial participants are highly desirable. Differential and large losses to follow-up may result in attrition bias as the groups may differ with regard to important characteristics, despite similarity at baseline. Hence, the advantages of randomization may have been lost.

Were the trial groups treated equally in all other respects apart from the intervention?

Ideally, each treatment group should be managed equally in terms of follow-up, outcome assessment, and parallel treatments, as this increases the validity of the results. Unequal handling of participants between treatment groups is a potential source of *performance bias*. For example, when assessing the periodontal effects related to treatment with competing bracket systems, bias towards one of the systems may lead to biased delivery of oral hygiene instructions and follow-up. Blinding, where feasible, along with standardization of treatment procedures, should help to mitigate this problem.

Analysis

Were participants analyzed according to randomization?

In trials where patients are lost to follow-up, it is important that outcomes are analyzed within the group to which those patients were randomized. This type of analysis is called *intention to treat (ITT)* and is usually less biased than a *per protocol analysis (PP)*, in which only patients for whom complete outcome data has been collected are considered. This is particularly important in orthodontic studies evaluating the comparative effectiveness of interventions reliant on compliance, such as removable appliances or headgears. In Table 5.1, failure of Class II correction with two types of functional appliance (FA-1 and FA-2) is illustrated with differential loss to follow-up, both in terms of numbers and also participant characteristics. In the FA-1 group, the lost patients were less cooperative compared to FA-2 group. As such, it may be inferred that the difference in Class II

Table 5.1 Intention to treat (ITT) versus per protocol (PP) analysis. The extreme assumption is made here that lost patients failed to comply. Other assumptions during missing data imputations are sensible.

	ITT analysis		PP analysis	
Treatment group	FA -1	FA-2	FA-1	FA-2
Numbers randomized	100	100	100	100
Lost to follow-up	20	30	20	30
Baseline characteristics	Least cooperative	More cooperative	Least cooperative	More cooperative
Number of patients failing to comply	20	28	20	28
Risk of failure	20/100 = 20%	28/100 = 28%	20/80 = 25%	28/70 = 40%
Risk difference	**8% (risk ratio = 1.4)**		**15% (risk ratio = 1.6)**	

correction failures is due to the differential performance of the appliance, rather than to the difference in patient baseline characteristics (cooperation) between trial arms. An ITT analysis that does not exclude patients with missing outcome data from the analysis reduces the chance of biased results and tends to dilute the treatment effect, whereas a PP analysis is more likely to be biased and tends to exaggerate the results (Table 5.1). A true ITT analysis in the presence of missing data is feasible only when a complete dataset can be constructed using some form of appropriate missing data imputations.

Were the analyses appropriate and prespecified?

RCT data can be assessed in many different ways, including: analysis of final values, analysis of changes from baseline to final values, analysis of final values adjusted for baseline values, analysis of subgroups, analysis using parametric or nonparametric tests, and analysis using data transformation such as the logarithmic scale, etc. Different approaches to data analysis may produce slightly different results and, unless the statistical analyses are prespecified, investigators may be tempted to resort to selective reporting of only "interesting" results. In orthodontic trials where multiple teeth are included, such as in bond failure studies, erroneously treating teeth nested within patients as independent and failing to account for clustering effects (similarity of results within the same patient) can be problematic. A report has indicated that only 25% of all studies published in major orthodontic journals account for clustering effects (Koletsi *et al.* 2012). Although it may be practically difficult to prespecify all analyses, a clear analysis plan should be drafted stipulating the indications for alternative analyses. Caution is required when interpreting results from subgroup analyses, especially if they have not been prespecified. Subgroup analyses and multiple testing may reveal significant differences between treatment groups that are false, and therefore carry the risk of overinterpretation. Guidelines for interpreting results indicating qualitative differences between subgroups are shown in Table 5.2.

Results

Size of effect

Depending on the type of data (binary or continuous), the effect size may be expressed in terms of an absolute difference or a relative risk ratio, such as risk ratio, odds ratio, or rate ratio. Caution should be exercised in interpreting effect size, as the same result in an *additive (absolute difference)* or *multiplicative scale (ratio)* may give erroneous impressions. For example, a small absolute difference of two risks (4% – 2% = 2%) equates to a risk ratio of 2 (risk ratio 4/2 = 2). However, a larger absolute difference between risks (40% – 20% = 20%) may present the same difference in a ratio scale (risk ratio = 40/20 = 2); interpretation based on absolute differences (2% vs. 20%) could be quite different.

Table 5.2 When the answer to the six questions in the table are all "yes" then qualitative differences in treatment effects between subgroups from subgroup analyses are likely.

Questions to ask when assessing results from subgroup analyses
1. Is the result clinically and biologically plausible?
2. Is the qualitative difference both clinically and statistically significant?
3. Was the subgroup analysis prespecified or the result of data dredging?
4. Was this analysis one of the many subgroup analyses conducted?
5. Is the difference suggested by within rather than between study comparisons?
6. Has the same result been confirmed in other independent studies?

Source: Adapted from Straus *et al.* 2007.

Precision of effect

The absence of a statistical difference related to an intervention in a trial may of course be related to a genuine lack of effect. However, false-negative findings may also arise due to bias in design, or insufficient power to show effect due to a small sample size. *The power of the study* is related to the precision of the estimate, with studies with low power yielding imprecise results and vice versa. *P* values, although indicative of a statistically significant result, depend on sample size and variance, and provide limited insight into the clinical relevance of the findings. A more clinically relevant and important piece of information obtained from the results is the actual difference/ effect size and its *range (confidence interval)* (Gardner and Altman; 1986 Goodman 1999).

Overreliance on *P* values when presenting and interpreting results is inappropriate and often misleading (Rothman 1978; Mainland 1984). Significant results, regardless of their clinical importance or plausibility, are labeled important, whereas any nonsignificant result is labeled unimportant. On the other hand, reporting of confidence intervals moves the interpretation of the results from the dichotomy of significant/ nonsignificant to the size of the effect or association and its range of plausible values derived from the data investigated (Chia 1997; Savitz 1993; Kloukos *et al.* 2014).

External validity or generalizability

The external validity of a study is the applicability of the trial results to other settings and populations. This is critical, as the clinician or patient may be interested in how the findings of the study may best be applied.

To whom do the results apply?

Although trial populations are unlikely to be the same, applicability of results to other settings and populations is often feasible as long as the inclusion and exclusion criteria are relevant and under the assumption of consistent biologic responses.

Are the results important to patients?

Apart from the information that allows the reader to answer the clinical question, other outcomes of importance to patients, such as adverse effects, should be considered. For example, the efficiency of orthodontic alignment and quality of posterior interdigitation may be important to clinicians; however, potential side effects, such as pain and impact of the appliances, are all important aspects that should be considered. Moreover, it is important that outcomes of importance to patients are assessed within clinical trials; for example, the impact of treatment on oral health-related quality of life. Metaepidemiological reviews scoping both the dental literature generally (Tsichlaki and O'Brien 2014) and the orthodontic literature specifically

(Fleming *et al.* 2016) have exposed a dearth of research focusing on patient-centered outcomes. A standardized set of key outcomes (a core outcome set) specific to orthodontics will remedy this (see Section Core outcomes in orthodontics).

Simple approaches to appraising RCTs, including scales, have been developed (Moher *et al.* 1995) in which a score is assigned based on certain features associated with RCT quality. The Cochrane Collaboration, however, cautions against using scores, as they may pertain more to quality of reporting rather than RCT quality. The Cochrane Risk of Bias Tool has been developed for assessment of the methodological quality of a RCT, and can be included in systematic reviews. The Risk of Bias Tool has identified key areas that should be evaluated, and gives a risk of bias judgment as low risk, high risk, or unclear risk, with the latter indicative of either lack of information or uncertainty over the potential risk for bias (Higgins *et al.* 2011a,b). The Centre for Evidence-based Medicine (CEBM) in Oxford (UK) has also developed an easy to follow checklist for assessing the quality of RCTs. The full document may be freely accessed at: http://www.cebm.net/index.aspx?o=1157 and used for RCT assessment (CEBM 2017).

Conflict of Interest

Robust prospective research is predicated on impartiality, which may be compromised by a conflict of interest. Conflict of interest refers to a set of conditions in which professional judgment concerning a primary interest (such as a patient's welfare or the validity of research) is unduly influenced by a secondary interest (such as financial gain). Investigators trying to advance their career or investigators who are passionate about their area of research may subconsciously lose objectivity. In biomedical research, preferential publication of positive and "interesting" research studies and outcomes are prevalent, leading to *publication bias* and selective outcome reporting, respectively. In turn, this may lead to biased systematic review conclusions (Thornton and Lee 2000; Koletsi *et al.* 2009; Fleming *et al.* 2015). Attending company sponsored conferences, workshops, and dinners, as well as receiving free products and travelling at a company's expense may all create conflicts of interest. Other sources of conflict of interest in orthodontics may stem from a researcher's role in the development of a technique or system (Katz 2010). The impact of this development remains unclear in the field of orthodontics, while in medicine it has been reported that studies funded by the pharmaceutical industry are more likely to produce results favoring the product made by the sponsoring company (Sismondo 2008). The updated CONSORT reporting guidelines require disclosure of "sources of funding and other support (such as supply of drugs) role of funders, etc." (Higgins *et al.* 2011).

Systematic reviews and meta-analyses for orthodontic interventions

Systematic reviews for interventions should identify and combine (where possible) the best available evidence concerning the effects of an intervention, in a systematic, transparent, and unbiased manner. Quantitative synthesis of data from individual primary studies may produce a more precise estimate of the efficacy and safety of a therapy. Depending on the volume and nature of related primary research, systematic reviews may reconcile controversies regarding therapies and expose knowledge gaps and unanswered questions, which may be addressed in future trials.

The validity of systematic review results is predicated on transparent and verifiable methodology (Figure 5.2), as arbitrary combination of potentially biased and mismatched data may result in recycling of poor research (garbage in, garbage out) (Borenstein *et al.* 2009), potentially giving unwarranted credence to unreliable primary research. In order for the results of a systematic to review to be valid, the review process should have low risk of bias (Higgins *et al.* 2011). The main biases encountered in systematic reviews are selective study inclusion (selection bias), publication bias (studies with significant results are more likely to be published than studies with nonsignificant results), and heterogeneity of quality of included studies. Inclusion of only a

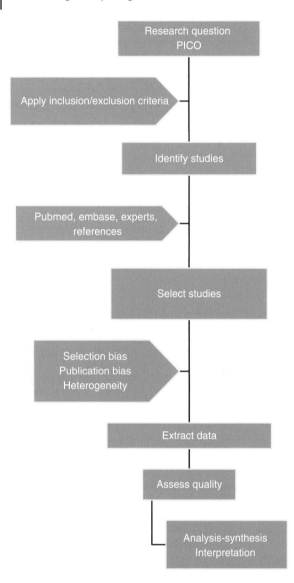

Figure 5.2 Main steps of a systematic review. Abbreviations: PICO, participants, intervention(s), comparators, outcome measures.

portion of the available studies in a systematic review, particularly if these are of variable quality and involve heterogeneous participants, interventions, and outcomes, may not yield valid results (Juni *et al.* 2001).

The results of meta-analysis (quantitative synthesis) from a systematic review assessing the effect of halogen, plasma, and light emitting diode (LED) curing lights in orthodontic bonding are shown in Table 5.3 (Fleming *et al.* 2013). The results of the individual studies, especially between halogen versus plasma and halogen versus LED, were considered similar enough and were therefore combined to give an overall estimate of effect (pooled effect), along with the 95% confidence and prediction intervals (applicable to random effects meta-analysis). Two main statistical methods (fixed effects and random effects) may be used to combine the data from individual studies using weights according to the size of the primary studies. Table 5.3 is called a forest plot and consists of:

- Individual studies with total sample size and events per treatment arm.

Table 5.3 Forest plot for halogen versus plasma, halogen versus led and halogen versus plasma and LED curing lights.

Authors	Halogen (events)	Halogen (N)	Plasma/LED (events)	Plasma/LED (N)	OR (95% CI)	% Weight
Plasma						
Manzo	12	304	12	304	1.00 (0.44, 2.26)	8.16
Pettemerides	13	176	12	176	0.92 (0.41, 2.08)	8.24
Cacciafesta	12	300	21	300	1.75 (0.85, 3.62)	10.27
Russel	31	354	22	354	0.71 (0.40, 1.25)	16.96
Sfondrini	39	717	31	717	0.79 (0.49, 1.29)	23.29
Subtotal (I-squared = 4.8%, p = 0.379) with estimated predictive interval.					0.92 (0.68, 1.23) . (0.54, 1.56)	66.92
LED						
Koupis	10	300	15	300	1.50 (0.66, 3.39)	8.16
Mirabella	19	577	15	575	0.79 (0.40, 1.57)	11.51
Krishnawamy	22	273	19	271	0.87 (0.46, 1.64)	13.41
Subtotal (I-squared = 0.0%, p = 0.463) with estimated predictive interval.					0.96 (0.64, 1.44) . (0.07, 13.32)	33.08
Overall (I-squared = 0.0%, p = 0.565) with estimated predictive interval.					0.93 (0.74, 1.17) . (0.69, 1.24)	100.00

.2   1   3

Plasma or LED   Halogen

Note: Weights are from random effects analysis.
Source: Fleming *et al.* 2013 with permission.

- A horizontal line next to each study: the rectangle in the middle of the line is the individual study estimate. The solid vertical line represents a "line of no difference" (in this case odds ratio = 1). The rectangle size varies according to the sample size of the individual study. Rectangles intersecting the solid vertical line of no difference indicate that the corresponding individual study did not favor either type of curing light. The whiskers extending from the rectangle indicate the 95% confidence interval of the estimate of the individual study. Wider whiskers indicate lower precision for the estimate and vice versa.
- The dotted vertical line indicates the pooled estimate after combining data from all studies. In this particular forest plot there are three results sections. The upper part compares studies using halogen or plasma curing lights, the middle part halogen versus LED, and the lower compares halogen versus plasma-LED combined. Within each analysis section there is a diamond representing the pooled estimate and its confidence interval and predictive interval per subgroup (halogen vs. plasma or halogen vs. LED) and overall.
- On the right side of the forest plot, the actual numerical estimates and 95% confidence intervals (and prediction intervals, where applicable) are shown per study, subgroup, and overall. When the confidence interval (for an odds ratio) includes 1 it indicates that the result is not significant at conventional levels ($P > 0.05$).

In a fixed effects meta-analysis, it is assumed that a single population effect exists and that differences in estimates between studies relates to random error. Under this assumption the pooled effect from the quantitative synthesis represents the best estimate of the true effect and the corresponding confidence interval for the given level (i.e., 95%) indicates the precision of the mean effect. The random effects model assumes that the effects of the intervention are not the same across studies, but that they follow a distribution. The pooled effect from the random effects model indicates the average treatment effect and the corresponding 95% confidence interval that in 95% of cases the mean pooled effect will be inside the diamond. On the other hand, the 95% prediction interval indicates the range of the different effect sizes, and therefore that in 95% the true effect of a new trial will lie within the prediction interval (Borenstein *et al.* 2009).

On the left side at the level of the diamonds, results of testing for individual study similarity are shown which indicate, from a statistical perspective, whether synthesis of the included studies is appropriate.

Checklists to appraise systematic review quality have been developed and often follow a question–answer format, such as that developed by the CEBM (CEBM 2017). Research on systematic reviews is expanding and new methods for assessing and synthesizing the existing evidence are constantly being developed. A relatively recent development in meta-analysis allows, under certain assumptions, the combination of direct and indirect comparisons of diverse interventions in trials using the same outcome, reducing the loss of information when calculating pooled estimates. This type of meta-analysis has been termed multiple interventions meta-analysis (MIM), or mixed treatments, or network meta-analysis. Applying MIM allows ranking of different interventions, even if direct comparisons between interventions do not exist, by utilizing the transitivity of the therapies, if the required assumptions are satisfied. For example, if therapies A, B, C are mainly compared with a control, network meta-analysis may allow ranking of A, B, and C in terms of efficacy (Salanti *et al.* 2008). This methodology has, for example, been utilized in orthodontics to permit comparison of the relative efficiency of orthodontic alignment associated with conventional, active, and passive self-ligating brackets (Pandis *et al.* 2014a).

Metaepidemiological findings from orthodontics

A wealth of research on research, also known as meta-epidemiology, focusing on the quality and reporting characteristics of a body of research has been carried out in biomedical research, and more recently has been applied to orthodontics. In particular, clinical trials and systematic reviews have been scrutinized in detail. The importance of transparent reporting of all research studies is well established. The Consolidated Standards of Reporting Trials (CONSORT) guidelines were directed at informing the reporting of RCTs (Higgins *et al.* 2011). CONSORT has been endorsed by most leading journals, with authors encouraged to adhere to recommendations within their submissions. Moreover, numerous extensions to CONSORT have been made to account for variations in trial design, setting, and outcomes. CONSORT for Abstracts also details correct reporting of abstracts of clinical trials. This is particularly important as consumers of research are known to focus on abstracts without always referring to the details provided in the body of the article.

The need for enhanced research reporting and conduct within biomedical research has intensified in recent years. One example of this is a recent, well-publicized series of articles published in The Lancet, alluding to the amount of money wasted on research (up to 85% of research funding, or about of $210 billion each year). The failure to publish and unclear reporting are significant reasons for this "waste" (Glasziou *et al.* 2014). It is therefore clear that while reporting guidelines do exist, robust implementation of these is required if research funding and efforts are to be fully realized. Overall, the conduct and reporting of orthodontic research seems to mirror that of biomedical research, although some improvement has been observed over the past 5 to 10 years (Table 5.4) (Pandis *et al.* 2010).

Table 5.4 Compliance with Consolidated Standards of Reporting Trials (CONSORT) subitems within a sample of dental journals.

Adequately reported	Inadequately reported
Sample calculation	Hypothesis or objectives
All parts of randomization	Eligibility criteria
Blinding	Settings
Intention to treat	Data collection
Effect estimates, confidence intervals (focus on *P* values)	Interventions
Multiple testing	Definition of outcome measures
Limitations, generalizability, funding	

Source: Adapted from Pandis *et al.* 2010.

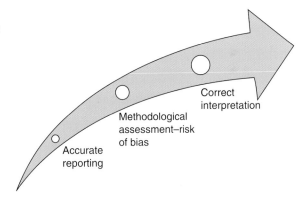

Figure 5.3 Relationship between reporting quality, methodological quality–risk of bias, and interpretation of trial results.

Accurate reporting

Methodological assessment–risk of bias

Correct interpretation

Other important reporting and quality assessment guidelines pertinent to orthodontics are: PRISMA (Preferred Reporting Items for Systematic Reviews and Meta-analyses) (Liberati *et al.* 2009), STROBE (Strengthening the Reporting of Observational Studies in Epidemiology) (Vandenbroucke *et al.* 2007), STARD (Standard for Reporting of Diagnostic Accuracy) (Bossuyt *et al.* 2003), and AMSTAR (A Measurement Tool to Assess Systematic Reviews) (Shea *et al.* 2007). It should be noted, however, that quality of reporting, study quality, and risk of bias are not synonymous (Figure 5.3). Study quality answers the question: "Did the investigators do the best they could?", whereas risk of bias answers the question: "Should I believe the result?" On the other hand, as Davidoff has suggested: "Accurate and transparent reporting is like turning the light on before you clean up a room; it does not clean for you, but it does tell you where the problems are" (Davidoff 2000). The potential benefits of developing and adopting reporting guidelines are shown in Figure 5.4.

Improving research reporting in orthodontics

Within orthodontics, initiatives have been undertaken to promote improved compliance with CONSORT and PRISMA. For example, publication templates have been developed mirroring these guidelines to facilitate better reporting, such as that of the *American Journal of Orthodontics and Dentofacial Orthopedics* (AJO-DO 2017). Moreover, a novel approach to the peer-review process has been implemented in AJO-DO, with respect

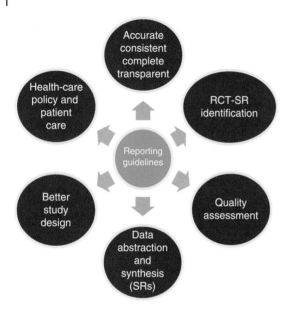

Figure 5.4 Benefits of reporting guidelines. Abbreviations: RCT, randomized controlled trial; SR, systematic review.

to clinical trial submissions. Specifically, from 2011, the AJO-DO adopted a systematic process involving the editor-in-chief, an associate editor, and RCT authors, whereby initial RCT submissions were first assessed by the associate editor to ensure all CONSORT items were reported completely following transfer from the editor-in-chief. The associate editor replied to the authors listing unreported items and highlighting ways to address incompletely reported items prior to resubmission. Resubmitted manuscripts were again scrutinized by the associate editor for CONSORT adherence, after which they were sent for standard peer review. This initiative led to near complete reporting of most CONSORT items in published articles, but did require significant input from the editorial team and added an additional cycle to the review process (Pandis *et al.* 2014b). More recently, in order to improve reporting at the level of submissions, the approach changed with the adoption of a publication template incorporating 20 subheadings corresponding to the 27 CONSORT items. A model clinical trial report providing the rationale for reporting of individual items was also published (AJO-DO 2017). A specialty-specific CONSORT document has also been developed to ensure that it resonates with prospective authors (Pandis *et al.* 2015). These initiatives have resulted in enhanced compliance within AJO-DO and may have wider utility.

Core outcomes in orthodontics

Research that does not address questions that are central to patients, including their experiences of care, treatment-related side effects, and patient-focused outcomes, may result in missed opportunities to consider important treatment parameters (Sinha *et al.* 2008). There is a resultant emphasis on involving patients and end users in the design and analysis of clinical research studies. This is evidenced by the prerequisite that funding applications for clinical studies increasingly involve patients in their planning and design (National Institute for Health Research 2017). In order to ensure that research questions lead to a holistic and meaningful conclusion, there is also an increasing drive to incorporate patient-related outcome measures. Moreover, accepted reporting guidelines have also been adapted in an effort to facilitate better reporting of these influential patient-reported outcomes (Calvert *et al.* 2013).

A further problem related to the failure to focus on common, important outcomes in clinical research is the risk that systematic reviews will be unable to synthesize data from the various studies. Moreover, the development and routine adoption of a standard set of outcomes may reduce the likelihood of preferential publication of interesting or statistically significant outcomes. This is known as outcome reporting bias, and is associated with the risk of distorted estimates of treatment effects, as well as hampering our ability to combine results within systematic reviews (Dwan *et al.* 2008).

A core outcome set (COS), which involves, but is not restricted to, the inclusion of important, core outcomes, has gained increasing traction in recent years, and over 200 are in existence throughout biomedical research areas. Within dentistry, and indeed, specifically within orthodontics, scoping reviews have exposed an undue focus on clinician-centered outcomes (Tsichlaki and O'Brien 2014; Fleming *et al.* 2016) with quality of life and functional aspects rarely considered. In particular, an undue emphasis on clinician-focused outcomes, including morphological features of malocclusion, such as cephalometric changes, has been exposed in orthodontic research. The development of a core outcome set in orthodontics is underway and likely to be completed by 2018 (Ebell *et al.* 2004).

Integration of evidence into daily practice

Research awareness

Further obstacles to the integration of orthodontic research findings into daily practice include lack of awareness among clinicians of contemporary evidence, but also a dearth of recommendations or guidance stemming from primary research or systematic reviews. Ultimately, the goal of evidence-based practice is to continually improve patient care in response to research developments (Rinchuse *et al.* 2008). Despite widespread acceptance of evidence-based approaches, a limited knowledge of evidence sources (including the Cochrane database), low utility of portals of evidence (including PubMed), and inadequate knowledge of scientific terms is commonplace among practicing clinicians (Madhavji *et al.* 2011). As such, enhanced education and accessibility to the best evidence remains important.

Efforts to improve accessibility to orthodontic research have been made in recent years, with open-access journals increasing in number. For example, the *Angle Orthodontist* and *Progress in Orthodontics* are both freely available on the Internet. Moreover, prominent research blogs have gained considerable traction with regular appraisal of influential papers (O'Brian 2017; Minervation 2017). Peer-to-peer sharing of research studies and findings has also become commonplace with websites (e.g., ResearchGate) becoming increasingly popular, although access does require a registered account (ResearchGate 2017).

Research transparency

The issue of publication bias, whereby negative results are less likely to be published than positive or interesting results, is a significant problem in biomedical research. Moreover, selective outcome reporting of specific data or outcomes within a study is recognized (Higgins *et al.* 2011). Selective reporting may manifest as preferential publication of either interesting or positive research findings, while less interesting, often negative, results are not published. The upshot of selective reporting is potentially misleading conclusions from research, which may translate into inappropriate or poorly informed health-care practices (Dwan *et al.* 2008). Within CONSORT, it has been suggested that primary and nonprimary outcomes should be defined clearly with presentation of both estimated effect size and associated precision. Post hoc adjustments should be described to allow potentially biased or data-driven alterations to be identified. There is also empirical evidence of both inconsistencies and selective outcome reporting in medical and surgical journals, with issues exposed in relation to primary and nonprimary outcomes (Rosenthal and Dwan 2013; Hannink *et al.* 2013; Killeen *et al.* 2014). Registration of clinical trials has been advocated to promote greater clarity. Clinical trial registries can be viewed to inspect the similarity between the planned study and the published article. This can aid in the identification of selective outcome reporting and other inconsistencies. Mandatory trial registration has been adopted widely, with the International Committee of Medical Journal Editors advocating registration prior to consideration for publication in a member journal (De Angelis *et al.* 2004). Trial registration is also encouraged within orthodontic journals, although mandatory registration is not yet stringently enforced.

A recent extension to the mandatory publication of research protocols is the commitment to publish clinical trials irrespective of the findings. AllTrials is an initiative geared at ensuring that publication of research findings is universal (AllTrials 2017). This would also mitigate against publication bias. Moreover, there is a recognition that clinical trial data should be made available on accessible databases to facilitate verification and replication of findings, and indeed to facilitate access for the purposes of systematic review. Again, these initiatives are focused on the surgical and pharmacological literature for now. However, in time, it would be intuitive and beneficial for these to become accepted practice within orthodontics.

Several tools have been developed to facilitate the translation of scientific evidence into clinical practice (Bossuyt *et al.* 2003; Shea *et al.* 2007). One of these to gain traction is GRADE (Grades of Recommendation, Assessment, Development, and Evaluation) (http://www.gradeworkinggroup.org; Guyatt *et al.* 2011), which has been incorporated into *Cochrane Systematic Reviews*, and has also been advocated for use in orthodontic trials (AJO-DO 2017). The GRADE approach considers the quality of the available evidence from systematic reviews, but also the values and preferences of patients, safety, and costs, and has only two recommendation levels: strong or weak. GRADE considers all outcomes of interest and classifies them as either critical, important but not critical, or not important. The evidence is graded for all outcomes and one of four possible ratings is assigned (high, moderate, low, and very low). Ultimately, a recommendation is given, either strong or weak, depending on the previous information and on whether one approach is accepted across the board (strong recommendation) or alternative options for patients are available, which are likely to be accepted and followed. If, based on the available evidence, it is certain that the benefits clearly outweigh the risks, then a strong recommendation regarding the therapy is likely, whereas if benefits and risks are balanced, or there is uncertainty about the benefits and risks, a weak recommendation is likely (Figure 5.5). Grade utilizes GRADEPro (http://gradepro.org/) specialized software developed to assist in producing summary of findings tables (Table 5.5), GRADE evidence tables, and overview of findings tables permit simple presentation of the findings of the review.

Collaboration/multicenter research and funding

There is an increasing recognition of the need for more and better clinical research in orthodontics with, for example, a recent metaepidemiological overview of orthodontic systematic reviews exposing that meta-analysis was possible in less than one-quarter of systematic reviews, and that each meta-analysis included a median of just four trials (Koletsi *et al.* 2015). These figures compare unfavorably with medical literature, where 63% of reviews have been found to involve meta-analysis, with each meta-analysis involving a median of 15 studies (Page *et al.* 2016). Arguably, some of these barren reviews may emanate from asking less important questions or undertaking reviews prematurely (Page and Moher 2016). Notwithstanding this, some of the aforementioned initiatives, including enhanced reporting and core outcome set development, should help to remedy this issue. There is also an appreciation that better clinical research is required in orthodontics. Some of the barriers to more meaningful research include difficulties in obtaining financial support for expensive clinical research, as well as the problems of identifying and involving suitable participants (Cunningham *et al.* 2011).

Several multicentre research studies have been undertaken successfully in orthodontics in the United Kingdom (O'Brien *et al.* 2009; Mandall *et al.* 2016). Additionally, the National Institute of Dental and Craniofacial Research in the United States has also been promoting orthodontic research within a network setting. From 2005 to 2012, several orthodontic studies were conducted in a network centered in the Pacific Northwest (Hyde *et al.* 2010; Huang *et al.* 2013; Kim *et al.* 2016). Currently, a National Dental Practice-based

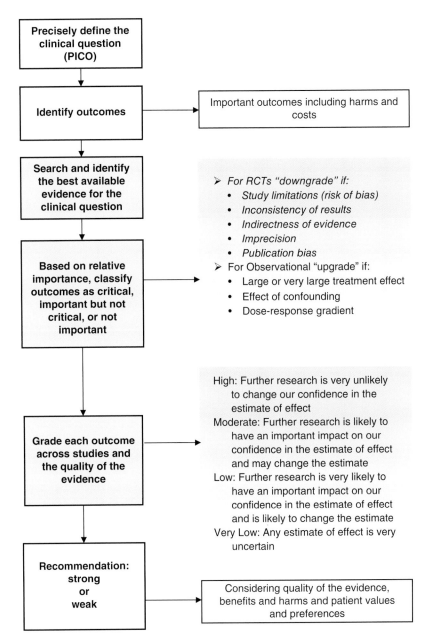

Figure 5.5 The Grades of Recommendation, Assessment, Development, and Evaluation (GRADE) process for assessing the evidence from systematic reviews and making recommendations. Abbreviations: PICO, participants, intervention(s), comparators, outcome measures; RCT, randomized controlled trial.

Research Network has been funded, and one of the studies within that network has enrolled over 300 patients to investigate the treatment and subsequent stability of adults with anterior open-bite (Huang 2016). Additionally, a network study investigating Class II treatment has been initiated in Iowa. Hopefully, these studies will assist with improving the evidence that exists in our specialty, and will foster additional network studies in the future.

Table 5.5 Grades of Recommendation, Assessment, Development, and Evaluation (GRADE) profile (American College of Chest Physicians, ACCP) table from the systematic review comparing bond failure of brackets bonded with halogen versus plasma curing lights.

							Study event rates (%)			Anticipated absolute effects *Time frame is 2000–2008*	
Should Plasma Arc Curing Light be used instead of Halogen Curing Light for Orthodontic Bonding?											
Participants (studies) Follow-up	Risk of bias	Inconsistency	Indirectness	Imprecision	Publication bias	Overall quality of evidence	With Halogen Curing Light	With Plasma Curing Light	Relative effect (95% CI)	Risk with Halogen Curing Light	Risk difference with Plasma Curing Light (95% CI)
Bond failure											
3702 (5 studies) 6–24 months	no serious risk of bias[a]	no serious inconsistency[b]	no serious indirectness[c]	no serious imprecision[d,e]	undetected	⊕⊕⊕⊕ **HIGH**[a,b,c,d,e]	107/1851 (5.8%)	98/1851 (5.3%)	**RR 0.92** (0.68 to 1.23)	**58 per 1000**	**5 fewer per 1000** (from 18 fewer to 13 more)

[a] Unclear allocation concealment and no blinding applied. Lack of allocation concealment and blinding was judged that are unlikely to influence the outcome of interest. No attrition or outcome reporting bias detected/suspected. It was decided not to rate down the evidence.
[b] Statistical heterogeneity was minimal (I^2 = 4.8%). It was decided not to rate down the evidence.
[c] No indirectness as all studies included head to head comparisons with similar inclusion/exclusion criteria. It was decided not to rate down the evidence.
[d] No explanation was provided.
[e] Confidence intervals overlap and although estimates were on both directions the difference was small. It was decided not to rate down the evidence.
Source: Adapted from Fleming *et al.* 2013.

Conclusions

Evidence-based orthodontics has developed greatly over the past 20 years, with an acceptance that clinical decision making should be supported by robust scientific evidence whenever possible. That being said, we need to dedicate our efforts to designing and conducting rigorous trials that will provide the evidence that we need to deliver the most efficient, effective, predictable, safe, and stable treatment. Over the next decade, an increasing emphasis on multicenter clinical trials focusing on meaningful and consistent outcomes should be prioritized. Better and more transparent communication of clinical evidence via open access publications and on-line mechanisms will reach and resonate with clinicians and their patients, thereby maximizing the yield from orthodontic research.

References

All Trials, 2017. Available at: www.alltrials.net (Accessed November 2017).

American Journal of Orthodontics and Dentofacial Orthopedics (AJO-DO), 2017. *Annotated RCT Sample Article.* Available at: http://cdn.elsevier.com/promis_misc/YMOD_Annotated_RCT_Sample_Article.pdf (accessed November 2017).

Borenstein M, Hedges LV, Higgins JPT, *et al.*, 2009. *Introduction to Meta-Analysis.* Chichester: Wiley, 127–132, 377–187.

Bossuyt PM, Reitsma JB, Bruns DE, *et al.*, 2003. Towards complete and accurate reporting of studies of diagnostic accuracy: the STARD initiative. *BMJ* 326, 41–44.

Boutron I, Moher D, Altman DG, *et al.*, 2008. Extending the CONSORT statement to randomized trials of no pharmacologic treatment: explanation and elaboration. *Ann Intern Med* 148, 295–309.

Calvert M, Blazeby J, Altman DG, *et al.*, 2013. Reporting of patient-reported outcomes in randomized trials: the CONSORT PRO extension. *J Am Med Assoc* 309, 814–822.

Centre for Evidence Based Medicine, Oxford University, (CEBM) 2017. *Critical Appraisal Tools*. Available at: http://www.cebm.net/index.aspx?o=1157 (accessed November 2017).

Chalmers TC, Levin H, Sacks HS, *et al.*, 1987. Meta-analysis of clinical trials as a scientific discipline. I: Control of bias and comparison with large co-operative trials. *Stat Med* 6, 315–328.

Chia KS, 1997. "Significant-itis" – an obsession with the P-value. *Scand J Work Environ Health* 23, 152–154.

Cunningham S, Bearn D, Benson P, *et al.*, 2011. In search of the sample: recent experiences of a trial team in orthodontics. *Contemp Clin Trials* 32, 530–534.

Davidoff F, 2000. News from the International Committee of Medical Journal Editors. *Ann Intern Med* 133, 229–231.

De Angelis C, Drazen JM, Frizelle FA, *et al.*, 2004. Clinical trial registration: a statement from the International Committee of Medical Journal Editors. *N Engl J Med* 351, 1250–1251.

Dwan K, Altman DG, Arnaiz JA, *et al.*, 2008. Systematic review of the empirical evidence of study publication bias and outcome reporting bias. *PLoS One* 3, e3081.

Ebell MH, Siwek J, Weiss BD, *et al.*, 2004. Strength of recommendation taxonomy (SORT): a patient-centered approach to grading evidence in the medical literature. *Am Fam Physician* 69, 548–556.

Fleming PS, Eliades T, Katsaros C, *et al.*, 2013. The choice of curing lights for orthodontic bonding: A systematic review and meta-analysis. *Am J Orthod Dentofacial Orthop* 143, S92–103.

Fleming PS, Koletsi D, Dwan K, *et al.*, 2015. Outcome discrepancies and selective reporting: impacting the leading journals? *PLoS One* 10, e0127495.

Fleming PS, Koletsi D, O'Brien K, *et al.*, 2016. Are dental researchers asking patient-important questions? A scoping review. *J Dent* 49, 9–13.

Gardner MJ, Altman DG, 1986. Confidence intervals rather than p values: estimation rather than hypothesis testing. *Br Med J* 292, 746–750.

Glasziou P, Altman DG, Bossuyt P, *et al.*, 2014. Reducing waste from incomplete or unusable reports of biomedical research. *Lancet* 383, 267–276.

Goodman SN, 1999. Toward evidence-based medical statistics I. The P value fallacy. *Ann Int Med* 130, 995–1004.

Guyatt G, Oxman AD, Akl EA, *et al.*, 2011. GRADE guidelines: 1. Introduction-GRADE evidence profiles and summary of findings tables. *J Clin Epidemiol* 64, 383–394.

Haag U, 1998. Technologies for automating randomized treatment assignment in clinical trials. *Drug Inf J* 32, 11.

Hannink G, Gooszen HG, Rovers MM, 2013. Comparison of registered and published primary outcomes in randomized clinical trials of surgical interventions. *Ann Surg* 257, 818–823.

Harbour R, Miller J, 2001. A new system for grading recommendations in evidence based guidelines. *BMJ* 323, 334.

Higgins JPT, Altman DG, Sterne JAC (eds), 2011a. Assessing risk of bias in included studies. In: Higgins JPT, Green S (eds). Cochrane Handbook for Systematic Reviews of Interventions, Version 5.1.0 (updated March 2011). The Cochrane Collaboration. Available at: http://handbook-5-1.cochrane.org/ (accessed November 2017).

Higgins JPT, Altman DG, Gøtzsche PC, *et al.*, 2011b. Cochrane Collaboration's tool for assessing risk of bias in randomised trials. *BMJ* 343, d5928.

Huang GJ, 2016. Giving back to our specialty: Participate in the national anterior open-bite study. *Am J Orthod Dentofacial Orthop* 149, 4–5.

Huang GJ, Roloff-Chiang B, Mills BE, *et al.*, 2013. Effectiveness of MI Paste Plus and PreviDent fluoride varnish for treatment of white spot lesions: a randomized controlled trial. *Am J Orthod Dentofacial Orthop* 143, 31–41.

Hyde JD, King GJ, Greenlee GM, *et al.*, 2010. Survey of orthodontists' attitudes and experiences regarding miniscrew implants. *J Clin Orthod* 44, 481–486.

Jadad AR, Moore RA, Carroll D, *et al.*, 1996. Assessing the quality of reports of randomized clinical trials: is blinding necessary? *Control Clin Trials* 17, 1–12.

Juni P, Altman DG, Egger M, 2001. Systematic reviews in health care: assessing the quality of controlled clinical trials. *BMJ* 323, 42–46.

Katz MI, 2010. Appearances count when industry underwrites research. *Am J Orthod Dentofacial Orthop* 137, 3–4.

Killeen S, Sourallous P, Hunter IA, *et al.*, 2014. Registration rates, adequacy of registration, and a comparison of registered and published primary outcomes in randomized controlled trials published in surgery journals. *Ann Surg* 259, 193–196.

Kim S, Katchooi M, Bayiri B, *et al.*, 2016. Predicting improvement of postorthodontic white spot lesions. *Am J Orthod Dentofacial Orthop* 149, 625–633.

Kloukos D, Papageorgiou SN, Fleming PS, *et al.*, 2014. Reporting of statistical results in prosthodontic and implantology journals: p values or confidence intervals? *Int J Prosthodont* 27, 427–432.

Koletsi D, Fleming PS, Eliades T, *et al.*, 2015. The evidence from systematic reviews and meta-analyses published in orthodontic literature. Where do we stand? *Eur J Orthod* 37, 603–609.

Koletsi D, Karagianni A, Pandis N, *et al.*, 2009. Are studies reporting significant results more likely to be published? *Am J Orthod Dentofacial Orthop* 136, 632.e1–632.e5.

Koletsi D, Pandis N, Polychronopoulou A, *et al.*, 2012 Does published orthodontic research account for clustering effects during statistical data analysis? *Eur J Orthod* 34, 287–292.

Lempesi E, Koletsi D, Fleming PS, *et al.*, 2014. The reporting quality of randomised controlled trials in orthodontics. *J Evid Based Dent Pract* 14, 46–52.

Liberati A, Altman DG, Tetzlaff J, *et al.*, 2009. The PRISMA statement for reporting systematic reviews and meta-analyses of studies that evaluate healthcare interventions: explanation and elaboration. *BMJ* 339, b2700.

Madhavji A, Araujo EA, Kim KB, *et al.*, 2011. Attitudes, awareness, and barriers toward evidence-based practice in orthodontics. *Am J Orthod Dentofacial Orthop* 140, 309–316.

Mainland D, 1984. Statistical ritual in clinical journals: is there a cure? *BMJ* 1984; 288, 841–843.

Mandall N, Cousley R, DiBiase A, *et al.*, 2016. Early class III protraction facemask treatment reduces the need for orthognathic surgery: a multi-centre, two-arm parallel randomized, controlled trial. *J Orthod* 43, 164–175.

Minervation Ltd, 2017. *National Elf Service.* Available at: www.nationalelfservice.net (accessed November 2017).

Moher D, Hopewell S, Schulz KF, *et al.*, 2010. CONSORT 2010 explanation and elaboration: updated guidelines for reporting parallel group randomised trials. *BMJ* 340, c869.

Moher D, Jadad AR, Nichol G, *et al.*, 1995. Assessing the quality of randomized controlled trials: An annotated bibliography of scales and checklists. *Control Clin Trials* 16, 62–73.

National Institute for Health Research, 2017. *INVOLVE Briefing notes for researchers.* Available at: http://www.invo.org.uk/resource-centre/resource-for-researchers/ (accessed November 2017).

O'Brian K, 2017. *Kevin O'Brian's Orthodontic Blog.* Available at: www.kevinobrienorthoblog.com (accessed November 2017).

O'Brien K, Wright J, Conboy F, *et al.*, 2009. Early treatment for Class II Division 1 malocclusion with the twin-block appliance: a multi-center, randomized, controlled trial. *Am J Orthod Dentofacial Orthop* 135, 573–579.

Page MJ, Moher D, 2016. Mass production of systematic reviews and meta-analyses: An exercise in mega-silliness. *Millbank Q* 94, 515–519.

Page MJ, Shamseer L, Altman DG, *et al.*, 2016. Epidemiology and reporting characteristics of systematic reviews in biomedical research: A cross-sectional study. *PLoS Med* 13, e1002028.

Pandis N, Fleming PS, Hopewell S, *et al.*, 2015. The CONSORT Statement: Application within and adaptations for orthodontic trials. *Am J Orthod Dentofacial Orthop* 147, 663–679.

Pandis N, Fleming PS, Spineli LM, *et al.*, 2014a. Initial orthodontic alignment effectiveness with self-ligating and conventional appliances: A network meta-analysis in practice. *Am J Orthod Dentofacial Orthop*145, S152–163.

Pandis N, Polychronopoulou A, Eliades T, 2010. An assessment of quality characteristics of randomized control trials published in dental journals. *J Dent* 38, 713–721.

Pandis N, Shamseer L, Kokich, V, *et al.*, 2014b. Implementation of a strategy to improve adherence to the CONSORT guidelines by a dental specialty journal. *J Clin Epidemiol* 67, 1044–1048.

Papageorgiou SN, Koretsi V, Jager A, 2016. Bias from historic controls used in orthodontic research: a meta-epidemiological study. *Eur J Orthod* 39, 98–105.

Pildal J, Hróbjartsson A, Jórgensen KJ, *et al.*, 2007. Impact of allocation concealment on conclusions drawn from meta-analyses of randomized trials. *Int J Epidemiol* 36, 847–857.

Pocock SJ, 1983. *Clinical Trials: a Practical Approach.* Chichester: Wiley.

ResearchGate, 2017. Available at: www.researchgate.net (accessed November 2017).

Rinchuse D, Kandasamy S, Ackerman M, 2008. Deconstructing evidence in orthodontics: making sense of systematic reviews, randomized clinical trials, and meta-analyses. *World J Orthod* 9, 167–176.

Rosenthal R, Dwan K, 2013. Comparison of randomized controlled trial registry entries and content of reports in surgery journals. *Ann Surg* 257, 1007–1015.

Rothman KJ, 1978. A show of confidence. *N Engl J Med* 299, 1362–1363.

Sackett DL, Haynes RB, Tugwell P, 1985. *Clinical Epidemiology: a Basic Science for Clinical Medicine.* Little, Brown and Company.

Salanti G, Higgins JP, Ades AE, *et al.*, 2008. Evaluation of networks of randomized trials. *Stat Methods Med Res* 17, 279e301.

Santoro MA, Gorrie TM (eds), 2005. *Ethics and the Pharmaceutical Industry.* Cambridge, UK: Cambridge University Press.

Sarkis-Onofre R, Cenci MS, Demarco FF, *et al.*, 2015. Use of guidelines to improve the quality and transparency of reporting oral health research. *J Dent* 43, 397–404.

Savitz D, 1993. Is statistical significance testing useful in interpreting data? *Reprod Toxicol* 7, 95–100.

Shea BJ, Grimshaw JM, Wells GA, *et al.*, 2007. Development of AMSTAR: a measurement tool to assess the methodological quality of systematic reviews. *BMC Med Res Methodol* 7, 10.

Sinha I, Jones L, Smyth RL, *et al.*, 2008. systematic review of studies that aim to determine which outcomes to measure in clinical trials in children. *PLoS Med* 5, e96.

Sismondo S, 2008. Pharmaceutical company funding and its consequences: a 300 qualitative systematic review. *Contemp Clin Trials* 29,109–113.

Straus SE, Glasziou P, Haynes RB, *et al.*, 2007. Misunderstandings, misperceptions and mistakes. *ACP J Club* 146, A8.

Straus SE, McAlister FA, 2000. Evidence-based medicine: a commentary on common criticisms. *CMAJ* 163, 837–841.

Thornton A, Lee P, 2000. Publication bias in meta-analysis: its causes and consequences. *J Clin Epidemiol* 53, 207–216.

Tsichlaki A, O'Brien K, 2014. Do orthodontic research outcomes reflect patient values? A systematic review of randomized controlled trials involving children. *Am J Orthod Dentofacial Orthop* 146, 279–285.

Vandenbroucke JP, von Elm E, Altman DG, *et al.*, 2007. STROBE initiative. Strengthening the reporting of observational studies in epidemiology (STROBE): explanation and elaboration. *Epidemiology* 18, 805–835.

Wood L, Egger M, Gluud LL, *et al.*, 2008. Empirical evidence of bias in treatment effect estimates in controlled trials with different interventions and outcomes: meta-epidemiological study. *BMJ* 336, 601–605.

6

Factors Influencing Facial Shape

Stephen Richmond, Caryl Wilson-Nagrani, Alexei Zhurov, Damian Farnell, Jennifer Galloway, Azrul Safuan Mohd Ali, Pertti Pirttiniemi, and Visnja Katic

Introduction

The systematic reviews and meta-analyses tend to focus on a particular anomaly or condition, making a comparison between interventions or controls. This chapter provides a brief overview of genetic and environmental factors that may contribute to the shape of the face, which may have an influence on the outcome of any intervention.

Identifying the etiology of a malocclusion and determining the most effective and efficient approach for the management of the presenting problem to achieve a satisfactory long-lasting outcome is often challenging. Some localized dental anomalies can be relatively easy to manage; however, when these minor anomalies are combined with anteroposterior, horizontal, or vertical discrepancies in the dentition and/or facial features the management is more complex, especially in a growing child, and the facial growth may unpredictably hinder or enhance the treatment process. Surprisingly, the precise etiology and morphologies of dental and facial features are not fully explained and it has only been the advent of life-course and longitudinal cohort studies that have helped the understanding of the relative importance of genetic and environmental contributions to facial shape, occlusion, malocclusion, and development (Golding *et al.* 2001; Nybo Andersen 2017).

The improved understanding of the relative contributions to dental and facial development will lead to more informative descriptions of population samples. The effect of traditional or novel treatment regimes on detailed homogenous etiologies and morphologies will yield invaluable treatment outcome information.

Robust outcome measures are best derived from sufficiently powered randomized controlled trials or observational longitudinal cohort studies. The background and observational data collected in outcome studies is usually hierarchical or clustered in nature. For example, a population group may present with an overjet of greater than 6 mm, but the etiology of the increased overjet may be a result of genetic, environment, or genetic–environmental interactions. The population group will have a proportion of male and females with different ethnicities/ admixture/ ancestries, at different stages of growth and development with differing chronological ages. One way to analyze hierarchical data is to employ multilevel statistical models, which are effective statistical tools that recognize the hierarchical structure of the data, allowing residual components to be derived at each level in the hierarchy (Farnell *et al.* 2017). Multilevel models are useful as they identify the various factors in determining the outcome, group effects, and group-level predictors, and infer the effects on population groups.

Facial development begins at conception and is influenced by genetic and environmental interactions, illnesses, and medical conditions through the life course (Paternoster *et al.* 2012; Liu *et al.* 2012; Fatemifar 2013; Adhikari *et al.* 2016; Shaffer *et al.* 2016; Cole *et al.* 2016; Pound *et al.* 2014; Al Ali *et al.* 2014a,b, 2015; Djordjevic *et al.* 2013).

Biological basis of facial variation and heritability

Craniofacial genetic research has understandably focused on significant craniofacial anomalies (Bailleul-Forestier *et al.* 2008; Hart and Hart 2009) and it has only been in the last 10 years that there has been a drive to determine the biological basis of normal facial variation (Paternoster *et al.* 2012; Liu *et al.* 2012; Fatemifar 2013; Adhikari *et al.* 2016; Shaffer *et al.* 2016; Cole *et al.* 2016; Toma *et al.* 2012; Roosenboom *et al.* 2016; Claes and Shriver 2014; Tsagkrasoulis *et al.* 2017). This initiative has been facilitated by the availability of low-cost three-dimensional facial capture systems, as well as computationally competent hardware and software to handle large data arrays needed to explore genotype–phenotype associations using Genome Wide Association Studies (GWAS). This work on normal variation is important as an identifiable facial traits will be associated with genetic variant or variants, which in turn can be influenced by environmental factors and can be the basis to determine specific evidenced-based treatment approaches at the optimal times to produce the best health outcomes.

There are 23 pairs of chromosomes, including one sex linked (XX and XY). The transmission of genes to offspring is the basis of inheritance of facial features (heritability/phenotype). There are about 20 000 genes and not all these genes work independently, as often one gene is dependent on the presence of one or more "modifier genes" that may not necessarily be in the same location on the genome (Attanasio *et al.* 2013). In addition, genes can interact with the environment and this is highlighted by maternal smoking and *GRID2* and *ELAVL2* genes, resulting in cleft lip and palate (Beaty *et al.* 2013) and the intake of maternal alcohol during pregnancy (Suttie *et al.* 2013).

The importance of heritability and facial appearance is often highlighted by the Habsburg dynasty (1438–1740), where the characteristic jaws and noses were inherited from one generation to the next. However, you can see heritability quite clearly daily in families where dental and facial characteristic similarities are common among siblings and passed on from parents to their offspring. These facial traits are likely to be dominant and have varying levels of penetrance and expressivity.

The relative effect of genetic and environmental factors on normal facial shape variation can be explored in twin studies. The twin studies rely on monozygotic (MZ) twins sharing 100% of their genes and dizygotic (DZ) twins sharing 50% of their genes (Visscher *et al.* 2008). Narrow-sense heritability (h^2) can be expressed as variation due to additive genetic effects divided by the total phenotypic variation and broad-sense heritability (H^2) reflects additive as well as dominant and epistatic effects, and is defined by the total genetic variance divided by the total phenotypic variation. Narrow-sense heritability is useful to explore resemblance between relatives (e.g., twins, siblings, parents, and offspring). In classical twin studies, the equation $h^2 = 2(r_{MZ} - r_{DZ})$ is used, assuming the twins share the same environment. h^2 values range from 0 to 1; the closer the h^2 value is to 1 the greater influence of genetics has on the facial feature compared to the influence of environmental factors. In a study of 263 MZ and 341 DZ female twins, the highly heritable facial features were: prominence of the upper lip relative to the chin (1); interocular distance (0.85); prominence of the nose (0.81); nose width (0.78); prominence of the nasal root (0.77); nose height (0.64); and upper lip height (0.61) (Djordjevic *et al.* 2016). These facial features contribute to 53% of facial variation. Facial size/height (0.77) contributes 20% of normal facial variation. Mandibular asymmetry has an $h^2 = 0.2$. Therefore, the seven facial features show high levels of heritability with reduced environmental influence and mandibular asymmetry shows low levels of heritability with greater chance of environmental influences. Similar levels of heritability have been reported in African Bantu children

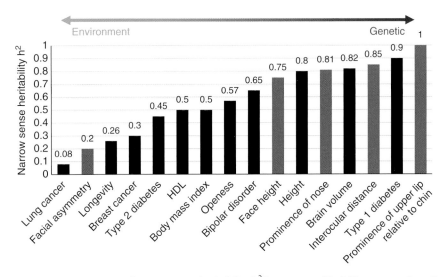

Figure 6.1 Comparison of narrow-sense heritability h² for a range of facial features and medical conditions. Abbreviation: HDL, high density lipid.

from the Mwanza region of Tanzania ($h^2 = 0.6$ to 0.8 for nasal root shape and mouth width, face width, centroid size, allometry, nasal width, midendocanthion to nasion, and face height) (Cole *et al.* 2017).

The h^2 values can be compared with other medical conditions (Figure 6.1) (Djordjevic *et al.* 2016; Bouchard and McGue 2003; Visscher *et al.* 2012; Marigota *et al.* 2016). Face height and overall height have similar levels of heritability. Interocular distance and relative prominence of upper lip and chin show similar levels of heritability to Type 1 diabetes and brain volume. Although brain volume is highly heritable, the constituent parts of the brain show different levels of heritability similar to the whole face and the individual facial components (Rentería *et al.* 2014).

The heritability of facial features was explored in 995 fathers and their offspring, 465 sons and 530 daughters (Mhani 2014). Highly heritable features ($h^2 > 0.65$) were associated around the eyes for sons and daughters. In addition, the nose tip and chin were highly heritable in sons and features around the nose and mouth highly heritable in daughters.

With reported high levels of heritability, it would be expected that these facial features should be related to genes and these can be explored through GWAS. Surprisingly, relatively few genes have been discovered and replicated (Table 6.1). Interestingly, pleiotropic effects have been noted in relation to facial distances, somatic height, and tooth eruption (Fatemifar 2013). Facial features have a hereditary basis, which informs us of our understanding of normal facial variation.

Facial shape can be derived from a series of facial landmarks, whole facial surface or part-face topography, or by direct characterization of specific facial morphological features. The use of facial landmarks and three-dimensional facial analyses are an important addition for the understanding of facial shape and facial development. However, the use of 20 or even 100 facial landmarks do not always capture the surface contour of subtle facial characteristics. A good example of this is the chin and cheek dimples, which are obvious facial features. The perioral characteristics have been captured in the Wilson–Richmond scale, which classifies subtle details of the lips, and many of these features have been linked to 20 candidate genes (Wilson *et al.* 2013; Wilson-Nagrani 2017).

Table 6.1 Currently reported phenotype-genotypes for various facial features for the normal population.

Facial phenotype/genotype	
Facial feature	**Gene**
Midendocanthion–nasion	*PAX 3*
Nose width and nose height	*PRDM16*
Interocular distance	*TP63*
Nasion position (prn alL)	*C5orf50*
Ocular–nasion distance	*COL17A1*
Midendocanthion–glabella	*AJUBA*
Inner/exocanthi	*HMGA2*
Subnasale to left alae	*ADK, VCL, AP3M1*
Columella inclination	*DCHS2*
Nose bridge breath	*SUPT3H/RUNX2*
Nose wing breath	*GLI3/PAX1*
Chin protrusion	*EDAR*
Cranial base width	*MAFB, PAX9, MIPOL1*
Intraocular	*GNA13, HDAC8, ALX3*
Nasal width	*PAX1*
Upper face depth	*TRPC6*
Nasal protrusion	*CHD8*
Centroid size	*SCHIP1*
Allometry	*PDE8A*

Source: data from Paternoster *et al.* 2012; Liu *et al.* 2012; Fatemifar 2013; Adhikari *et al.* 2016; Shaffer *et al.* 2016; Cole *et al.* 2016.

Environmental influences on facial shape

The environment has an influence on facial shape and development, and can be listed (Table 6.2). The clear environmental influences on face shape are trauma/surgery, infections, and burns, the other environmental influences will be a likely combination of environmental–genetic interactions. There is no doubt that these environmental factors influence face shape; however, the effect is often subtle, with small submillimetre facial differences, but these may have a greater influence on the dentition (Al Ali *et al.* 2014a,b, 2015; Djordjevic *et al.* 2013; Beaty *et al.* 2013; Pirilä-Parkkinen *et al.* 2009; Carvalho *et al.* 2014).

Assessment of normal facial variation

A study of facial variation in a large population-based sample of 15-year-old children (2514 females and 2233 males) identified 14 principal components that explained 82% of the total variance (Toma *et al.* 2012). The first four principal components accounted for 51% of facial variation and these were face height (28.8%), width of the eyes (10.4%), nose prominence (6.7%), and relative protrusion of upper lip to chin (5.3%)

Table 6.2 Environmental influences on facial growth and development.

Altitude	Higher altitudes associate with delayed menarche (Jansen *et al.* 2017).
Asthma	Inter ala distance 0.4 mm wider and midface 0.4 mm shorter in asthmatic females (Al Ali *et al.* 2014a).
Atopy	Total and midface height were 0.6 mm and 0.4 mm longer in atopic children (Al Ali *et al.* 2014b).
Childhood illnesses	Facial fluctuating asymmetry was initially found to be associated with longitudinal measures of childhood health; however, when a Bonferroni correction was undertaken no association was found. However, there was a very small negative association between facial fluctuating asymmetry and IQ that remained significant after correcting for a positive allometric relationship between fluctuating asymmetry and face size (Pound *et al.* 2014).
Geography	Different ethnicities and geographic locations can affect pubertal timings (Motlagh *et al.* 2011).
Maternal alcohol intake	Smooth philtrum, hypertelorism, small head size, lower levels of IQ (Suttie M *et al.* 2013; Zuccolo *et al.* 2013).
Metabolic factors (fasting insulin, glucose, cholesterol, triglycerides, high and low density lipids)	All metabolic factors studied (apart from fasting glucose) had an effect on face shape. However, when using the Bonferroni correction these no longer had a significant effect on facial shape (Djordjevic *et al.* 2013).
Nutrition	Caloric–protein malnutrition can slow growth and delay puberty (Muñoz-Calvo and Argente 2016).
Obesity	Can accelerate pubertal onset (Zhai *et al.* 2015).
Physical activity	Menarche is delayed in athletes and ballet dancers (Malina 1983).
Sleep disorder breathing	Increase in face height 0.3 mm, decrease in ANB 0.9 degrees, decrease in nose prominence and width (Al Ali *et al.* 2015; Pirilä-Parkkinen *et al.* 2009).
Socioeconomic	Earlier puberty associated with higher socioeconomic status (Sabageh *et al.* 2015).
Trauma, infection, burns, surgery, etc.	Localized restriction of facial growth due to scarring and treatment (Fricke *et al.* 1996).

(Figure 6.2). Principal component analysis is a method that helps explore patterns in the data and aims to explain the maximum facial variation with the fewest facial characteristics, either in isolation or in association with other facial features. Certainly, the first four principal components are commonly used diagnostic assessments, traditionally determined either from direct patient observation or from cephalometric radiographs. Facial variation is likely to be similar in different ethnic populations although there are subtle variations even within Caucasian population groups, highlighted in the comparison of population groups in the Netherlands and UK (Hopman *et al.* 2014).

Pubertal timing

The timing of puberty is the result of a combination of genetic and environmental factors incorporating metabolic factors (Figure 6.3a) (Cousiner *et al.* 2013). Hundreds of common genetic variants have been implicated in the coordinated timing of the pubertal transition (Perry *et al.* 2014). Simple methods to clinically determine the onset of puberty have been proposed that correlate well with skeletal maturation ($r = 0.7$ to 0.8), these include standing height (Figure 6.3b), self-reported secondary sexual characteristics, cervical maturation, and hand–wrist radiographs (Perinetti and Contardo 2017). However, there is a lack of precision in identifying growth spurts and insufficient evidence that intraoral or extraoral appliances can effect sufficiently consistent

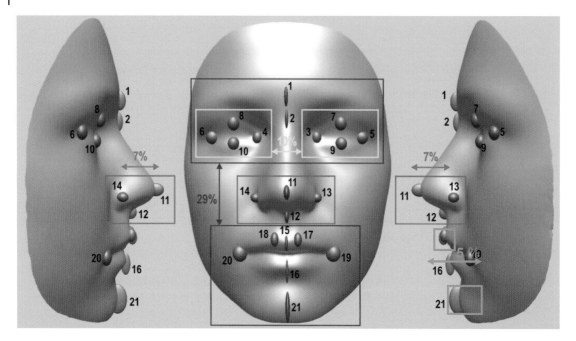

Figure 6.2 Standard deviation ellipsoids for 21 facial landmarks, highlighting facial morphology variation revealed by the first three principal components (PCs): PC1 explains 29% of total variance (red); PC2 10% (yellow); PC3 7% (green); PC4 5% (blue). Facial landmarks: 1, glabella; 2, nasion; 3 and 4, endocanthion (left and right); 5 and 6, exocanthion (left and right); 7 and 8, palpebrale superius (left and right); 9 and 10, palpebrale inferius (left and right); 11, pronasale; 12, subnasale; 13 and 14, alare (left and right); 15, labiale superius; 16, labiale inferius; 17 and 18, crista philtri (left and right); 19 and 20, cheilion (left and right); 21, pogonion. *Source:* Toma *et al.* 2012. Reproduced with permission of Oxford University Press.

and directional controllable promotion or retardation of growth of the maxilla or mandible. In addition, not all children grow at the same time and puberty may manifest as early or late onset (Figure 6.3c) (Tanner *et al.* 1966). The growth velocities (Figure 6.3d) for hard and soft tissue face heights (male and female) are shown based on a cross-sectional longitudinal study (n = 5 to 58, from 5 to 20 years of age) (Bhatia and Leighton 1993). Peaks in upper face height are observed for boys at the age of 14 and for lower face height peaks are present at 13 years of age for girls and 14 years of age for boys. The magnitude of the annual growth velocity is 0.6 mm greater for males compared to females. Not surprisingly, the soft and hard tissue landmarks follow a similar pattern, which allows noninvasive facial soft-tissue surface analyses that can be combined with hereditary and genetic studies.

Observing facial growth velocities in two different population groups

The various systematic reviews and meta-analyses use a variety of craniofacial and dental landmarks to determine the effect of health-care interventions. The use of appropriate facial landmarks are important as there is a tendency for most of the traditional cephalometric facial landmarks to move relatively to each other during the growth period. This is illustrated in Figure 6.4, where facial growth velocities were plotted monthly for seven facial distances for Finnish (female n = 25, male n = 23) and Welsh (female n = 23, male n = 27) population groups from the age of 12.8 to 15.3 years of age. The relative movement of the seven facial landmarks are based on distances to three landmarks: midendocanthion, nasion, and subnasale. From our knowledge of

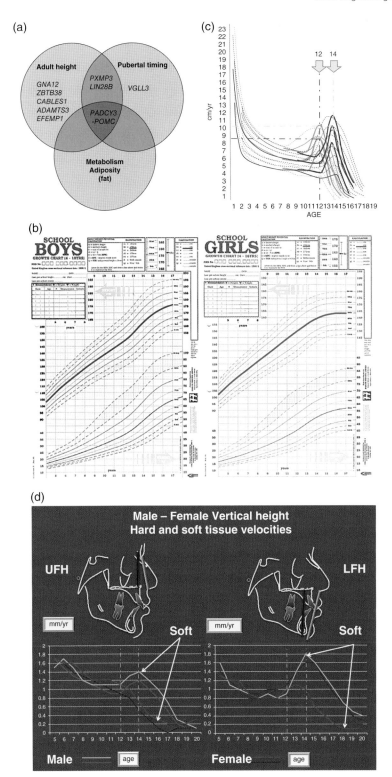

Figure 6.3 (a) Association of adult height, pubertal timing, and fat levels. *Source:* Cousiner *et al.* 2013. (b) Height and weight growth charts. (c) Early and late patterns of pubertal growth (height velocities). *Source:* Adapted from Hopman *et al.* 2014. (d) Soft and skeletal facial height growth velocities from 5 to 20 years of age. *Source:* Al Ali 2014b. Reproduced with permission of Oxford University Press.

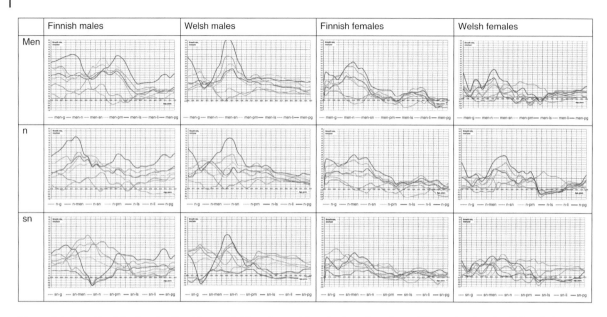

Figure 6.4 Growth of the face for Finnish and Welsh males and females based on three different landmarks. Abbreviations: men, midendocanthion; g, glabella; n, nasion; sn, subnasale; prn, pronasale; ls, labiale superius; li, labiale inferius; pg, pogonion.

the genotype–phenotype associations, we know that there is a valid genetic basis for the midendocanthion to nasion distance (*Pax3* gene) (Paternoster *et al.* 2012) and this constructed landmark is less likely to move as it is close to the anterior cranial base compared to nasion and subnasale. Interestingly, the growth velocity curves for Finnish and Welsh males showed different patterns, with two surges of growth for midendocanthion to pogonion at 13.2 and 14.2 years of age for Finnish males and prior to 12.8 and 13.6 years of age for Welsh males. The magnitude of the surges were similar in the Finnish males (3.6 and 3.8 mm/year) and Welsh males (3.6 and 5 mm/year). The peaks for these growth velocities were also observed for the distances based on nasion and subnasale but obviously the magnitudes were different as the points are relatively closer. The two peaks indicate that there are two surges of growth associated with the pogonion. These are distances only and do not determine the direction of growth (anteroposterior or vertical). The contrast between the Finnish and Welsh populations was highlighted when using the midendocanthion; all the facial growth spurts for the Welsh cohort aligned at 13.6–13.7 years of ages, but this was less obvious for the Finnish cohort. The differences between the Welsh and the Finnish males may be a result of puberty being more aligned in the Welsh population group compared to the Finnish population group. The Finnish and Welsh females showed smaller repetitive surges in midendocanthion to pogonion distances and again this may reflect different stages in puberty or that this distance is subject to fluctuations during the 3-year period of observation. These observations suggest that there are significant variations in facial growth within and between populations and these are different for males and females. Certainly, these fluctuations in growth velocities should be accounted for in any longitudinal observational study assessing health-care interventions. The patterns of growth velocities are very different to those previously reported (Bhatia and Leighton 1993), and as a result the whole Finnish and Welsh cohort were remeasured several years apart with different examiners, which yielded very similar results. The differences between the growth velocity curves from the Finnish–Welsh study and an English study (described in Section Pubertal timing) may be the result of a consistent Finnish–Welsh cohort, which were followed through, and the English study, which was a longitudinal cross-sectional study with varying sample sizes (n = 5 to 58) (Bhatia and Leighton 1993). The surges of facial growth in Finnish and Welsh individuals have been visualized (Richmond 2015).

Determining differences in population groups using a multilevel principal component analysis

Principal component analysis (PCA) is a method of data reduction identifying a combination of key facial characteristics to explain robust variation in a population. In any observational study, data is usually hierarchical or clustered in nature. For the example shown in Figure 6.5, there are four ethnic groups (Croatian: female n = 38, males n = 35; English: female n = 40, male n = 40; Finnish: female n = 23, male n = 24; and Welsh: female n = 23, male n = 24).

A single-level PCA and a multilevel PCA (mPCA) for each set of facial landmarks for each subject are plotted as principal component 1 versus principal component 2 (Figure 6.5a). PC1 represents face height and PC2 face width. There is some evidence of clustering for the different groups. Centroids for males are on the right hand side and those for females are on the left hand side. Furthermore, centroids by country tend to be quite close to each other for PC1 versus PC2 and this is shown by the solid lines connecting centroids of the different sexes for the same country. However, there is considerable overlap between the groups in the scores for individual subjects for single-level PCA for these component scores.

Results for between-groups components of mPCA are also shown and it is remarkable that males and females are connected by a vector that is of similar direction and magnitude for all countries (Figure 6.5b). This result is shown by the solid lines connecting centroids of the different sexes for the same country. Furthermore, we see that centroids are being separated quite strongly by country more clearly for the between-group mPCA. The centroids of each group are certainly much easier to resolve compared with the single-level PCA. Although there is overlap in the individual scores between the groups, this overlap appears to be less than for single-level PCA.

Looking at the three-level model (subject, sex and ethnicity; Figure 6.5c) the scree plot shows the eigenvalue magnitude associated with the principal components (n = 30). The steepness of the curve followed by a flattening identifies the important components associated with face shape variation. Therefore, the scree plot highlights the importance of sex over ethnicity, followed by subject variation (Figure 6.5d), showing subtle but nevertheless distinct facial differences between females, males, and ethnicities (Farnell *et al.* 2017). The sex variation will be associated with sexual dimorphism and the ethnicities are likely to be associated with genetic variation and different ancestries (Paternoster *et al.* 2012; Liu *et al.* 2012; Fatemifar 2013; Adhikari *et al.* 2016; Shaffer *et al.* 2016; Cole *et al.* 2016; Hopman *et al.* 2014; Ralph and Coop 2013).

Multiple comparison tests

When evaluating differences between case–control or phenotypes, multiple hypothesis tests are often performed. Multiple comparison testing can present a problem as if 20 hypotheses are tested at a significance level of $P = 0.05$ there is a 64% chance of observing at least one significant result even if the tests are not significant. There are many methods to reduce the chance of observing one significant result below the desired significance level and two are commonly used (Sham and Purcell 2014). The Bonferroni correction method is a procedure for correcting multiple testing by reducing the critical significance level according to the number of independent tests carried out in the study. The Bonferroni correction method tends to be too conservative and may lead to a high rate of false negatives. In two studies looking at childhood illnesses related to asymmetry and cardiometabolic factors influencing face shape, significant differences were found but these were dismissed when the Bonferroni correction method was employed (Pound *et al.* 2014; Djordjevic *et al.* 2013). An alternative approach is to use the permutation method, which is less conservative than Bonferroni but computationally much more demanding. With the permutation method the statistical values (case–control or phenotype) are randomly shuffled based on the hypothesis that there is no relationship between the case–control or phenotype. The smallest P value of these multiple tests is recorded. The procedure is repeated many times to construct an empirical adjusted P value.

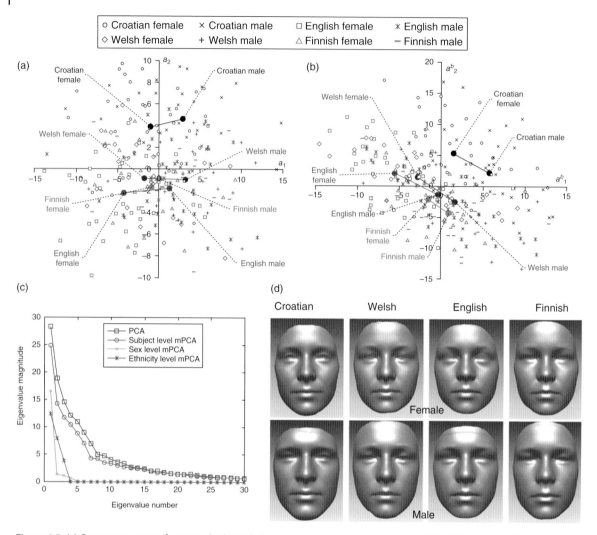

Figure 6.5 (a) Component scores from standard (single-level) principal component analysis (PCA) (PC1 against PC2). (b) Component scores from between-group multilevel PCA (PC1 against PC2). The filled circles indicate the centroids, and results for females and males from the same country are linked by a line, all following a similar trajectory. (c) Eigen vectors for three-level model: subject, sex and ethnicity. (d) Three-dimensional facial scans averaged over all subjects in each group (country and gender). *Source*: Zhurov *et al.* 2012.

It is important that any study supporting or rejecting a hypothesis should be replicated in different populations to determine the validity of the result. The use of multilevel modeling and permutation tests will reduce the number of false negatives and some of the findings of previous studies should be revisited using these relatively new statistical approaches.

Conclusions

One of the important aspects of improving our knowledge of orthodontic care outcomes is to undertake research when all the possible factors that could possibly influence the outcome are accounted for and recorded prior to undertaking the research. With the advent of more detailed information of genetic and environmental influences on dental and face shape with appropriate statistical management of the hierarchical nature of the data, more robust outcomes will be derived.

If the heritability of a facial feature is high it should be possible with sufficient sample sizes to determine the biological/genetic basis of that feature. If the heritability of the facial feature is low the likely environmental factors should be evaluated through life-course studies. Where there are midheritability estimates, the relative genetic contributions of the parents and environment contributions should be explored.

It is important for clinicians to understand the etiology of dental and facial features to determine the causative factors that will influence dental and facial variation. Large life-course cohort populations are now being collected with three-dimensional facial data alongside full genome sequencing, which potentially enables researchers to explain the etiology (genetic and environmental influences) of facial variation in greater detail. This will then inform the best timing of interventions (preventative, invasive/noninvasive) to produce long-lasting outcomes.

References

Adhikari K, Fuentes-Guajardo M, Quinto-Sánchez M, *et al.*, 2016. A genome-wide association scan implicates DCHS2, RUNX2, GLI3, PAX1 and EDAR in human facial variation. *Nat Commun* 7, 11616.

Al Ali A, Richmond S, Popat H, *et al.*, 2014a. The influence of asthma on face shape: a three-dimensional study. *Eur J Orthod* 36, 373–380.

Al Ali A, Richmond S, Popat H, *et al.*, 2014b. A three-dimensional analysis of the effect of atopy on face shape. *Eur J Orthod* 36, 506–511.

Al Ali A, Richmond S, Popat H, *et al.*, 2015. The influence of snoring, mouth breathing and apnoea on facial morphology in late childhood: a three-dimensional study. *BMJ Open* 5, e009027.

Attanasio C, Nord AS, Zhu Y, *et al.*, 2013. Fine tuning of craniofacial morphology by distant-acting enhancers. *Science* 342, 1241006.

Bailleul-Forestier I, Berdal A, Vinckier F, *et al.*, 2008.The genetic basis of inherited anomalies of the teeth. Part 2: syndromes with significant dental involvement. *Eur J Med Genet* 51, 383–408.

Beaty TH, Taub MA, Scott AF, *et al.*, 2013. Confirming genes influencing risk to cleft lip with/without cleft palate in a case-parent trio study. *Hum Genet* 132, 771–781.

Bhatia SN, Leighton BC, 1993. *A Manual of Facial Growth*. Oxford Medical Publications.

Bouchard TJ Jr, McGue M, 2003. Genetic and environmental influences on human psychological differences. *J Neurobiol* 54, 4–45.

Carvalho FR, Lentini-Oliveira DA, Carvalho GM, *et al.*, 2014. Sleep-disordered breathing and orthodontic variables in children--pilot study. *Int J Pediatr Otorhinolaryngol* 78, 1965–1969.

Claes P, Shriver MD, 2014. Establishing a multidisciplinary context for modeling 3D facial shape from DNA. *PLoS Genet* 10, e1004725.

Cole JB, Manyama M, Kimwaga E, *et al.*, 2016. Genomewide association study of african children identifies association of SCHIP1 and PDE8A with facial size and shape. *PLoS Genet* 12, e1006174.

Cole JB, Manyama M, Larson JR, *et al.*, 2017. Human facial shape and size heritability and genetic correlations. *Genetics* 205, 967–978.

Cousiner DL, Berry DJ, Timpson NJ, *et al.*, 2013. Genome-wide association and longitudinal analyses reveal genetic loci linking pubertal height growth, pubertal timing and childhood adiposity. *Hum Mol Genet* 22, 2735–2747.

Djordjevic J, Lawlor DA, Zhurov AI, *et al.*, 2013. A population-based cross-sectional study of the association between facial morphology and cardiometabolic risk factors in adolescence. *BMJ Open* 3, e002910.

Djordjevic J, Zhurov AI, Richmond S; Visigen Consortium, 2016. Genetic and environmental contributions to facial morphological variation: a 3D population-based twin study. *PLoS One* 11, e0162250.

Farnell DJJ, Galloway J, Zhurov A, *et al.*, 2017. Initial results of multilevel principal components analysis of facial shape. In: Valdes Hernandez M, González-Castro V (eds). *Medical Image Understanding and Analysis*. Proceedings 21st Annual Conference, Medical Image Understanding and Analysis 2017, Edinburgh, UK, July 11–13, 2017. Springer, 674–685.

Fatemifar G, Hoggart CJ, Paternoster L, *et al.*, 2013. Genome-wide association study of primary tooth eruption identifies pleiotropic loci associated with height and craniofacial distances. *Hum Mol Genet* 22, 3807–3817.

Fricke NB, Omnell ML, Dutcher KD, *et al.*, 1996. Skeletal and dental disturbances after facial burns and pressure garments. *J Burn Care Rehabil* 17, 338–345.

Golding J, Pembrey M, Jones R, Alspac Study Team, 2001. ALSPAC--the Avon Longitudinal Study of Parents and Children. I. Study methodology. *Paediatr Perinat Epidemiol* 15, 74–87.

Hart TC, Hart PS, 2009. Genetic studies of craniofacial anomalies: clinical implications and applications. *Orthod Craniofac Res* 12, 212–220.

Hopman SM, Merks JH, Suttie M, *et al.*, 2014. Face shape differs in phylogenetically related populations. *Eur J Hum Genet* 22, 1268–1271.

Jansen EC, Herrán OF, Fleischer NL, *et al.*, 2017. Age at menarche in relation to prenatal rainy season exposure and altitude of residence: results from a nationally representative survey in a tropical country. *J Dev Orig Health Dis* 8, 188–195.

Liu F, van der Lijn F, Schurmann C, *et al.*, 2012. A genome-wide association study identifies five loci influencing facial morphology in Europeans. *PLoS Genet* 8, e1002932.

Malina RM, 1983. Menarche in athletes: a synthesis and hypothesis. *Ann Hum Biol* 10, 1–24.

Marigota UM, Rodriguez JA, Navarro A, 2016. GWAS: a milestone in the road from genotypes to phenotypes. In: Appasani K (ed). *Genome-Wide Association Studies: From Polymorphism to Personalized Medicine*. Cambridge University Press, 12–25.

Mhani NA, 2014. *The Heritability of Facial Features: Fathers and their Offspring*. MSc thesis, Cardiff University.

Motlagh ME, Rabbani A, Kelishadi R, *et al.*, 2011. Timing of puberty in Iranian girls according to their living area: a national study. *J Res Med Sci* 16, 276–281.

Muñoz-Calvo MT, Argente J, 2016. Nutritional and pubertal disorders. *Endocr Dev* 29, 153–173.

Nybo Andersen A-M, 2017. Birthcohorts.net. Available at: http://www.birthcohorts.net/about-birthcohorts-net/ (accessed November 2017).

Paternoster L, Zhurov AI, Toma AM, *et al.*, 2012. Genome-wide association study of three-dimensional facial morphology identifies a variant in PAX3 associated with nasion position. *Am J Hum Genet* 90, 478–485.

Perinetti G, Contardo L, 2017. Reliability of growth indicators and efficiency of functional treatment for skeletal class II malocclusion: current evidence and controversies. *Biomed Res Int* 2017, 1367691.

Perry JR, Day F, Elks CE, *et al.*, 2014. Parent-of-origin-specific allelic associations among 106 genomic loci for age at menarche. *Nature* 514, 92–97.

Pirilä-Parkkinen K, Pirttiniemi P, Nieminen P, *et al.*, 2009. Dental arch morphology in children with sleep-disordered breathing. *Eur J Orthod* 31, 160–167.

Pound N, Lawson DW, Toma AM, *et al.*, 2014. Facial fluctuating asymmetry is not associated with childhood ill-health in a large British cohort study. *Proc Biol Sci* 281, 20141639.

Ralph P, Coop G, 2013. The geography of recent genetic ancestry across Europe. *PLoS Biology* 11, e1001555.

Rentería ME, Hansell NK, Strike LT, *et al.*, 2014. Genetic architecture of subcortical brain regions: common and region-specific genetic contributions. *Genes Brain Behav* 13, 821–830.

Richmond S, 2015. *3D Imaging group*. https://itunes.apple.com/gb/book/3d-imaging/id974985609?mt=13 (accessed November 2017).

Roosenboom J, Hens G, Mattern BC, *et al.*, 2016. Exploring the underlying genetics of craniofacial morphology through various sources of knowledge. *Biomed Res Int* 2016, 3054578.

Sabageh AO, Sabageh D, Adeoye OA, *et al.*, 2015. Pubertal timing and demographic predictors of adolescents in southwest Nigeria. *J Clin Diagn Res* 9, LC11–3.

Shaffer JR, Orlova E, Lee MK, *et al.*, 2016. Genome-wide association study reveals multiple loci influencing normal human facial morphology. *PLoS Genet* 12, e1006149.

Sham PC, Purcell SM, 2014. Statistical power and significance testing in large-scale genetic studies. *Nat Rev Genet* 15, 335–346.

Suttie M, Foroud T, Wetherill L, *et al.*, 2013. Facial dysmorphism across the fetal alcohol spectrum. *Pediatrics* 131, e779–788.

Tanner JM, Whitehouse RH, Takaishi M, 1966. Standards from birth to maturity for height, weight, height velocity, and weight velocity: British children, 1965 Part II. *Arch Dis Child* 41, 613.

Toma AM, Zhurov AI, Playle R, *et al.*, 2012. The assessment of facial variation in 4747 British school children. *Eur J Orthod* 34, 655–664.

Tsagkrasoulis D, Hysi P, Spector T, *et al.*, 2017. Heritability maps of human face morphology through large-scale automated three-dimensional phenotyping. *Sci Rep* 7, 45885.

Visscher PM, Brown MA, McCarthy MI, *et al.*, 2012. Five years of GWAS discovery. *Am J Hum Genet* 90, 7–24.

Visscher PM, Hill WG, Wray NR, 2008. Heritability in the genomics era – concepts and misconceptions. Heritability in the genomics era--concepts and misconceptions. *Nat Rev Genet* 9, 255–266.

Wilson CE, Playle R, Toma A, *et al.*, 2013. The prevalence of lip vermillion morphological traits in a 15 year old population. *Am J Med Genet A* 161A, 4–12.

Wilson-Nagrani CE, 2017. *Matching Genotype to Phenotype in Detailed Assessment of Lip Morphology*. PhD thesis, Cardiff University.

Zhai L, Liu J, Zhao J, *et al.*, 2015. Association of obesity with onset of puberty and sex hormones in Chinese girls: A 4-year longitudinal study. *PLoS One* 10, e0134656.

Zhurov A, Richmond S, Kau CH, *et al.*, 2012. Averaging facial images. In: CH Kau, S Richmond (eds). *Three-Dimensional Imaging for Orthodontics and Maxillofacial Surgery*. Wiley-Blackwell, 126–144.

Zuccolo L, Lewis SJ, Smith GD, *et al.*, 2013. Prenatal alcohol exposure and offspring cognition and school performance. A 'Mendelian randomization' natural experiment. *Int J Epidemiol* 42, 1358–1370.

Summaries of Selected Systematic Reviews

Summaries Contents

Preface to Summaries

In the next section, we have assembled and summarized key systematic reviews and meta-analyses on various orthodontic topics. In most cases, the two-page summaries have been prepared by one or more of the systematic review/meta-analysis authors, and these individuals are indicated by asterisks in the title. Each summary follows the same format, beginning with the title (which also serves as the reference for the paper), the rationale for the review, the PICO question (population, intervention, comparison, outcome), the search parameters, and the search findings. The bubblegrams provide a quick summary of the quality of the included studies, and the main results are typically presented in one or two forest plots or tables. Additionally, a description of the key findings is highlighted, along with commentary to place the information in perspective. At the end of some summaries, there may be some additional references. These are often articles that have been published since the systematic review/meta-analysis was published.

Of course, the 56 summaries we include in this section are only a fraction of the roughly 300 orthodontic systematic reviews/meta-analyses that have been published. Therefore, at the end of the book, we have compiled lists of systematic reviews and meta-analyses by each topic. These reference lists (current through June 2017) will allow you to see what questions have and have not been addressed for a certain topic, and for those who are interested in more detailed information, many of these reviews can be accessed online.

We hope you will find the summaries and the reference lists to be helpful in accessing information quickly and efficiently, and that the evidence will be useful to you every day as you discuss treatment options with your patients.

S1

Curing lights for orthodontic bonding: a systematic review and meta-analysis

Fleming PS, Eliades T, Katsaros C, Pandis N. Am J Orthod Dentofacial Orthop 2013;143:S92–103.*

Background

In recent years, alternatives to halogen lights, including light emitting diodes (LEDs) and plasma lights, have been developed. These have superior longevity to halogen lights and plasma arc lasers have shorter curing times. However, there is limited evidence concerning the relative effect of choice of curing light on attachment failure rate and chairside time.

Study Information

Population – orthodontic patients treated with fixed appliances
Intervention – LED or plasma arc light
Comparison – LED or plasma arc versus halogen lamp
Outcomes – attachment failure, chairside time, and demineralization.

Search Parameters

Inclusion criteria – randomized and controlled clinical trials, with split-mouth designs included
Databases searched – MEDLINE, Embase, Cochrane
Dates searched – 1966 to April 2012
Other sources of evidence – gray literature and reference lists
Language restrictions – none.

Search Results

496 references were identified, eight of which were suitable for meta-analysis.

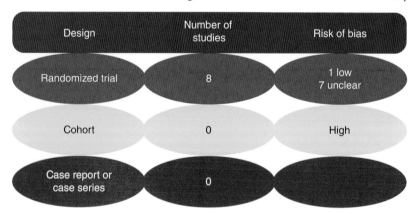

Design	Number of studies	Risk of bias
Randomized trial	8	1 low 7 unclear
Cohort	0	High
Case report or case series	0	

Study Results

The risks of bond failures using (A) plasma and (B) LED curing lights are shown in Table S1.1.

Table S1.1 Risk of bond failure comparing halogen to (A) plasma and (B) light emitting diode (LED) curing lights.

Authors	Halogen		Plasma/LED			Odds ratio, 95% CI		
	Events	n	Events	n	Weight %		Favors plasma or LED	Favors halogen
A, Plasma								
Manzo *et al.* 2004	12	304	12	304	8.16	1.00 (0.44, 2.26)		
Pettemerides *et al.* 2004	13	176	12	176	8.24	0.92 (0.41, 2.08)		
Cacciafesta *et al.* 2004	12	300	21	300	10.27	1.75 (0.85, 3.62)		
Russell *et al.* 2008	31	354	22	354	16.96	0.71 (0.40, 1.25)		
Sfondrini *et al.* 2004	39	717	31	717	23.29	0.79 (0.49, 1.29)		
Subtotal $I^2 = 4.8\%$, $P = 0.379$	107	1851	98	1851	66.92	0.92 (0.68, 1.23)		
Estimated predicted interval						(0.54, 1.56)		
B, LED								
Koupis *et al.* 2008	10	300	15	300	8.16	1.50 (0.66, 3.39)		
Mirabella *et al.* 2008	19	577	15	575	11.51	0.79 (0.40, 1.57)		
Krishnaswamy and Sunitha, 2007	22	273	19	271	13.41	0.87 (0.46, 1.64)		
Subtotal $I^2 = 0.0\%$, $P = 0.463$					33.08	0.96 (0.64, 1.44)		
Estimated predicted interval						(0.07, 13.32)		
Overall $I^2 = 0.0\%$, $P = 0.565$						0.93 (0.74, 1.17)		
Estimated predicted interval						(0.69, 1.24)		

Source: Fleming *et al.* 2013. Reproduced with permission of American Association of Orthodontists.

Key Finding

- There was no significant difference in the risk of bond failure with conventional halogen, plasma arc, or LED curing light systems.

Commentary

This review contained a reasonable number of randomized trials. While further research would be welcome, it appears that there is little to choose between curing lights from a clinical perspective. As such, the choice of curing light system should be based on clinical preferences, accounting for factors such as chairside time, purchase costs, and longevity.

S2

Self-etch primers and conventional acid-etch technique for orthodontic bonding: a systematic review and meta-analysis

Fleming PS,* Johal A, Pandis N. Am J Orthod Dentofacial Orthop 2012;142:83–94.

Background

Self-etch primers streamline the bonding process combining enamel etch and bonding phases. This may result in time saving and reduce inventory requirements. However, there is limited evidence concerning the relative effect of self-etch priming to traditional bonding techniques on attachment failure rate and chairside time.

Study Information

Population – orthodontic patients treated with fixed appliances
Intervention – self-etch primer
Comparison – Conventional etch and bond
Outcomes – attachment failure, chairside time, and demineralization.

Search Parameters

Inclusion criteria – randomized and controlled clinical trials, with split-mouth designs included
Databases searched – MEDLINE, Embase, Cochrane
Dates searched – 1966 to July 2011
Other sources of evidence – gray literature and reference lists
Language restrictions – none.

Search Results

48 references were identified, five of which were suitable for meta-analysis.

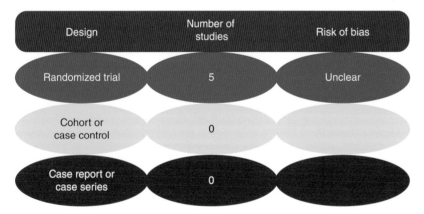

Design	Number of studies	Risk of bias
Randomized trial	5	Unclear
Cohort or case control	0	
Case report or case series	0	

Study Results

The comparison of self-etch primer and acid etch in relation to bracket failure and chairside time is shown in Table S2.1.

Table S2.1 Comparison of self-etching primer versus acid etch (A) bracket failure and (B) difference in time.

A, Assessment of bracket failure comparing self-etching primer versus acid etch

Authors	Acid etch		Self-etching primer		Weight %	Mean difference, Odds ratio, 95% CI	
	Events	n	Events	n		Favors self-etching primer	Favors acid-etching
Aljubouri *et al.* 2004	11	388	6	380	9.32	0.56 (0.20, 1.52)	
Cal-neto *et al.* 2009	13	272	19	276	17.90	1.44 (0.70, 2.97)	
Manning *et al.* 2006	13	298	21	299	18.66	1.61 (0.79, 3.27)	
Banks and Thirvenkatachari 2007	15	433	21	438	20.60	1.38 (0.70, 2.72)	
Murfitt *et al.* 2006	25	331	37	330	33.52	1.48 (0.87, 2.52)	
Total	77	1722	85	1723	100	1.35 (0.99, 1.83)	
Estimated predicted interval						(0.82, 2.22)	

Overall I^2 = 0%, *P* = 0.497

.2   1   3

B, Difference in time (seconds per tooth) required to bond with self-etching primer versus acid etch

	Mean difference	Standard error	Weight %	Mean difference, ES 95% CI	
Aljubouri *et al.* 2004	24.9	1.424	38.11	24.90 (22.11, 27.69)	
Banks and Thirvenkatachari 2007	22.2	0.542	61.89	22.20 (21.14, 23.26)	
Total			100	23.32 (20.66, 25.80)	

Overall I^2 = 0%, *P* = 0.497

30   20   10   0

Source: Fleming *et al.* 2012. Reproduced with permission of American Association of Orthodontists.

Key Findings

- There is weak but statistically insignificant evidence that the likelihood of attachment failures is higher with self-etch primers.
- Use of a one-step bonding technique may lead to a modest time saving compared with two-stage techniques. To free up 1 hour, eight bond-ups (each involving 20 teeth) would need to be undertaken in 1 day using the self-etch primer.

Commentary

Only one trial evaluating the whole course of treatment was identified. Given the absence of clear evidence to favor either system, the choice of bonding modality remains at the discretion of each operator. However, further research, ideally covering the course of treatment while accounting for the incidence of demineralization, would be welcome.

S3

Adhesives for bonded molar tubes during fixed brace treatment

Millett DT,* Mandall NA, Mattick RC, Hickman J, Glenny AM. Cochrane Database Syst Rev 2011;(6):CD008236.

Background

Molar teeth may either be banded or have a tube bonded as part of fixed appliance treatment. Failure of either attachment type impedes treatment progress and has cost implications for clinical time and materials, as well as patient inconvenience. Decalcification is a common risk of fixed appliance treatment and may occur in relation to either form of attachment. This review assessed the first-time failure rate and decalcification of types of adhesives used to attach bonded molar tubes during fixed appliance treatment.

Study Information

Population – patients with full arch fixed orthodontic appliances
Intervention – metal molar tubes bonded with any adhesive
Comparison – different types of adhesives for bonds, or metal molar tubes on bands cemented with any adhesive
Outcome – primary: first-time bond (or band) failure, presence or absence of decalcification associated with or around the tubes or bands. Secondary: adverse events (i.e., illness, allergy, bad taste, mucosal trauma), damage to teeth on attachment removal, length of treatment, treatment cost, and time to replace tubes with an adhesive.

Search Parameters

Inclusion criteria – randomized controlled trials (RCTs) comparing different adhesives for molar bonds, as well as comparing molar bonds to molar bands
Databases searched – the Cochrane Oral Health Group's Trials Register, CENTRAL (*The Cochrane Library*, 2010, Issue 3), MEDLINE via OVID, EMBASE
Dates searched – various start dates to 16 December 2010
Other sources of evidence – no additional hand searching of journals was undertaken. Proceedings and abstracts of: British Orthodontic Conferences, European Orthodontic Conferences and IADR Conferences
Language restrictions – none.

Search Results

Two parallel group RCTs were included.

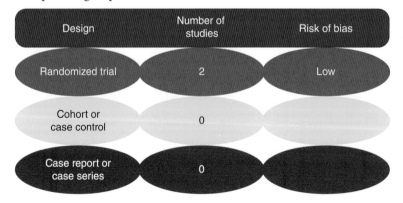

Study Results

The results for (A) failure at tooth level, (B) participant level, and (C) decalcification are shown in Table S3.1.

Table S3.1 Bonded molar tubes versus bands (A) failure at tooth level, (B) failure at participant level and (C) decalcification.

A, Failure at tooth level

Study	Log (Hazard ratio) (SE)	Weight %	Mean difference	Hazard ratio, Fixed, 95% CI
				Favors molar tubes — Favors molar bands
Banks and Macfarlane 2007	0.88 (0.275)	79.8	2.41 (1.41, 4.13)	
Nazir *et al*. 2011	1.82 (0.546)	20.2	6.17 (2.12, 18.00)	
Total		100	2.92 (1.80, 4.72)	

Heterogeneity: Chi^2 = 2.36, df = 1, P = 0.12, I^2 = 58%
Test for overall effect: z = 4.36, P = 0.000013

B, Failure at participant level

Study	Molar tubes n/N	Molar bands	Weight %	Risk ratio M–H, fixed, 95% CI	
				Favors molar tubes	Favors molar bands
Banks *et al*. 2007	34/55	19/55	82.6	1.79 (1.18, 2.72)	
Nazir *et al*. 2011	19/38	4/38	17.4	4.75 (1.78, 12.66)	
Total	93	93	100	2.30 (1.56, 3.41)	

Heterogeneity: Chi^2 = 2.70, df = 1, P = 0.10, I^2 = 63%
Test for overall effect: z = 6.10, P = 0.00001

C, Decalcification

Study					
Nazir *et al*. 2011	28/36	16/38	100	1.85 (1.22, 2.79)	
Total	36	38	100	1.85 (1.22, 2.79)	

Heterogeneity: N/A
Test for overall effect: z = 2.92, P = 0.0035

Abbreviations: M-H, Mantel-Haenszel; SE, standard error; n/N, number affected over total number.

Key Findings

Well-designed low risk of bias trials indicated:

- A greater first-time failure rate of molar tubes bonded with either a chemically-cured or light-cured adhesive compared to bands cemented with glass ionomer cement (GIC).
- Banded molars with GIC exhibited less decalcification than molars where tubes were bonded with a light-cured adhesive.
- Additional high-quality studies with different adhesives/molar tubes are required.

Commentary

Both of the included studies (Banks and Macfarlane 2007; Nazir *et al*. 2011) made comparisons of bonded tubes or cemented bands on first permanent molars only. Limited comparative data (one trial) exists on decalcification in relation to bonded tubes or cemented bands on first permanent molars (Nazir *et al*. 2011).

Additional references for Summary 3 can be found on page 205.

Acknowledgement

This Cochrane Review was published in the Cochrane Database of Systematic Reviews 2011, Issue 6. Cochrane Reviews are regularly updated as new evidence emerges and in response to feedback, and the Cochrane Database of Systematic Reviews should be consulted for the most recent version of the Cochrane Review.

S4

Adhesives for fixed orthodontic brackets

Mandall NA, Hickman J, Macfarlane TV, Mattick RCR, Millett DT,* Worthington HV.
Cochrane Database Syst Rev 2003;(2):CD002282.

Background

The reliability of an orthodontic adhesive for bonding is important, as replacing brackets during treatment delays progress, takes up clinical time, uses additional materials, and is inconvenient to the patient. Additionally decalcification around bonded brackets is a common risk of orthodontic treatment with a reported prevalence of 2–95%. This review assessed the reliability of orthodontic adhesives and if any adhesive was better at preventing decalcification during treatment.

Study Information

Population – patients receiving fixed appliances. Patients with cleft lip and/or palate or any other syndrome and those who received surgery (orthognathic or surgical exposure of impacted teeth) were excluded
Intervention – stainless steel brackets bonded to all teeth (except molars)
Comparison – adhesive groups, and then within groups according to polymerization mechanism (chemically or light-cured)
Outcome – primary: failure of the orthodontic adhesive; secondary: decalcification around the orthodontic bracket.

Search Parameters

Inclusion criteria – randomized clinical trials (RCTs) and controlled clinical trials (CCTs) that compared two or more different adhesives
Databases searched – Medline, Embase Electronic Registers, Cochrane Clinical Trials Register (CCTR), and Cochrane Oral Health Group Specialized Register
Dates searched – 1970 to 2000
Other sources of evidence – hand searching of European Journal of Orthodontics, American Journal of Orthodontics, Journal of Orthodontics and Angle Orthodontist for years not then included on Cochrane Oral Health Group Register. First authors of trials were contacted to identify any unpublished studies and seek clarification regarding published trials. Reference lists of identified studies were screened. Proceedings and abstracts of: British Orthodontic Conferences and European Orthodontic Conferences
Language restrictions – none.

Search Results

Three trials fulfilled the review criteria (two RCTs and one CCT).

Design	Number of studies	Risk of bias
Randomized trial	2	High
Controlled trial	1	High
Case report or case series	0	

Study Results

Failure of the orthodontic adhesive: Reported as number of teeth with debonded brackets and the percentage debond by all trials. Although the number of debonded brackets was reported for the same adhesive by two trials, brackets with different bases (mesh foil versus either Dynalok cut groove base or GAC Microloc) were compared.

Decalcification around the orthodontic bracket: Reported by one trial as a secondary outcome but for the other two trials it was either not an appropriate outcome or not reported.

Key Findings

It is difficult to draw any conclusions from this review due to the heterogeneity of the included trials. Suggestions are given for future research:

- RCT comparing all generic groups of adhesive with patients followed to the end of fixed appliance treatment.
- Sample size calculation (involving statistician regarding this and study design) with explicit inclusion and exclusion criteria.
- Withdrawals and dropouts described with appropriate modification of statistical analyses.
- Assessment of occlusal interferences possibly affecting bond failure.
- Single (patient) or double blind (patient and operator) studies if possible.
- All patients treated similarly except for intervention.
- Mean *and standard deviation* given for bond failures with appropriate statistical analyses.
- Decalcification measured as a secondary outcome as appropriate.

Commentary

Stronger evidence is required regarding which orthodontic adhesive is most reliable for bonding and most effective at preventing decalcification.

Additional Reference

Mandall NA, Millett DT, Mattick CR, Hickman J, Worthington HV, Macfarlane TV, 2002. Orthodontic adhesives: a systematic review. *J Orthod* 29, 205–210.

Acknowledgement

This Cochrane Review was published in the Cochrane Database of Systematic Reviews 2003, Issue 2. Cochrane Reviews are regularly updated as new evidence emerges and in response to feedback, and the Cochrane Database of Systematic Reviews should be consulted for the most recent version of the Cochrane Review.

S5

Determinants for success rates of temporary anchorage devices in orthodontics: a meta-analysis (n >50)

Dalessandri D,* Salgarello S, Dalessandri M, Lazzaroni E, Piancino M, Paganelli C, Maiorana C, Santoro F. Eur J Orthod 2014;36:303–313.

Background

Temporary anchorage devices (TADs) were recently introduced for better anchorage control. This review sought to analyze the influence of the various elements on the success rate of TADs.

Study Information

Population – orthodontic patients treated with fixed appliances
Intervention – temporary anchorage devices
Comparison – patient, implant, and management related factors
Outcome – TADs success rate.

Search Parameters

Inclusion criteria – clinical studies analyzing factors affecting TADs stability
Databases searched – PubMed, Scopus, and Web of Knowledge
Dates searched – up to December 2012
Other sources of evidence – hand searching of reference lists
Language restrictions – studies published in English, German, French, Spanish, and Italian.

Search Results

244 references were identified, 26 of which met the inclusion criteria.

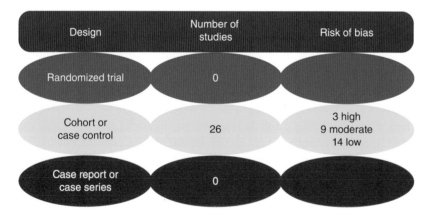

Design	Number of studies	Risk of bias
Randomized trial	0	
Cohort or case control	26	3 high 9 moderate 14 low
Case report or case series	0	

Study Results

The outcomes for TADs placed in (A) associated with healthy/inflamed gingiva and (B) placed in the maxilla/mandible are shown in Table S5.1.

Table S5.1 Temporary anchorage devices (TADs) failure rates (A) associated with healthy and inflamed tissues and (B) in maxilla or mandible.

A, Association of healthy and inflamed tissues with TADs failure rates

Authors	Maxilla Events	Total	Mandible Events	Total	Weight %	Odds ratio M-H, Random, 95% CI	Favors inflamed / Favors healthy
Chen *et al.* 2008	33	272	14	220	24.3	2.03 (1.06, 3.90)	
Cheng *et al.* 2004	5	7	10	133	16.2	30.75 (5.28, 179.08)	
Miyawaki *et al.* 2003	5	11	15	113	19.6	5.44 (1.48, 20.08)	
Sharma *et al.* 2011	9	18	8	121	20.7	14.13 (4.39, 45.49)	
Viwattanatipa *et al.* 2009	16	19	16	78	19.3	20.67 (5.36, 70.72)	
Total	68	327	63	665	100	8.92 (2.86, 27.82)	

Heterogeneity: Tau^2 = 1.27, Chi^2 = 18.87 df = 4 (*P* = 0.0008), I^2 = 79%
Test for overall effect: Z = 3.77 (*P* = 0.0002)

B, The influence of insertion site (maxilla or mandible) on TADs failure rates

Author	Maxilla Events	Total	Mandible Events	Total	Weight %	Odds ratio M-H, Random, 95% CI	Favors maxilla / Favors mandible
Chen *et al.* 2007	31	263	22	96	8.8	0.45 (0.25, 0.82)	
Chen *et al.* 2008	26	399	11	90	7.5	0.71 (0.35, 1.46)	
Cheng *et al.* 2004	7	105	8	35	4.4	0.24 (0.08, 0.72)	
Lim *et al.* 2009	40	286	22	92	9.1	0.52 (0.29, 0.93)	
Luzi *et al.* 2007	5	41	8	99	3.9	1.58 (0.48, 5.15)	
Manni *et al.* 2011	18	137	39	163	8.7	0.48 (0.26, 0.89)	
Miyawaki *et al.* 2003	10	63	10	61	5.3	0.96 (0.37, 2.51)	
Moon *et al.* 2008	46	279	32	201	10.4	1.04 (0.64, 1.71)	
Moon *et al.* 2010	67	345	60	270	11.9	0.84 (0.57, 1.25)	
Motoyoshi *et al.* 2009	13	115	11	94	6.1	0.96 (0.41, 2.26)	
Park *et al.* 2006	5	124	14	103	4.6	0.27 (0.09, 0.77)	
Sharma 2011	12	97	7	42	4.9	0.71 (0.26, 1.94)	
Viwattanatipa *et al.* 2009	32	97	0	0		-	
Wiechmann *et al.* 2007	12	90	19	43	6.1	0.19 (0.08, 0.46)	
Wu 2009	25	268	17	135	8.2	0.71 (0.37, 1.37)	
Total	359	2709	280	1524	100	0.61 (0.47, 0.80)	

Heterogeneity: Tau^2 = 0.12, Chi^2 = 25.46 df = 13 (*P* = 0.02), I^2 = 49%
Test for overall effect: Z = 3.56 (*P* = 0.0004)

Source: Dalessandri *et al.* 2014. Reproduced with permission of Oxford University Press.

Key Findings

- Good oral hygiene around the implant site is very important because it prevents soft tissue inflammation, which is associated with higher TAD failure rates.
- TADs were more successful when inserted in the alveolar bone of the maxilla compared with the alveolar bone of the mandible and when they are used in patients older than 20 years of age.

Commentary

The conclusions of this analysis must be interpreted cautiously because of the disparate nature of the studies reviewed and the heterogeneity of the data. Nevertheless, all the studies indicate rates of TAD success greater than 80%.

S6

The effectiveness of laceback ligatures during initial orthodontic alignment: a systematic review and meta-analysis

Fleming PS,* Johal A, Pandis N. Eur J Orthod 2013;35:539–546.

Background

Stainless steel lacebacks extending from the first molars to canines have been advocated to control the position of the incisors during the initial alignment phase by controlling the angulation of the canines. They are believed to be particularly useful where the canines are upright or distally angulated at the outset, as in these cases, significant mesial crown movement is likely to be accompanied by advancement of the incisors. While many clinicians routinely use lacebacks, their effectiveness has been disputed. Moreover, they may induce loss of posterior anchorage, lead to plaque stagnation, and additional chairside time and complexity.

Study Information

Population – orthodontic patients treated with fixed appliances
Intervention – laceback ligatures
Comparison – no laceback ligatures
Outcomes – molar and incisor position, periodontal effects and appliance breakages.

Search Parameters

Inclusion criteria – randomized controlled trials
Databases searched – MEDLINE, Embase, Cochrane
Dates searched – 1966 to January 2012
Other sources of evidence – gray literature and reference lists
Language restrictions – none.

Search Results

194 references were identified, 2 of which were suitable for meta-analysis.

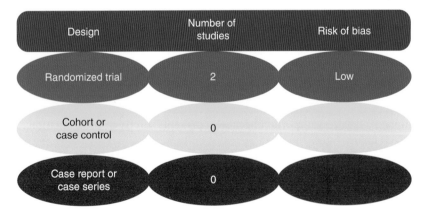

Design	Number of studies	Risk of bias
Randomized trial	2	Low
Cohort or case control	0	
Case report or case series	0	

Study Results

The effect of lacebacks on (A) incisor and (B) molar positions is shown in Table S6.1.

Table S6.1 The use of lacebacks and their effect on (A) incisor and (B) molar positions.

A, Change in the position of incisors with and without laceback

Authors	Lacebacks			No lacebacks			Weight	WMD, 95% CI	Favors laceback	Favors no laceback
	n	Mean	SD	n	Mean	SD				
Usmani *et al.* 2002	16	−0.5	1.06	19	0.36	1.09	53.34	−0.86 (−1.57, −0.15)		
Irvine *et al.* 2004	30	−0.53	1.9	32	−0.44	1.29	46.66	−0.09 (−0.90, 0.72)		
Total	46			51			100	−0.50 (−1.25, 0.25)		

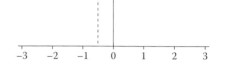

$I^2 = 48.5\%$, $P = 0.163$

B, Change in anteroposterior position of molars with and without laceback.

Authors	Lacebacks			No lacebacks			Weight	WMD, 95% CI	Favors laceback	Favors no laceback
	n	Mean	SD	n	Mean	SD				
Usmani *et al.* 2002	16	0.49	1.34	19	0.5	1.37	42.60	−0.01 (−0.91, 0.89)		
Irvine *et al.* 2004	30	0.75	1.08	32	−0.05	1.55	57.40	0.80 (0.14, 1.46)		
Total	46			51			100	0.45 (−0.33, 1.24)		

$I^2 = 50.5\%$, $P = 0.155$

Source: Fleming *et al.* 2013. Reproduced with permission of Oxford University Press.

> **Key Findings**
>
> - The use of lacebacks has neither a clinically nor a statistically significant effect on the anteroposterior molar or incisor position.
> - There is no evidence concerning the use of lacebacks on chairside time or periodontal health.

Commentary

Further high-quality randomized controlled trials on the impact of lacebacks during orthodontic alignment would be welcome. However, on the basis of limited evidence it appears that they may represent an unnecessary complexity in many cases.

S7

Mini-implants in orthodontics: a systematic review of the literature

Meursinge Reynders R,* Ronchi L, Bipat S. Am J Orthod Dentofacial Orthop 2009;135:564.e1–19.

Background

When considering the use of orthodontic mini-implants (OMIs) orthodontists need to know the success rates of these devices. This systematic review quantified these rates. The eligible studies of this review were also used to identify and quantify evidence on variables that influence these success rates, and on the adverse effects of using OMIs.

Study Information

Population – orthodontic patients of any age and sex treated with OMIs
Intervention – OMIs with diameters <2.5 mm and more than 120 days of orthodontic force application. Bone plates were excluded.
Comparison – various implant and patient parameters
Outcome – success rates of OMIs according to prespecified definitions of success.

Search Parameters

Inclusion criteria – randomized and nonrandomized clinical studies that (1) measure success rates of OMIs, (2) defined success, and (3) defined the duration of the application of orthodontic force to OMIs
Databases searched – PubMed (MEDLINE), Google Scholar Beta, Embase, Science Direct, all 7 Evidence Based Medicine Reviews (EBMR), Web of Science, Ovid, and Bandolier
Dates searched – through March 31 2008
Other sources of evidence – hand searching of journals and reference lists
Language restrictions – English, French, German, and Italian.

Search Results

3364 abstracts were identified. Of the 52 retrieved full-text articles only 19 met the inclusion criteria.

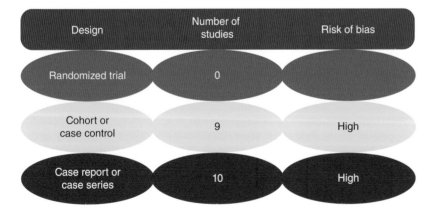

Design	Number of studies	Risk of bias
Randomized trial	0	
Cohort or case control	9	High
Case report or case series	10	High

Study Results

The success rates for mini-implants are shown in Table S7.1.

Table S7.1 Success rates of orthodontic mini-implants.

Authors	Time of success measurement	Success rate
Freudenthaler *et al.* 2001	ARTT. Average: 11 months (range: 7–20 months)	75% (NSS)
Miyawaki *et al.* 2003	1 year or ARTT	76.1% (NSS) (range: 0–85%)
Liou *et al.* 2004	9 months	56.25% (score 0) 43.75% (score 2)
Motoyoshi *et al.* 2006	6 months	85.5% (NSS)
Thiruvenkatachari *et al.* 2006	ARTT. 3.5–5.5 months	100% (score 0)
Park *et al.* 2006	ARTT. Mean (SD): 15 months (6.16 months)	91.6% (score 0 and 1) (range: 80–93.6%)
Tseng *et al.* 2006	ARTT. Average: 16 months	91.1% (score 0 and 1) (range: 80–100%)
Chen *et al.* 2006	ARTT. Mean 19.5 months	84.7% (score 0) (range: 72.2–90.2%)
Berens *et al.* 2005	ARTT. Average: 235 days Maximum: 733 days	Protocol 1: 68.4% (score 0) 8.3% (score 1) 23.3% (score 3) Protocol 2: 4.7% (score 3)
Luzi *et al.* 2007	ARTT. Minimum:120 days and maximum: 37 months	84.3% (score 0) 6.4% (score 1)
Wiechmann *et al.* 2007	180 days	76.7% (score 0) (range: 69.6–87%)
Kuroda *et al.* 2007	1 year or ARTT	86.4% (NSS) (range: 35.3–100%)
Motoyoshi *et al.* 2007	6 months	85.2% (score 0) (range: 63.8% to 97.3%)
Kurod *et al.* 2007	1 year or ARTT	86.2% (NSS) (range: 81.1–88.6%)
Motoyoshi *et al.* 2007	ARTT. 6 months or more	87.4 (score 0)
Hedayati *et al.* 2007	ARTT. Average: 5.4 months (range: 4–6.5 months)	81.5% (score 0, 1, and 2)
Chaddad *et al.* 2008	150 days	87.5% (score 0) (range: 82.5–93.5%)
Moon *et al.* 2008	8 months	83.8 (score 0)
Kinzinger *et al.* 1991	ARTT. 6.5 months	100% (score 2)

Abbreviation: ARTT, anchorage for required treatment time. Success score 0, success without mobility; score 1, success with mobility; score 2, success with displacement; NSS, not specified success (includes scores 0–2).
Source: Reynders *et al.* 2009. Reproduced with permission of American Association of Orthodontists.

Key Findings

- Most studies found success rates greater than 80% (range 0–100%) if usable, mobile, and displaced implants were considered successful (Table S7).
- 70 associations between specific variables such as patient, implant, location, surgery, orthodontics, and implant maintenance-related factors were identified, but were rejected because of confounding.
- Few articles reported on adverse effects of OMIs.

Commentary

- The validity of the outcomes of this study was hampered by: (1) the wide variation and poor definition of success of OMIs, (2) different time points for assessing success, (3) poor research methodology, and (4) poor reporting.
- Poor quality of primary research on OMIs is widespread as was identified in another systematic review on OMIs (Meursinge Reynders 2016).
- An update of this systematic review is indicated, which should also apply a new (2016) risk of bias tool for nonrandomized studies (ROBINS-I) (Sterne JA *et al.*, 2016).
- When using OMIs, clinicians should consider: (1) the low quality evidence in this systematic review, (2) similarities between their patients and those included in this review, (3) patient values and preferences, (4) alternative interventions, (5) whether the benefits of OMIs outweigh the adverse effects, (6) the cost of OMIs, and (7) the quality of this systematic review. This latter issue is particularly important because many systematic reviews are poorly conducted (Ioannidis 2016).

Additional references for Summary 7 can be found on page 205.

S8

Initial arch wires for tooth alignment during orthodontic treatment with fixed appliances

Jian F, Lai W, Furness S, McIntyre GT, Millett DT,* Hickman J, Wang Y.* Cochrane Database Syst Rev 2013;(4):CD007859.

Background

Initial arch wires are those first inserted in fixed appliance orthodontic treatment, primarily to align teeth. Several types are available. It is important to understand which wire is most efficient as well as which causes least root resorption and pain during initial tooth alignment.

Study Information

Population – participants with upper and/or lower full arch fixed orthodontic appliances. Excluded concurrent use of palatal expansion devices, extraoral appliances, previous orthodontic treatment, or relevant medical history

Intervention – first arch wires inserted at start of treatment

Comparison/ control group – another type of initial arch wire

Outcome – primary: alignment rate/ month; incidence/ prevalence and amount of root resorption. Secondary: time to next/working arch wire; time to alignment; intensity and duration of pain.

Search Parameters

Inclusion criteria – randomized controlled trials (RCTs) comparing initial arch wires

Databases searched – MEDLINE via OVID, Cochrane Oral Health Group's Trials Register, Cochrane Central Register of Controlled Trials (CENTRAL) (The Cochrane Library 2012, Issue 7), EMBASE via OVID

Dates searched – various start dates to Aug 2012

Other sources of evidence – conference proceedings and abstracts from British and European orthodontic conferences (to 2012) and International Association for Dental Research. Hand searched: *American Journal of Orthodontics and Dentofacial Orthopedics* to 2012, 153(1); the *Angle Orthodontist* to 2011, 81(6); *European Journal of Orthodontics* to 2011, 33(6); *Journal of Orthodontics* (and the predecessor, the *British Journal of Orthodontics*) to 2011, 38(4); *Seminars in Orthodontics* from 1995 to 2011, 17(4); *Clinical Orthodontics and Research* from 1998 to 2011, 14(4); *Australian Orthodontic Journal* from 1956 to 2011, 27(2). Checked reference lists of potential clinical trials to identify any additional studies. Contacted corresponding authors of included trials to identify unpublished or ongoing studies and to clarify trial details, if required. Contacted manufacturers to confirm arch wire type and knowledge of any unpublished and/or ongoing clinical trials

Language restrictions – none.

Search Results

Nine RCTs fulfilled the inclusion criteria.

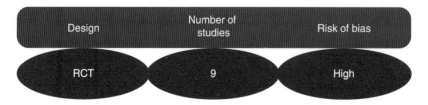

Design	Number of studies	Risk of bias
RCT	9	High

Study Results

- Multistrand stainless steel initial arch wires compared to superelastic nickel titanium (NiTi) initial arch wires: Insufficient evidence for rate of alignment and pain.
- Conventional (stabilized) NiTi compared to superelastic NiTi initial arch wires: Insufficient evidence for rate of alignment and pain.
- Single-strand superelastic NiTi compared to other NiTi (coaxial, copper NiTi [CuNiTi] or thermoelastic): Weak unreliable evidence that coaxial superelastic NiTi may produce greater tooth movement over 12 weeks, but no information on associated pain. Insufficient evidence to determine if there is a difference between either thermoelastic or CuNiTi and superelastic NiTi initial arch wires.

None of the trials reported on root resorption.

Key Findings

- No reliable evidence that a specific initial arch wire material is better or worse than another for speed of alignment or reduction of pain.
- No evidence regarding the effect of initial arch wire material on root resorption.

Commentary

Well-designed and conducted, adequately powered, RCTs are needed to assess if the laboratory performance of initial arch wire materials results in a clinically important difference in initial tooth alignment.

Acknowledgement

This Cochrane Review was published in the Cochrane Database of Systematic Reviews 2013, Issue 4. Cochrane Reviews are regularly updated as new evidence emerges and in response to feedback, and the Cochrane Database of Systematic Reviews should be consulted for the most recent version of the Cochrane Review.

S9

Initial orthodontic alignment effectiveness with self-ligating and conventional appliances: a network meta-analysis in practice

Pandis N,* Fleming PS, Spineli LM, Salanti G. Am J Orthod Dentofacial Orthop 2014; 145(4 Suppl.):S152–163.

Background

An extension of the traditional meta-analysis is network meta-analysis (NMA) allowing, under certain assumptions, the quantitative synthesis of all evidence under a unified framework and across a network of all eligible trials. This review aims to raise awareness of this type of synthesis and to compare and rank the effectiveness of conventional and self-ligating appliances in terms of initial alignment efficiency.

Study Information

Population – orthodontic patients treated with full fixed appliances
Intervention – self-ligating appliances
Comparison group – conventional appliances
Outcome – millimeters of crowding resolved during initial orthodontic alignment.

Search Parameters

Inclusion criteria – randomized and controlled clinical trials, including split-mouth, comparing any self-ligating and conventional appliances
Databases searched – PubMed, Embase, Cochrane, Trial and Thesis registries, conference proceedings
Dates searched – 1966 to December 2012
Other sources of evidence – hand searching of reference lists and contact of authors
Language restrictions – none.

Search Results

132 references were identified, 11 of which met the inclusion criteria.

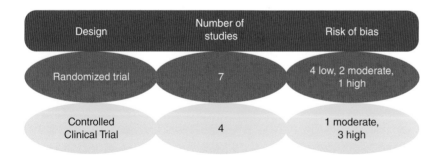

Design	Number of studies	Risk of bias
Randomized trial	7	4 low, 2 moderate, 1 high
Controlled Clinical Trial	4	1 moderate, 3 high

Figures from Publication

The bar plot of the SUCRA (surface under the cumulative ranking) values for the outcome "overall efficacy" indicates the ranking of the bracket systems in terms of efficiency (Figure S9.1). Larger values indicate greater efficiency.

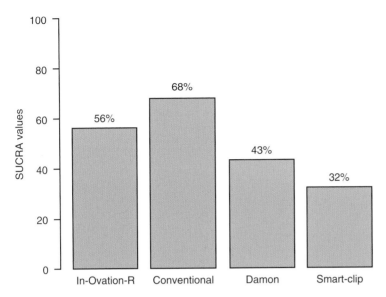

Figure S9.1 Bar plot of the SUCRA (surface under the cumulative ranking) values for the outcome "overall efficacy".
Source: Pandis *et al.* 2014. Reproduced with permission of Elsevier.

Key Finding

- There is no evidence that self-ligating appliances are more efficient than conventional appliances during initial alignment.

Commentary

NMA is a relatively new advancement with the potential for significant applications in orthodontics. NMA combines evidence from direct and indirect information via common comparators; interventions, therefore, can be ranked in terms of the analyzed outcome. The key values of NMA are:

1) to compare treatments, untested in primary studies, by using common comparators;
2) to strengthen the evidence base by combining direct and indirect effects, where applicable;
3) to rank the available interventions for the studied outcomes.

S10

Systematic review of self-ligating brackets

Chen S,* Greenlee G, Kim K, Smith C, Huang GJ.* Am J Orthod Dentofacial Orthop 2010;137: 726.e1–726.e18.

Background

Many claims have been made about the superiority of self-ligating brackets with respect to treatment efficiency, effectiveness, and stability. However, many of these claims are supported by limited evidence. This review sought to identify and summarize the existing evidence.

Study Information

Population – orthodontic patients treated with fixed appliances
Intervention – self-ligating brackets
Comparison – conventional brackets
Outcome – treatment efficiency, effectiveness, and stability.

Search Parameters

Inclusion criteria – clinical studies comparing self-ligating and conventional fixed appliances
Databases searched – PubMed, Web of Science, Embase, Cochrane
Dates searched – 1966 to May 2009
Other sources of evidence – hand searching of reference lists
Language restrictions – none.

Search Results

114 references were identified, 16 of which met the inclusion criteria.

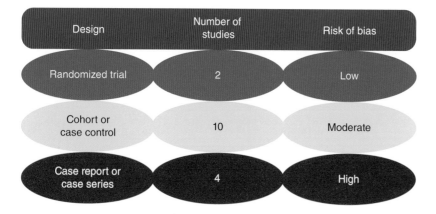

Design	Number of studies	Risk of bias
Randomized trial	2	Low
Cohort or case control	10	Moderate
Case report or case series	4	High

Study Results

The effects of self-ligating brackets on (A) total treatment time and (B) rate of movement are shown in Table S10.1.

Table S10.1 The effect of self-ligating brackets on (A) total treatment time and (B) rate of incisor alignment.

Authors	Self-ligating			Conventional				Standardized mean differences (A) random, (B) fixed 95% CI		
	Mean	SD	Total	Mean	SD	Total	Weight (%)		Favors self-ligating	Favors conventional
A, Total treatment time (months)										
Eberting *et al.* 2001	24.5	6.5	108	30.9	7.9	107	34.4	−0.88 (−1.16, −0.60)		
Hamilton *et al.* 2008	15.6	5.2	379	15.9	6.1	383	36.2	−0.05 (−0.19, 0.09)		
Harradine 2001	19.4	5.9	30	23.5	5.2	30	29.4	−0.73 (−1.25, −0.20)		
Total			517			520	100	−0.54 (−1.17, −0.09)		

Heterogeneity: Tau² = 0.28, Chi² = 30.13, df = 2 ($P < 0.00001$), I² = 93%
Test for overall effect: Z = 1.67 (p = 0.10)

B, Rate of incisor alignment (change of irregularity index at 20 weeks)										
Miles 2005	−4.3	2.7	29	−4.4	2.9	29	33.3	0.04 (−0.48, 0.55)		
Miles *et al.* 2006	−1.4	1.5	58	−1.5	1.8	58	66.7	0.06 (−0.30, 0.42)		
Total			87			87	100	0.05 (−0.25, 0.35)		

Heterogeneity: Chi² = 0.01, df = 1 ($P = 0.94$), I² = 0%
Test for overall effect: Z = 0.34 ($P = 0.73$)

Source: Chen *et al.* 2010. Reproduced with permission of Elsevier.

Key Findings

- Self-ligating brackets do appear to have an advantage in efficiency, when measured by chair time. However, time for alignment and total treatment time were not found to be significantly faster.
- Incisor proclination was found to be less with self-ligating brackets, but the difference was only 1.5 degrees.
- No studies could be found that addressed stability after treatment.

Commentary

Generally, there is a lack of evidence indicating any difference between effectiveness and overall efficiency of conventional and self-ligating brackets. Additional randomized controlled trials have been published since this systematic review appeared, and they indicate no significant differences in treatment efficiency or effectiveness (Celikoglu *et al.* 2015; da Costa Monini *et al.* 2014; Johansson and Lundström 2012; O'Dywer *et al.* 2016).

Additional References

Celikoglu M, Bayram M, Nur M, *et al.*, 2015. Mandibular changes during initial alignment with SmartClip self-ligating and conventional brackets: A single-center prospective randomized controlled clinical trial. *Korean J Orthod* 45, 89–94.

da Costa Monini A, Júnior LG, Martins RP, *et al.*, 2014. Canine retraction and anchorage loss: self-ligating versus conventional brackets in a randomized split-mouth study. *Angle Orthod* 84, 846–852.

Johansson K, Lundström F, 2012. Orthodontic treatment efficiency with self-ligating and conventional edgewise twin brackets: a prospective randomized clinical trial. *Angle Orthod* 82, 929–934.

O'Dywer L, Littlewood SJ, Rahman S, *et al.*, 2016. A multi-center randomized controlled trial to compare a self-ligating bracket with a conventional bracket in a UK population: Part 1: Treatment efficiency. *Angle Orthod* 86, 142–148.

S11

Impacted and transmigrant mandibular canines incidence, aetiology, and treatment: a systematic review

Dalessandri D,* Parrini S, Rubiano R, Gallone D, Migliorati M. Eur J Orthod 2017;39:161–169.

Background

The incidence of impacted and transmigrant canines in the mandible is not as high as that in the maxilla; consequently, it is more difficult to find clinical guidelines derived from sound studies based on large patient samples. The aim of this systematic review was to summarize currently available data pertaining to the incidence and etiology of impacted and transmigrant mandibular canines and the success rates of different treatment strategies.

Study Information

Population – patients with impacted and transmigrant mandibular canines
Intervention – orthodontic treatment or autotransplantation
Comparison – surgical removal or monitoring
Outcome – success and complications rates.

Search Parameters

Inclusion criteria – prospective and retrospective original studies on human subjects with impacted and transmigrant mandibular canines
Databases searched – PubMed, Medline, Google Scholar, Cochrane Central Register of Controlled Trials (issue 1, 2015), ISI Web of Knowledge, Scopus
Dates searched – various initial dates, all up to 2016
Other sources of evidence – authors' personal libraries and the references lists of all selected articles
Language restrictions – none.

Search Results

630 unique citations were identified. Application of the inclusion and exclusion criteria identified 13 relevant publications that were included in the qualitative analysis.

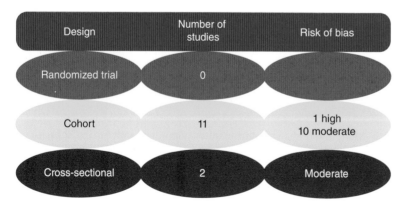

Design	Number of studies	Risk of bias
Randomized trial	0	
Cohort	11	1 high 10 moderate
Cross-sectional	2	Moderate

Study Results

The incidence of impacted and transmigrant mandibular canines and treatment outcomes are shown in Tables S11.1 and S11.2.

Table S11.1 The incidence of impacted and transmigrant mandibular canines.

Author	Study design	Population	Screened	Males Impacted Uni	Bi	Males Transmigrant Uni	Bi	Females Impacted Uni	Bi	Females Transmigrant Uni	Bi	Overall Impacted Uni	Bi	Overall Transmigrant Uni	Bi
Sajnani 2014	Observational	Southern Chinese										62	1		
Sajnani 2014	Observational	Southern Chinese										74			
Kamiloglu 2014	Observational	Cypriot										4	0		
Jain 2014	Cross-sectional	Indian		10	2			27	3			37	5		
Topkara 2012	Cross-sectional	Turkish		7	5			7				14	5		
Aras 2011	Cohort	Turkish	5100									19	4		
Kara 2011	Observational	Turkish		37				51				88			
Aktan 2010	Cohort	Turkish		3		5		6		12		9		17	
Celikoglu 2010	Observational	Turkish		3		1		6		4		9		5	
Gündüz	Cohort	Turkish				7				5				12	
González-Sánchez 2001	Observational	Spanish				8				6	1			14	1
Yavuz 2007	Cohort	Turkish		32	3			33	3			65	6		
Aydin 2004	Cohort	Turkish		9		6		11		2		20		8	

Abbreviations: Bi, bilateral; Uni, unilateral. *Source:* Dalessandri *et al.* 2017. Reproduced with permission of Oxford University Press.

Table S11.2 Treatment success and outcome of impacted and transmigrant mandibular canines.

Author	Study design	% Orthodontic traction and success Impacted	Transmigrant	% Autotransplantation and success Impacted	Transmigrant	% Surgical removal and complication Impacted	Transmigrant	% Monitored and complications Impacted	Transmigrant
Sajnani 2014	Observational					89.0			
Aras 2011	Cohort	6.6/17.4		4.3		9.0			
Kara 2011	Observational							2.2	
Aktan 2010	Cohort								
Celikoglu 2010	Observational	21.4/14.3	28.5			28.6			14.3
Gündüz	Cohort						25.0		75.0
González-Sánchez 2001	Observational					53.3		40.0	
Yavuz 2007	Cohort	32.0		1.4		58.0			
Aydin 2004	Cohort								

Abbreviations: Bi, bilateral; Uni, unilateral. *Source:* Dalessandri *et al.* 2017. Reproduced with permission of Oxford University Press.

Key Findings

- The incidence of mandibular canines impaction ranges between 0.92 and 5.1%, while that of transmigration ranges from 0.1 to 0.31%.
- Although the precise etiology remains unknown, odontomes (4–20%), cysts, and lateral incisor anomalies (5–17%) are more likely to play a role.
- The most common treatment strategies are surgical extraction and orthodontic traction for impacted mandibular canines, while surgical extraction and radiographic monitoring are most common for transmigrant mandibular canines.

Commentary

A radiological screening with a dentopantomograph is appropriate in late mixed dentition in the presence of teeth morphology anomalies, family history of teeth impaction or transmigration, presence of aggressive caries destruction, or poorly restored deciduous teeth with possible presence of inflammatory cysts. From a therapeutic point of view, the time of diagnosis plays a crucial role in treatment options and prognosis. During the mixed dentition phase the extraction of the deciduous canine and, if present, of the adjacent first deciduous molar could stimulate the impacted canine to spontaneously erupt.

S12

Effectiveness of early orthopaedic treatment with headgear: a systematic review and meta-analysis

Papageorgiou SN,* Kutschera E, Memmert S, Gölz L, Jäger A, Bourauel C, Eliades T. Eur J Orthod 2017;39:176–187.

Background

Although headgear has been used extensively to correct anteroposterior discrepancies, its treatment effects have not yet been adequately assessed in an evidence-based manner. The aim of this systematic review was to assess the therapeutic and adverse effects of early headgear treatment in an evidence-based approach.

Study Information

Population – patients of any age or sex with Class II malocclusion
Intervention – early treatment with headgear
Comparison – untreated matched Class II patients
Outcome – lateral cephalometric measurements, treatment effectiveness, adverse events like dental trauma or temporomandibular joint (TMJ) pain.

Search Parameters

Inclusion criteria – randomized clinical trials and prospective controlled non-randomized studies
Databases searched – MEDLINE, Cochrane Library, Scopus, Web of Knowledge, and Virtual Health Library
Dates searched – from inception to December 2015
Other sources of evidence – hand searching of reference/citation lists and author communications
Language restrictions – none.

Search Results

830 references were identified; 15 unique studies from 44 papers met the inclusion criteria.

Design	Number of studies	Risk of bias
Randomized trial	5	High
Cohort or case control	10	High
Case report or case series	0	

Study Results

The outcome measures for use of headgear versus controls for (A) phase 1 and (B) phase 2 treatments are shown in Table S12.1.

Table S12.1 Outcome measures for use of headgear versus controls for (A) phase 1 and (B) phase 2 treatments.

A, Directly after early treatment with headgear (phase 1)

Outcome measure	Number of patients and (studies)	Summaries	Absolute effect (increase/decrease, +/−)		Relative effects (95% CI)	Quality of evidence (GRADE)
			Control	Headgear		
SNA angle (dg)	607 (12)	Probably decreases the SNA angle	+0.33°/yr	−1.30°/yr	MD −1.63 (−2.20 to −1.06)	⬤◯◯◯ Very low
SN-NL angle (dg)	667 (12)	Probably increases the SN-NL angle	+0.16°/yr	+0.60°/yr	SMD 0.54 (0.09 to 1.00)	⬤◯◯◯ Very low
N perpendicular - A distance (mm)	427 (8)	Probably decreases the N perp-A distance	+2.11 mm/yr	−0.71 mm/yr	SMD −0.61 (−0.95 to −0.26)	⬤◯◯◯ Very low
Nasolabial angle (dg)	287 (4)	There may be little or no difference in the nasolabial angle	+1.38°/yr	+1.95°/yr	MD 0.57 (−0.58 to 1.72)	⬤◯◯◯ Very low

B, After phase 1 and subsequent fixed appliance treatment (phase 2)

Outcome measure	Number of patients and (studies)	Summaries	Control	Headgear	Relative effects (95% CI)	Quality of evidence (GRADE)
PAR reduction (phase 2)	240 (1)	There may be little or no difference in PAR reduction	19.6 points	20.2 points	MD −0.69 (−2.83 to 1.46)	⬤⬤⬤◯ Moderate
Incidence of dental trauma (overall)	140 (1)	May decrease the incidence of dental trauma	33.3%	22.6% (13.0 to 39.0)	RR 0.68 (0.39 to 1.17)	⬤⬤◯◯ Low
Incidence of new TMJ pain (phase 1)	83 (1)	May decrease the incidence of TMJ pain	28.9%	15.6% (6.6 to 36.1)	RR 0.54 (0.23 to 1.25)	⬤⬤◯◯ Low
Incidence of TMJ pain in patients with existing pain (phase 1)	48 (1)	May eliminate existing TMJ pain	54.5%	46.3% (26.2 to 81.2)	RR 0.85 (0.48 to 1.49)	⬤⬤◯◯ Low

CI, confidence interval; dg, degree; GRADE, Grading of Recommendations Assessment, Development and Evaluation; MD, mean difference; PAR, peer assessment rating; RR, relative risk; SMD, standardized mean difference.
Source: Adapted from Papageorgiou *et al.* 2017.

Key Findings

- Early headgear treatment is associated with a short-term reduction of the SNA angle, which is independent of confounding effects on the subspinale point and is proportional to the degree of the initial discrepancy in the SNA angle.
- Therefore, headgear might be a viable and effective option for the early management of Class II malocclusion with maxillary prognathism.
- Early treatment with headgear might decrease the risk of dental trauma during the subsequent years, which would be favorable for high-risk patients.

Commentary

The effect of headgear on maxillary rotation, nasolabial angle, reduction in PAR scores, and signs of temporomandibular disorders could not be robustly assessed due to limited evidence of low quality.

S13

Early orthodontic treatment for Class II malocclusion reduces the chance of incisal trauma: results of a Cochrane systematic review

Thiruvenkatachari B,* Harrison J, Worthington H, O'Brien K. Am J Orthod Dentofacial Orthop 2015;148:47–59.

Background

This form of malocclusion affects nearly a quarter of 12 year olds in the United Kingdom and 15% of 12 to 15 year olds in the United States. Prominent front teeth can lead to higher incidence of incisal trauma.

Study Information

Population – children or adolescents (≤16 years) or both receiving orthodontic treatment to correct Class II malocclusion
Intervention – early treatment (7–11 years) in two phases
Comparison – late/ adolescent treatment (10–14 years) in one phase
Outcome – overjet, skeletal relationship, self-esteem, patient satisfaction, any injury to the upper front teeth, jaw joint problems.

Search Parameters

Inclusion criteria – randomized controlled trials (RCTs) comparing early versus late treatment for Class II malocclusion
Databases searched – Medline Ovid, Embase Ovid, Cochrane Oral Health Trials Register, Cochrane Central Register Of Controlled Trials, Clinical Trials.gov, WHO International Clinical Trials Registry
Dates searched – 1946 to April 17 2013
Other sources of evidence – hand searching of all orthodontic journals including personal reference lists
Language restrictions – none.

Search Results

1572 references were identified, three of which met the inclusion criteria.

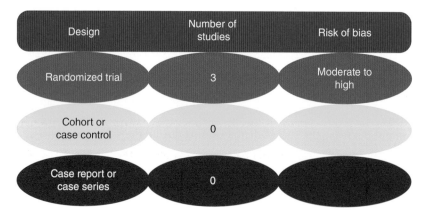

Design	Number of studies	Risk of bias
Randomized trial	3	Moderate to high
Cohort or case control	0	
Case report or case series	0	

Study Results

The incidence of incisal trauma in patients for (A) early treatment/ adolescence and (B) headgear/ functional appliance is shown in Table S13.1.

Table S13.1 The incidence of trauma (A) early treatment and adolescence only and (B) headgear or functional appliance.

A, Incidence of incisor trauma in patients receiving early treatment with a functional appliance compared with phase 1 treatment during adolescence only

Study	Functional		Adolescent treatment		Weight	Mean difference Odds ratio M-H, Fixed, 95% CI	
	Events	Total	Events	Total			
Florida, 1998	19	67	23	69	42.0	0.79 (0.38, 1.64)	
North Carolina, 2004	11	42	24	51	41.4	0.40 (0.17, 0.96)	
UK (mixed), 2009	4	63	7	65	16.7	0.56 (0.16, 2.02)	
Total	34	172	54	185	100	0.59 (0.35, 0.99)	

Favors functional   Favors adolescent

0.001 0.1 1 10 100

Heterogeneity: Chi^2 = 1.38 df = 2 (*P* = 0.50), I^2 = 0% Test for overall effect: Z = 2.02 (*P* = 0.04)

B, Effect of early treatment with either a functional appliance or headgear and the incidence of incisal trauma

Study	Headgear		Functional		Weight	Mean difference Odds ratio M-H, Fixed, 95% CI	
	Events	Total	Events	Total			
Florida, 1998	16	71	19	67	63.4	0.73 (0.34, 1.59)	
North Carolina, 2004	11	46	11	42	36.6	0.89 (0.34, 2.33)	
Total	27	117	30	109	100	0.79 (0.43, 1.44)	

Favors headgear   Favors functional

0.1 0.2 0.5 1 2 5 10

Heterogeneity: Chi^2 = 0.09 df = 1 (*P* = 0.77), I^2 = 0% Test for overall effect: Z = 0.77 (*P* = 0.44)

Abbreviation: M-H, Mantel-Haenszel.
Source: Thiruvenkatachari *et al.* 2015. Reproduced with permission of Elsevier.

Key Findings

- Two of the three studies showed high risk of bias. Orthodontic treatment for young children, followed by a later phase of treatment when the child is in early adolescence, appears to reduce the incidence of new incisal trauma significantly compared with treatment in one phase when the child is in early adolescence.
- However, the numbers needed to treat (NNT) showed we needed to treat 10 patients early (II phase) to prevent one episode of trauma (confidence interval [CI] 5–175).
- Due to the high degree of uncertainty (wide CI) in NNT, the data should be interpreted with caution.

Commentary

Several RCTs on Class II malocclusion have been published since this review but none of them have looked at early treatment benefits or incisal trauma.

Additional Reference

Thiruvenkatachari B, Harrison JE, Worthington HV, *et al.*, 2013. Orthodontic treatment for prominent upper front teeth (Class II malocclusion) in children. *Cochrane Database Syst Rev* (11), CD003452.

S14

Efficacy of molar distalization associated with second and third molar eruption stage

Flores Mir C,* McGrath L, Heo G, Major PW. Angle Orthod 2013;83:735–742.

Background

Among treatment alternatives to address Class II malocclusions, maxillary molar distalization is a commonly used one. This systematic review aimed to assess the efficacy of molar distalization based on second and third molar eruption stage.

Study Information

Population – orthodontic patients that require upper molar distalization
Intervention – second molar fully erupted
Comparison – partially erupted or no second molar erupted at all or partially erupted or no third molar erupted at all
Outcome – magnitude and direction of dental movement.

Search Parameters

Inclusion criteria – articles were upper molar distalization was assessed through cephalometry in patients with Class II malocclusion
Databases searched – Medline, PubMed, Embase, EMB reviews, PubMed, and Web of Science
Dates searched – various initial dates, all up to April 2012
Other sources of evidence – reference lists of included studies
Language restrictions – none.

Search Results

A total of 588 unique citations were identified. Four publications remained after inclusion criteria applied. Due to differences in their methodologies to assess molar distalization, a meta-analysis was not possible.

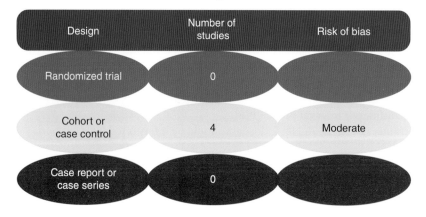

Design	Number of studies	Risk of bias
Randomized trial	0	
Cohort or case control	4	Moderate
Case report or case series	0	

Study Results

The molar distalization and distal crown tip for four studies are outlined in Table S14.1.

Table S14.1 Molar movement (distalization and distal crown tip) at various stages of second and third molar eruption.

Study	Group classifications based on molar eruption	Sample size	Mean duration (weeks)	Age	Appliance used	Movement to reference	Mean linear distalization -mm (SD)	P value	Mean crown tip degrees (SD)	P value
Kinzinger et al. 2004	**Group 1** = 2nd molars incompletely erupted or unerupted	18	12.8	12	Pendulum K	Pterygoid vertical	1st molar = 3.16 (0.77)	NS	1st molar = 5.36 (3.49) 2nd molar = 4.06 (2.15)	P < 0.01 P < 0.05
	Group 2 = 2nd molars erupted to level of occlusal plane and 3rd molars at budding stage	15	17.6			Pterygoid vertical	1st molar = 3.21 (1.01) 2nd molar = 2.26 (0.84)	NS	1st molar = 0.80 (3.40)	P < 0.01 P < 0.05
	Group 3 = 2nd molars erupted and germectomy of 3rd molars	13	24			Pterygoid vertical	1st molar = 2.70 (1.55) 2nd molar = 2.27 (0.75)	NS	2nd molar = 7.92 (5.83) 1st molar = 0.67 (2.08) 2nd molar = 2.00 (1.73)	NS NS
Karlsson and Bondemark 2006	**Group 1** = 2nd molars not erupted (2nd and 3rd molars were present in alveolar bone)	20	22	11.4	NiTi coil with Nance	Sella to occlusal plane	1st molar = 3 (0.64)	P ≤ .001	1st molar = 3	NS
	Group 2 = 2nd molars erupted and distalized simultaneously with 1st molars (3rd molars were present, but unerupted, in the left and right side of all patients)	20	26			Sella to occlusal plane	1st molar and 2nd molar = 2.2 (0.84)	P ≤ .001	1st molar and 2nd molar = 3	NS
Bussick and McNamara 2000		57	28	12.1	Pendulum K		1st molar and 2nd molar = 5.7 (1.6)	NS	1st molar = 11.7 (5.6)	NS
		44	28			Registration on repeated points	1st molar and 2nd molar = 5.6 (2.0)	NS		NS
Gosh and Nanda 1996	**Group 1** = 2nd molars unerupted	18	24.8	12	Pendulum K	(ant. and post. cranial base, maxilla and mandible)	1st molar = 3.37 (2.1) 2nd molar = 2.27 3rd molar = not reported	NS	1st molar = 9.8 (5.6)	NS
	Group 2 = 2nd molars erupted	23				Pterygoid vertical			1st molar = 8.36 (8.37) 2nd molar = 11.99 3rd molar = 2.49	
	Group 1 = erupted 2nd molars									
	Group 2 = unerupted 2nd molars									

Source: Adapted from Flores-Mir *et al.* 2013.

Key Findings

- The effect of the stage of second and third molar eruption appears to have minimal clinical effect on molar distalization and molar rotation.
- No meta-analysis was undertaken as the methodologies were not comparable.

Commentary

1) There is inconsistency in the outcome assessments and therefore the findings should be considered cautiously in respect to clinical practice.
2) The effect of including more dental units to be distalized among the anterior anchorage unit was not investigated.
3) Three of the studies used a pendulum appliance and one nickel-titanium (NiTi) coil springs in similar age groups. Other forms of distalization were not assessed.
4) The detail of the magnitude of the initial molar Class II was not clearly stated in the included studies.

S15

Orthodontic treatment for prominent upper front teeth (Class II malocclusion) in children

Thiruvenkatachari B,* Harrison JE, Worthington HV, O'Brien KD. Cochrane Database Syst Rev 2013;(11):CD003452.

Background

If a child with prominent upper front teeth (Class II) is referred at a young age, the orthodontist is faced with the dilemma of whether to treat the patient early or to wait until the child is older and provide treatment in early adolescence.

Study Information

Population – children or adolescents (≤16 years) or both receiving orthodontic treatment to correct Class II malocclusion

Intervention – (i) early treatment (7–11 years) in two phases or (ii) late treatment with an orthodontic appliance

Comparison – (i) late/ adolescent treatment (10–14 years) in one phase or (ii) late treatment with another type of orthodontic appliance or untreated control

Outcome – overjet (primary outcome), skeletal relationship, self-esteem, patient satisfaction, any injury to the upper front teeth, jaw joint problems.

Search Parameters

Inclusion criteria – randomized controlled trials (RCTs) on Class II malocclusion treatment

Databases searched – Medline Ovid, Embase Ovid, Cochrane Oral Health Trials Register, Cochrane Central Register of Controlled Trials

Dates searched – 1946 to April 17, 2013

Other sources of evidence – hand searching of all orthodontic journals including personal reference lists

Language restrictions – none.

Search Results

1572 studies were identified, of which 17 RCTs were included. Three RCTs compared early versus late treatment and 14 RCTs compared a type of appliance with untreated control or another type of appliance in adolescence.

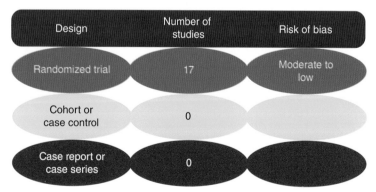

Design	Number of studies	Risk of bias
Randomized trial	17	Moderate to low
Cohort or case control	0	
Case report or case series	0	

Study Results

The outcomes for OJ, ANB, PAR score and self-concept are shown in Table S15.1.

Table S15.1 Outcomes for orthodontic treatment of prominent teeth (A) two-phase (early) and (B) one-phase (adolescent) in terms of OJ, ANB, PAR score and self-concept.

Study	A, 2-phase (early)		B, 1-phase (delayed treatment)			Mean difference, Fixed, 95% CI	
	n	Mean (SD)	n	Mean (SD)	Weight	Favors 2-phase (early)	Favors 1-phase (delayed)
1, Final overjet (mm) 3 studies Florida 1988; North Carolina 2004; and UK (mixed) 2009							
Subtotal	162	3.54 (1.77)	181	3.31 (1.44)	100	0.21 (−0.10, 0.51)	
Heterogeneity: $Chi^2 = 5.23$ df = 2 ($P = 0.07$), $I^2 = 62\%$ Test for overall effect: Z = 1.34 ($P = 0.18$)							
2, Final ANB (degrees) 3 studies Florida, 1988; North Carolina, 2004 and UK (mixed), 2009							
Subtotal	166		181		100	−0.02 (−0.47, 0.43)	
Heterogeneity: $Chi^2 = 2.62$ df = 2 ($P = 0.27$), $I^2 = 24\%$ Test for overall effect: Z = 0.10 ($P = 0.92$)							
3, PAR score 3 studies Florida, 1988; North Carolina, 2004 and UK (mixed), 2009							
Subtotal	169	8.27 (7.71)	191	7.25 (6.24)	100	0.62 (−0.66, 1.91)	
Heterogeneity: $Chi^2 = 6.43$ df = 2 ($P = 0.04$), $I^2 = 69\%$ Test for overall effect: Z = 0.95 ($P = 0.34$)							
4, Self concept 1 study UK (mixed), 2009							
Subtotal	62	−68.87 (8.32)	70	−68.04 (10.09)	100	−0.83 (−3.97, 2.31)	
Test for overall effect: Z = 0.52 ($P = 0.60$) Test for subgroup differences: $Chi^2 = 1.59$ df = 3 ($P = 0.66$), $I^2 = 0.0\%$							

Source: Thiruvenkatachari *et al.* 2013. Reproduced with permission of John Wiley & Sons.

Key Findings

- There were no differences in treatment outcome between the groups of children who had received treatment at a younger age or treatment as usual for all variables except for the incidence of new incisal trauma.
- When functional appliance treatment is provided in early adolescence, it appears that there are minor beneficial changes in skeletal pattern. However, these are probably not clinically significant.

Commentary

Consideration needs to be given to forming a consensus on the type of measures that are used in orthodontic trials; this is particularly relevant for cephalometric measurement and analysis.

Additional Reference

Thiruvenkatachari B, Harrison J, Worthington H, *et al.*, 2015. Early orthodontic treatment for class II malocclusion reduces the chance of incisal trauma: results of a Cochrane systematic review. *Am J Orthod Dentofacial Orthop* 148, 47–59.

Acknowledgement

This Cochrane Review was published in the Cochrane Database of Systematic Reviews 2013, Issue 11. Cochrane Reviews are regularly updated as new evidence emerges and in response to feedback, and the Cochrane Database of Systematic Reviews should be consulted for the most recent version of the Cochrane Review.

S16

Efficacy of orthopedic treatment with protraction facemask on skeletal Class III malocclusion: a systematic review and meta-analysis

Cordasco G, Matarese G, Rustico L, Fastuca S, Caprioglio A, Lindauer SJ, Nucera R. Orthod Craniofac Res 2014;17:133–143.*

Background

This meta-analysis aimed to evaluate the best literature evidence in order to assess the short-term skeletal effects of protraction facemask treatment on growing Class III patients. The results of the study can help clinicians to evaluate what Class III patients can be successfully treated with protraction facemask.

Study Information

Population – patients with skeletal Class III malocclusion
Intervention – orthopedic protraction facemask treatment
Comparison – untreated patients with skeletal Class III
Outcome – the following cephalometric angles: ANB, SNA, SNB, SN-mandibular plane and SN-palatal plane were evaluated (only ANB shown in Table 16.1).

Search Parameters

Inclusion criteria – randomized controlled trials (RCTs), growing patients, no additional therapeutic intervention
Databases searched – PubMed, Ovid, Embase, Cochrane Central Register of Controlled Trials, Web of Science, LILACS, Google Scholar
Dates Searched – all electronic searches were performed on November 22, 2012
Other sources of evidence – references of previously published systematic review performed on the same topic were hand searched
Language restrictions – none.

Search Results

807 unique citations were identified; seven trials remained after preliminary evaluation of title and abstract, three trials were considered after evaluation of full text. These three RCTs were used to perform qualitative trial evaluation and quantitative results synthesis (Kilicoglu and Kirlic 1998; Mandall *et al.* 2010; Vaughn *et al.* 2005).

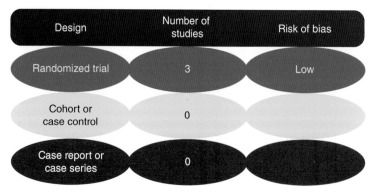

Study Results

The ANB changes with (A) facemask standalone and (B) facemask and RME protocols are shown in Table S16.1.

Table S16.1 The effect of the facemask on the ANB angle (degrees) (A) facemask alone and (B) facemask and rapid maxillary expansion (RME).

Authors	Intervention			Controls			Weight %	Mean difference, Random, 95% CI	
	Mean	SD	Total	Mean	SD	Total		Favors Control	Favors facemask/RME
A, Facemask standalone protocol									
Kiliçoglu and Kirliç 1998	4.34	1.81	16	−0.28	1.58	10	27.3	4.62 (3.30, 5.94)	
Vaughn *et al.* 2005	3.95	2.93	21	−0.05	2.09	8	18.8	4.00 (2.08, 5.92)	
Subtotal			37			18	46.1	4.42 (3.33, 5.51)	
Heterogeneity: Tau^2 = 0.00, Chi^2 = 0.27, df = 1 (P < 0.60), I^2 = 0%									
Test for overall effect: Z = 7.97 (P < 0.00001)									
B, Facemask and RME protocol									
Mandall *et al.*	2.1	2.3	33	−0.5	1.5	36	34.5	2.60 (1.67, 3.53)	
Vaughn *et al.* 2005	3.82	2.81	22	−0.05	2.22	9	19.4	3.87 (2.00, 5.74)	
Subtotal			55			45	53.9	2.97 (1.84, 4.09)	
Heterogeneity: Tau^2 = 0.24, Chi^2 = 1.43, df = 1 (P < 0.23), I^2 = 30%									
Test for overall effect: Z = 5.16 (P < 0.00001)									
Total			92			63	100	3.66 (2.58, 4.74)	
Heterogeneity: Tau^2 = 0.65, Chi^2 = 6.76, df = 1 (P = 0.08), I^2 = 56%									
Test for overall effect: Z = 6.66 (P < 0.00001)									
Test for subgroup differences: Chi^2 = 3.31, df = 1 (P < 0.07), I^2 = 69.8%									

Source: Cordasco et al. 2014. Reproduced with permission of John Wiley & Sons.

Key Findings

Evidence suggests that facemask treatment in growing Class III patients causes, in the short term, the following significant annual changes:

- correction of skeletal discrepancy (ANB, +3.66°);
- A point anterior projection increase (SNA, +2.1°);
- B point anterior projection reduction (SNB, −1,54°);
- mandibular plane clockwise rotation (SN-mandibular plane; +1.51°);
- slight anterior rotation of maxillary plane (SN-maxillary plane, −0.82°).

Commentary

1) Protraction facemask seems able to correct Class III malocclusion by stimulating maxillary growth and promoting a clockwise rotation of the mandibular plane.
2) The modifications lead to a tendency for bite opening.
3) The perfect candidate for facemask treatment would be a mild Class III growing patient with deep bite and low mandibular plane angle.
4) The subgroup analysis seems to show that preliminary rapid palatal expansion does not improve the effectiveness of facemask.
5) No recent evidence is available from RCTs to supplement these findings.

Additional References

Kilicoglu H, Kirlic Y, 1998. Profile changes in patients with Class III malocclusions after Delaire mask therapy. *Am J Orthod Dentofacial Orthop* 113, 453–462.

Mandall N, DiBiase A, Littlewood S, *et al.* 2010. Is early Class III protraction facemask treatment effective? A multicentre, randomized, controlled trial: 15-month follow-up. *J Orthod* 37, 149–161.

Vaughn GA, Mason B, Moon HB, *et al.* 2005. The effects of maxillary protraction therapy with or without rapid palatal expansion: a prospec- tive, randomized clinical trial. *Am J Orthod Dentofacial Orthop* 128, 299–309.

Class III

S17

Orthodontic treatment for prominent lower front teeth (Class III malocclusion) in children

Watkinson S, Harrison JE,* Furness S, Worthington HV. Cochrane Database Syst Rev 2013;(9):CD003451.

Background

Class III malocclusion may be due to a combination of skeletal or dental positions or both. Various treatment approaches have been described to correct Class III malocclusions in children and adolescents. There is, however, little consensus as to which of these approaches may be best. Also, little is known about the long-term effects of these approaches and their impact on the need for surgical treatment when the patient is older.

Study Information

Population – children and adolescents with a Class III malocclusion

Intervention – any orthodontic appliance (removable, fixed, functional, intraoral or extraoral) aimed at correcting a Class III malocclusion

Comparison group – no, delayed, or any another active intervention

Outcomes – overjet, ANB, psychosocial, patient satisfaction, TMD.

Search Parameters

Inclusion criteria – randomized controlled trials (RCTs) of orthodontic treatments to correct Class III malocclusions in children and adolescents

Databases searched – CENTRAL, MEDLINE, and EMBASE

Dates searched – 1966 to January 2013 as appropriate

Other sources of evidence – hand searching of reference lists

Language restrictions – none.

Search Results

440 references were identified. Eight papers, relating to seven RCTs, met the inclusion criteria.

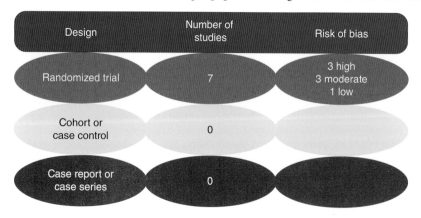

Design	Number of studies	Risk of bias
Randomized trial	7	3 high 3 moderate 1 low
Cohort or case control	0	
Case report or case series	0	

Study Results

The comparisons between facemask and controls at (A) 1 year follow-up and (B) 2–3 year follow-up are shown in Table S17.1.

Table S17.1 Comparison of ANB for facemask and untreated controls (A) 1 year follow-up and (B) 2–3 year follow-up.

A, 1 year follow-up

Study	Control N	Control Mean (SD)	Facemask n	Facemask Mean (SD)	Weight	Mean difference fixed, 95% CI
Vaughn 2005	17	−0.05 (1.98)	29	3.88 (1.83)	16.4	3.93 (2.78, 5.08)
Mandall 2010	36	−0.5 (1.5)	33	2.1 (2.3)	25.3	2.60 (1.67, 3.53)
Xu 2001	20	−1.5 (0.89)	20	3 (1.07)	58.3	4.50 (3.89, 5.11)
Subtotal	73		82		100	3.93 (3.46, 4.39)

Heterogeneity: $Chi^2 = 11.29$ df = 2 ($P = 0.004$), $I^2 = 82\%$
Test for overall effect: Z = 16.52 ($P < 0.00001$)

B, 2–3 year follow-up

Study	Control N	Control Mean (SD)	Facemask n	Facemask Mean (SD)	Weight	Mean difference fixed, 95% CI
Mandall 2010	33	0.1 (1.9)	30	1.5 (2)	100	1.40 (0.43, 2.37)
Subtotal	33		30		100	1.40 (0.43, 2.37)

Test for overall effect: Z = 2.84 ($P = 0.0045$)
Test for subgroup differences: $Chi^2 = 21.31$ df = 1 ($P = 0.00$), $I^2 = 95\%$

Source: Adapted from Watkinson 2013.

Key Findings

- There is some evidence that the use of a facemask to correct Class III malocclusion in children is effective when compared to no treatment on a short-term basis.
- However, in view of the general poor quality of the included studies, these results should be viewed with caution. Further RCTs, with long follow-up, are required.

Commentary

Although this review found some evidence that the use of a facemask appliance can help to correct Class III malocclusions in children on a short-term basis, there was no evidence available to show whether or not these changes were maintained until the child is fully grown.

Additional References

Since 2013, four new RCTs and a 6-year follow-up have been published (Mandall *et al.* 2016). The new RCTs are unlikely to change the original conclusions but the 6-year follow-up will provide valuable data on the long-term implications of facemask treatment.
Mandall N, Cousley R, DiBiase A, *et al.*, 2016. Early class III protraction facemask treatment reduces the need for orthognathic surgery: a multi-centre, two-arm parallel randomized, controlled trial. *J Orthod* 43,164–175.

Acknowledgement

This Cochrane Review was published in the Cochrane Database of Systematic Reviews 2013, Issue 9. Cochrane Reviews are regularly updated as new evidence emerges and in response to feedback, and the Cochrane Database of Systematic Reviews should be consulted for the most recent version of the Cochrane Review.

S18

Effectiveness of pre-surgical infant orthopedic treatment for cleft lip and palate patients: a systematic review and meta-analysis

Papadopoulos M,* Koumpridou E,* Vakalis M, Papageorgiou SN. Orthod Craniofac Res 2012;15:207–236.

Background

The effectiveness of presurgical infant orthopedic (PSIO) treatment for cleft lip and palate (CLP) patients remains controversial. This meta-analysis sought to assess the existing literature and provide the best evidence available on PSIO treatment outcomes in the short and long term.

Study Information

Population – complete CLP patients younger than 1 year old at treatment start
Intervention – PSIO appliances
Comparison - complete CLP infants with no PSIO treatment
Outcome – general developmental, craniofacial, and dentoalveolar treatment outcomes.

Search Parameters

Inclusion criteria – randomized or prospective controlled clinical trials (RCTs and pCCTs, respectively)
Databases searched – PubMed, Embase, Cochrane, Web of Science, Scopus, Lilacs, Ovid, and 10 other databases
Dates searched – from inception to September 2010
Other sources of evidence – hand searching of reference lists
Language restrictions – none.

Search Results

24 of 885 original studies met the inclusion criteria, whereas 10 of them were included in the meta-analysis.

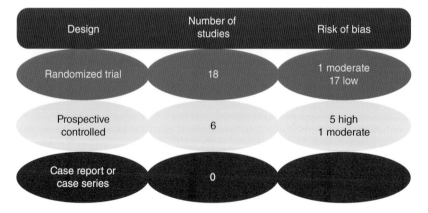

Design	Number of studies	Risk of bias
Randomized trial	18	1 moderate 17 low
Prospective controlled	6	5 high 1 moderate
Case report or case series	0	

Study Results

The details of the included studies are shown in Table S18.1 and the outcomes in Table S18.2.

Table S18.1 Study details on which the outcomes have been based.

Study/authors	Design	Sample size	Diagnosis (complete)	PSIO appliance	Treatment initiation (weeks)	Follow-up (weeks)	Risk of bias
Dutchcleft[a] project	RCT	54	UCLP	Passive (Zurich type)	Within 2	288	Low
Lohmander et al. 2004	pCCT	20	UCLP	Passive (intraoral palate-obturator)	About 2	72	Moderate-high
Masarei et al. 2007	RCT	34	UCLP	Active	Before 2	48	Moderate
Mishima et al. 1996 collated	pCCT	20	UCLP	Passive (Hotz plate)	At 2 or 3	192	High
Peat 1982	pCCT	40	BCLP	Passive (split-expansion appliance)	At 2	440	High

[a] Dutchcleft project: Bongaarts et al. 2004, 2006, 2008, 2009; Konst et al. 1999, 2000, 2003, 2004; Prahl et al. 2001, 2003, 2005, 2006, 2008; Severens et al. 1998.

Source: Papadopoulos et al. 2012. Reproduced with permission of John Wiley & Sons.

Table S18.2 Outcome for the angle (degrees) between the midpoint of the tuberosities, tuberosity, and the most occlusal point on the cusp of the canine M-T-C (5).

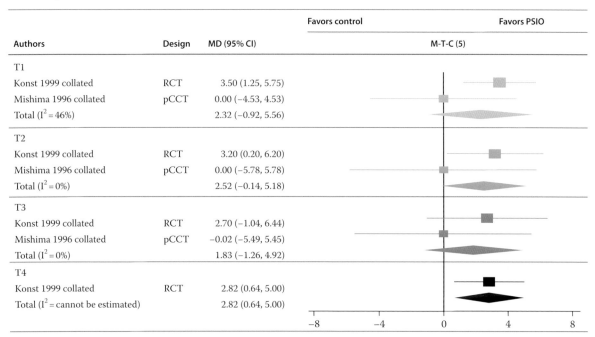

Authors	Design	MD (95% CI)
T1		
Konst 1999 collated	RCT	3.50 (1.25, 5.75)
Mishima 1996 collated	pCCT	0.00 (−4.53, 4.53)
Total ($I^2 = 46\%$)		2.32 (−0.92, 5.56)
T2		
Konst 1999 collated	RCT	3.20 (0.20, 6.20)
Mishima 1996 collated	pCCT	0.00 (−5.78, 5.78)
Total ($I^2 = 0\%$)		2.52 (−0.14, 5.18)
T3		
Konst 1999 collated	RCT	2.70 (−1.04, 6.44)
Mishima 1996 collated	pCCT	−0.02 (−5.49, 5.45)
Total ($I^2 = 0\%$)		1.83 (−1.26, 4.92)
T4		
Konst 1999 collated	RCT	2.82 (0.64, 5.00)
Total ($I^2 =$ cannot be estimated)		2.82 (0.64, 5.00)

Source: Papadopoulos et al. 2012. Reproduced with permission of John Wiley & Sons.

Key Findings

- In general, PSIO treatment seems to have no significant clinical effect.
- The only significant effect of PSIO found was on the maxillary arch form, as measured by one of the variables M-T-C(5), presenting a small but significant improvement.

Commentary

- The results of this study are valid mainly for passive PSIO appliances used mainly on unilateral CLP (UCLP) patients.
- All comparisons included a maximum of two compatible studies
- More RCTs are needed with long-term follow-up, investigating also active appliances and bilateral CLP patients.

Additional Reference

Noverraz RL, Disse MA, Ongkosuwito EM, *et al.*, 2015. Transverse dental arch relationship at 9 and 12 years in children with unilateral cleft lip and palate treated with infant orthopedics: a randomized clinical trial (DUTCHCLEFT). *Clin Oral Investig* 19, 2255–2265.

S19

Prevalence of dental anomalies in nonsyndromic individuals with cleft lip and palate: a systematic review and meta-analysis

Tannure PN, Oliveira CA, Maia LC, Vieira AR, Granjeiro JM, Costa MC. Cleft Palate Craniofac J 2012;49:194–200.*

Background

It appears to be clear that individuals born with cleft lip and palate have more dental anomalies, in particular tooth agenesis. A more precise estimate of the magnitude of the effect on the dentition of individuals born with cleft lip and palate would be relevant.

Study Information

Population – individuals born with cleft lip and palate
Intervention – assessment of the presence of dental anomalies
Comparison – individuals born without cleft lip and palate
Outcome – presence of dental anomalies.

Search Parameters

Inclusion criteria – clinical studies comparing frequency of dental anomalies in individuals born with cleft lip and palate to individuals born without clefts
Databases searched – PubMed, Web of Science, Embase, Cochrane
Dates searched – 1966 to May 2009
Other sources of evidence – hand searching of reference lists
Language restrictions – none.

Search Results

505 references were identified, six of which met the inclusion criteria.

Design	Number of studies	Risk of bias
Randomized trial	0	
Cohort or case control	6	4 moderate 2 high
Case report or case series	0	

Study Results

The prevalence of (A) tooth agenesis, (B) supernumeraries, and (C) abnormal crown formation are shown in Table S19.1.

Table S19.1 The prevalence of (A) tooth agenesis, (B) supernumerary teeth, and (C) irregularities of crown morphology.

A, Comparison of cleft versus control: prevalence of tooth agenesis

Study	Control Events	Total	Cleft Events	Total	Weight %	Means, Odds ratio M-H, Random, 95% CI	
Jordan et al. 1996	2	87	35	105	19.9	21.25 (4.94, 91.47)	
Schroeder and Green 1975	1	94	23	56	15.5	64.82 (8.42, 499.05)	
Quezada et al. 1988	0	38	79	100	10.9	284.72 (16.80, 4825.40)	
Eerens et al. 2007	39	250	15	50	26.0	2.32 (1.16, 4.64)	
Letra et al. 2007	36	500	131	500	27.7	4.58 (3.09, 6.78)	
Total	78	969	283	811	100	12.31 (3.75, 40.36)	

Heterogeneity: Tau^2 = 1.29, Chi^2 = 25.84 df = 4 (P < 0.0001), I^2 = 85%
Test for overall effect: Z = 4.14 (P < 0.0001)

B, Comparison cleft versus controls: Prevalence of supernumerary teeth

Means, Peto Odds ratio M-H, Fixed, 95% CI

Study							
Jordan et al. 1996	0	87	6	105	16.4	6.54 (1.28, 33.33)	
Schroeder and Green 1975	4	94	4	56	20.1	1.76 (0.41, 7.66)	
Letra et al. 2007	1	500	22	500	63.5	6.47 (2.83, 14.79)	
Total	5	681	32	661	100	4.99 (2.58, 9.64)	

Heterogeneity: Chi^2 = 2.41, df = 2 (P < 0.30), I^2 = 17%
Test for overall effect: Z = 4.78 (p < 0.00001)

C, Comparison of cleft versus control: Prevalence of morphological irregularities of the crown

Means, Peto Odds ratio M-H, Fixed, 95% CI

Study							
Jordan et al. 1996	13	87	57	105	38.2	5.42 (3.01, 9.76)	
Schroeder and Green 1975	11	94	30	56	24.2	8.12 (3.87, 17.01)	
Letra 2007	1	500	11	500	10.2	5.39 (1.73, 16.83)	
Rawashdeh 2009	6	60	42	100	27.3	4.55 (2.27, 9.12)	
Total	31	741	140	761	100	5.69 (3.96, 8.19)	

Heterogeneity: Chi^2 = 1.32, df = 3 (P < 0.72), I^2 = 0%
Test for overall effect: Z = 9.36 (P < 0.00001)

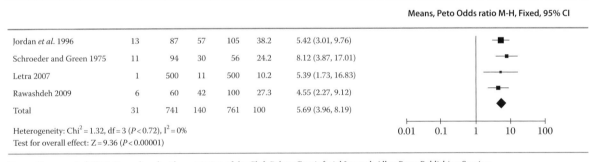

Source: Tannure et al. 2012. Reproduced with permission of the Cleft Palate-Craniofacial Journal, Allen Press Publishing Services.

Key Findings

- Three distinct subgroup analyses were carried out in terms of dental anomalies. In the tooth agenesis meta-analysis, a random effects model was used because of heterogeneity and showed a significant association between tooth agenesis and oral clefts (odds ratio [OR] = 12.31; 95% confidence interval [CI] = 3.75 to 40.36).
- In the remaining analyses, the fixed effects model revealed a positive association between supernumerary (OR = 4.99; 95% CI, 2.58 to 9.64) and crown morphologic abnormalities (OR = 5.69; 95% CI, 3.96 to 8.19) with oral clefts.

Commentary

It is conclusive that individuals born with cleft lip and palate have more dental anomalies. They are 12 times more likely to have tooth agenesis, five times more likely to have supernumerary teeth, and almost six times more likely to have crown morphologic anomalies.

Additional references for Summary 19 can be found on page 205.

S20

Long-term effects of presurgical infant orthopedics in patients with cleft lip and palate: a systematic review

Uzel A,* Alparslan ZN. Cleft Palate Craniofac J 2011;48:587–595.

Background

There is no a definitive conclusion about efficiency of presurgical infant orthopedics (PSIO) in the treatment of patients with cleft lip and palate (CLP). This systematic review aimed to assess the scientific evidence on the efficiency of PSIO appliances in patients with CLP to shed light on a specific, contemporary discussion of whether these appliances have long-term advantages with respect to treatment outcomes.

Study Information

Population – patients with cleft lip and palate
Intervention – presurgical infant orthopedics
Comparison/control group – no presurgical infant orthopedics
Outcome – motherhood satisfaction, feeding, speech, facial growth, maxillary arch, occlusion, nasal symmetry, and nasolabial appearance.

Search Parameters

Inclusion criteria – randomized controlled trials (RCTs) and nonrandomized controlled clinical trials (CCTs) with follow-up periods of a minimum of 6 years that reported data on treatment effects of PSIO and controls without PSIO
Databases searched – Medline/PubMed, National Library of Medicine Gateway, Web of Science, Cumulative Index to Nursing and Allied Health Literature, and Cochrane
Dates searched – various initial dates, all up to 2010
Other sources of evidence – the reference lists of the retrieved articles were hand-searched for possible missing articles from the database searches
Language restrictions – English, French.

Search Results

The survey strategy resulted in 319 articles, of which 12 qualified for the final analysis (eight RCTs, four nonrandomized CCTs). Differences in the methodologies and reporting results made statistical comparisons impossible.

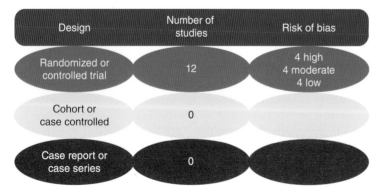

Design	Number of studies	Risk of bias
Randomized or controlled trial	12	4 high 4 moderate 4 low
Cohort or case controlled	0	
Case report or case series	0	

Study Findings

The outcome measures for PSIO in terms of age, appliance, and method/measurements are shown in Table S20.1.

Table S20.1 The outcome measures for PSIO in patients with cleft lip and palate.

Authors	Study design	Intervention PSIO (UCLP, BCLP)	Control	Age	Appliance	Method/measurement	Conclusion
Prahl *et al.* 2008	RCT	27	27	58 weeks	Passive moulding plate	Motherhood satisfaction questionnaire	PSIO had no influence on motherhood satisfaction
Masarei *et al.* 2007	RCT	17 8	16 8	3 months, 1 year	Active moulding plate with UCLP. Passive moulding plate with ICP	Feeding NOMAS, GOSMIF, videofluoroscopy, anthropometry at 3 months: SOMA, anthropology at 12 months	PSIO did not improve feeding efficiency
Prahl *et al.* 2005	RCT	24	25	3, 6, 15, 24 weeks	Passive moulding plate	Feeding log/ questionnaire anthropology	PSIO had no significant effect on feeding or consequent nutritional status
Karling *et al.* 1993	Nonrandomized	45	39	13.7 years	T-traction	Speech recording listening judgements	No differences between groups
Konst *et al.* 2003	RCT	6	6	2, 2.5, 3, 6 years	Passive moulding plate	Speech recording, Reynell Developmental scales	PSIO had no long-lasting effects on language development
Bongaarts *et al.* 2008	RCT	24 21	22 24	4, 6 years	Passive moulding plate	Nasolabial appearance Photographs, JS (Magnitude estimation method) VAS scale 1-100)	IO had a positive effect at 4 years of age but at 6 years there is an irrelevant difference between groups
Ross *et al.* 1994	Nonrandomized	20[a]	20	15.6/14.8 years	Passive plate + rubber band	Nasolabial appearance Photographs, JS score assignment (rating scale 1-10)	PSIO had no lasting effect on the esthetics of the lip and nose
Bongaarts *et al.* 2009	RCT	21 21	20 22	4, 6 years	Passive moulding plate	Facial growth. Lateral ceph 23 variables	No clinically relevant effect
Bongaarts *et al.* 2006	RCT	23 22	22 23	4, 6 years	Passive moulding plate	Maxillary arch dimension. 3D cast analysis	No differences on maxillary arch dimensions
Chan *et al.* 2003	Nonrandomized	19	21	7.3	Active moulding plate (Letham)	Occlusion. GOSLON Index	Active IO does not affect the dental arch relationship
Bongaarts *et al.* 2004	RCT	24 22	21 24	4, 6 years	Passive moulding plate	Occlusion. 5-year index	IO did not influence the occlusion at the age of 4 and 6 years of age
Barillas *et al.* 2009	Nonrandomized	15	10	9 years	Nam appliance	Nasal asymmetry. Stone cast measurements	The improvement of the symmetry of the nose maintained at 9 years of age.

Abbreviations: JS, judges system; VAS, visual analog score; NOMAS, Neonatal Oral Motor Assessment Scale; GOSMIF, Great Ormond Street Measurement of Infant Feeding; GOSLON, Great Ormond Street London and Oslo; SOMA, Schedule Of Oral Motor Assessment; NAM, nasoalveolar molding; IO, infant orthopedics; PSIO, presurgical infant orthopedics; UCLP, unilateral cleft lip and palate; ICP, isolated cleft palate; RCT, randomized controlled trial.
[a] BCLP, bilateral cleft lip and palate.
Source: Uzel *et al.* 2011. Reproduced with permission of the Cleft Palate-Craniofacial Journal, Allen Press Publishing Services.

Key Findings

- Infant orthopedic appliances have no positive effects on the seven treatment outcomes in patients with UCLP until the age of 6 years.
- There is limited evidence with high risk of bias on the improvement of nasal symmetry in patients with UCLP using nasal alveolar molding (NAM) appliances.

Commentary

No new evidence contradicting original findings was found.

Additional references for Summary 20 can be found on page 205.

S21

Secondary bone grafting for alveolar cleft in children with cleft lip or cleft lip and palate

Guo J, Li C, Zhang Q, Wu G, Deacon SA,* Chen J, Hu H, Zou S, Ye Q. Cochrane Database of Systematic Reviews 2011; (6):CD008050.

Background

Secondary alveolar bone grafting has been widely used to reconstruct alveolar clefts. However, there is still some controversy about which is the best technique, timing, and donor site for this procedure.

Study Information

Population – children older than 5 years with diagnosed clefting of the alveolus

Intervention – alveolar bone graft with autologous donor material

Comparison/ control group – alveolar bone graft using alternative techniques, donor material, or timing

Outcome – primary outcomes: radiographic/ clinical assessment of bone. Secondary outcomes: (i) morbidity of donor site; (ii) the successful rate of insertion of an implant or integration of denture in the alveolar cleft region; (iii) the rate of tooth eruption in the line of the alveolar cleft; (iv) gingival health; (v) quality of life after the surgery; (vi) length of hospital stay; (vii) adverse events of the secondary bone grafting.

Search Parameters

Inclusion criteria – human randomized controlled trials (RCTs)

Databases searched – Cochrane Oral Health Group's Trials Register, Cochrane Central Register of Controlled Trials, MEDLINE, EMBASE, Chinese Biomedical Literature Database, and WHO International Clinical Trials Registry Platform

Dates searched – various initial dates, all up to February 2011

Other sources of evidence – nonelectronic journals were hand searched including conference proceedings and abstracts

Language restrictions – none.

Search Results

582 unique citations were identified. Two publications, of two trials, remained after inclusion criteria applied.

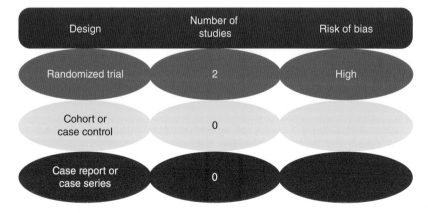

Design	Number of studies	Risk of bias
Randomized trial	2	High
Cohort or case control	0	
Case report or case series	0	

Study Results

Two small studies were found, one comparing traditional graft with a new material and the other looking at the benefit of applying a special type of glue to the graft. Both studies were considered to be of poor quality so no conclusions can be made.

Key Findings

- Currently there is no evidence that a particular technique, donor site, or timing of the procedure confers a superior outcome.

Commentary

1) Newer evidence from RCTs since the review include small prospective trials (n = 19–60 range), which may demonstrate some benefits to technique, different donor materials, or pain management of the donor site.
2) Other trends could not be substantiated because of small subject numbers.
3) Standard reporting methods of future clinical trials are recommended so data can be pooled and stronger clinical recommendations made.

Additional References

Alonso N, Risso GH, Denadai R, *et al.,* Effect of maxillary alveolar reconstruction on nasal symmetry of cleft lip and palate patients: a study comparing iliac crest bone graft and recombinant human bone morphogenetic protein-2. *J Plast Reconstr Aesthet Surg* 67, 1201 –1208.

Chang CS, Wallace CG, Hsiao YC, *et al.,* 2016. Difference in the surgical outcome of unilateral cleft lip and palate patients with and without pre-alveolar bone graft orthodontic treatment. *Sci Rep* 6, 23597.

Cunha MJ, Esper LA, Sbrana MC, *et al.,* 2013. Evaluation of the effectiveness of diode laser on pain and edema in individuals with cleft lip and palate submitted to secondary bone graft. *Cleft Palate Craniofac J* 50, e92–97.

de Ruiter A, Dik E, van Es R, *et al.,* 2014. Micro-structured calcium phosphate ceramic for donor site repair after harvesting chin bone for grafting alveolar clefts in children. *J Craniomaxillofac Surg* 42, 460–468.

Kumar Raja D, Anantanarayanan P, Christabel A, *et al.,* 2014. Donor site analgesia after anterior iliac bone grafting in paediatric population: a prospective, triple-blind, randomized clinical trial. *Int J Oral Maxillofac Surg* 43, 422–427.

Raposo-Amaral CA, Denadai R, Chammas DZ, *et al.,* 2015. Cleft patient-reported postoperative donor site pain following alveolar autologous iliac crest bone grafting: comparing two minimally invasive harvesting techniques. *J Craniofac Surg* 26, 2099–2103.

Takemaru M, Sakamoto Y, Sakamoto T, *et al.,* 2016. Assessment of bioabsorbable hydroxyapatite for secondary bone grafting in unilateral alveolar cleft. *J Plast Reconstr Aesthet Surg* 69, 493–496.

Acknowledgement

This Cochrane Review was published in the Cochrane Database of Systematic Reviews 2011, Issue 6. Cochrane Reviews are regularly updated as new evidence emerges and in response to feedback, and the Cochrane Database of Systematic Reviews should be consulted for the most recent version of the Cochrane Review.

S22

The effectiveness of non-surgical maxillary expansion: a meta-analysis

Zhou Y, Long Hu, Ye N, Xue J, Yang X, Liao L, Lai W. Eur J Orthod 2014;36:233–242.*

Background

Both rapid maxillary expansion (RME) and slow maxillary expansion (SME) could be applied to expand the constricted dental arches. However, whether they are effective for transverse maxillary discrepancy and which is superior is still poorly understood. This systematic review is aimed to evaluate and compare the effectiveness of RME and SME.

Study Information

Population – healthy adults or children who had a transverse discrepancy and required maxillary expansion
Intervention – RME, SME, or both
Comparison – untreated patients versus expansion appliance in subjects of similar age and type of malocclusion
Outcome – the changes of maxillary intermolar, intercanine, interpremolar, and mandibular intermolar widths.

Search Parameters

Inclusion criteria – clinical studies that evaluated the outcomes of RME and SME and comparative studies
Databases searched – PubMed, Embase, Web of Science, CENTRAL, ProQuest Dissertations and Theses, Clinical Trial.gov, and SIGLE
Dates searched – January 1980 to October 2012
Other sources of evidence – hand searching of reference lists
Language restrictions – none.

Search Results

2931 studies were identified, 14 of which met the inclusion criteria.

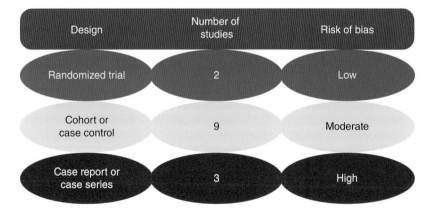

Design	Number of studies	Risk of bias
Randomized trial	2	Low
Cohort or case control	9	Moderate
Case report or case series	3	High

Study Results

The treatment effects for slow maxillary molar width expansion are shown in Table S22.1.

Table S22.1 Outcome measures for slow maxillary molar width expansion compared to control (mm).

Authors	Mean	SD	Total	Mean	SD	Total	Weight	Mean difference, Fixed 95% CI	
A, SME versus RME based on intermolar width									
Akkaya 1998	9.05	0.4	12	9.81	0.57	12	54.1	−0.76 (−1.15, −0.37)	
Ladner 1995	6	6.26	30	5.4	2	30	33	0.60 (−0.57, 1.77)	
Sandikcioglu 1997	5.5	3	10	5.6	2.7	10	12.9	−0.10 (−2.60, 2.40)	
Total			52			52	100	−0.23 (−1.24, 0.79)	

Heterogeneity: Tau^2 = 0.46, Chi^2 = 4.80, df = 2 (*P* = 0.09); I^2 = 58%
Test for overall effect: Z = 0.43 (*P* < 0.66)

B, Retention									
Akkaya 1998	−0.22	0.19	12	−0.2	0.06	12	98.9	−0.02 (−1.13, 0.09)	
Sandikcioglu 1997	−0.1	1.2	10	−0.5	1.2	10	1.1	0.40 (−0.65, 1.45)	
Total			22			22	100	−0.02 (−0.13, 0.10)	

Heterogeneity: Chi^2 = 0.61, df = 1 (*P* = 0.44); I^2 = 0%
Test for overall effect: Z = 0.27 (*P* < 0.79)

C, Net change									
Akkaya 1998	8.83	0.32	12	9.6	0.53	12	97.9	−0.77 (−1.12, −0.42)	
Sandikcioglu 1997	5.4	2.3	10	5.1	3.1	10	2.1	0.30 (−2.09, 2.69)	
Total			22			22	100	−0.75 (−1.09, −0.40)	

Heterogeneity: Chi^2 = 0.75, df = 1 (*P* = 0.39); I^2 = 0%
Test for overall effect: Z = 4.23 (*P* < 0.0001)

Source: Zhou *et al.* 2014. Reproduced with permission of Oxford University Press.

Key Findings

- SME is effective in expanding maxillary arch, although its effectiveness in mandibular arch expansion cannot be determined.
- RME is effective in expanding both maxillary and mandibular arches.
- SME is superior to expanding the molar region of maxillary arch, while similar to RME in mandibular arch expansion. However, we cannot compare their effectiveness in maxillary anterior region.

Commentary

1) More studies are needed to produce high-quality evidence with standard measurement methods and similar treatment strategies.
2) Further studies using more reliable outcome criteria and precise image capture techniques (e.g., cone-beam computed tomography) are recommended.

Additional References

Akkaya S, Lorenzon S, Ucem TT, 1998. Comparison of dental arch and arch perimeter changes between bonded rapid and slow maxillary expansion procedures. *Eur J Orthod* 20, 255–261.

Ladner PT, Muhl ZF, 1995. Changes concurrent with orthodontic treatment when maxillary expansion is a primary goal. *Am J Orthod Dentofacial Orthop* 108, 184–193.

Sandikcioglu M, Hazar S, 1997. Skeletal and dental changes after maxillary expansion in the mixed dentition. *Am J Orthod Dentofacial Orthop* 111, 321–327.

Crossbite (posterior)

S23

Orthodontic treatment for posterior crossbites

Agostino P, Ugolini A, Signori A, Silvestrini-Biavati A, Harrison JE, Riley P. Cochrane Database Syst Rev 2014;(8):CD000979.*

Background

A posterior crossbite occurs when the top back teeth bite inside the bottom back teeth. Several treatment approaches have been recommended to correct this problem; some expand the maxillary arch while others are directed at treating the cause of the posterior crossbite (e.g., breathing problems or sucking habits). The aim of the present review is to assess the effects of orthodontic treatment for posterior crossbites.

Study Information

Population – children and adults with a posterior crossbite
Intervention – orthodontic or dentofacial orthopedic
(nonsurgical) treatment used to correct posterior crossbite
Comparison – different expansion techniques
Outcome – correction of the posterior crossbite, molar and canine expansion.

Search Parameters

Inclusion criteria – randomized controlled trials (RCTs) of parallel design that assessed orthodontic treatments to correct a posterior crossbite
Databases searched – PubMed, Medline, Embase, Cochrane Library
Dates searched – 1984 to May 2014
Other sources of evidence – hand searching of reference lists
Language restrictions – none.

Search Results

517 studies were identified, of which 15 RCTs met the inclusion criteria.

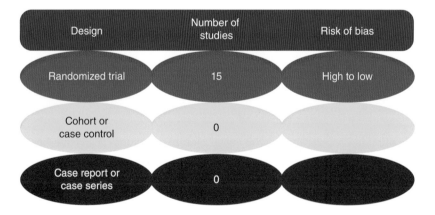

Design	Number of studies	Risk of bias
Randomized trial	15	High to low
Cohort or case control	0	
Case report or case series	0	

Study Results

The outcomes for two different appliances comparisons (A, B) to correct lateral crossbites are shown in Table S23.1.

Table S23.1 Comparison of different appliances and outcomes to correct lateral crossbites.

A, Comparison fixed rapid (Haas) versus rapid Hyrax – outcome molar expansion 3 months after completion of expansion phase

						Mean difference, fixed 95% CI		
Authors	Haas (n)	Mean (SD) (mm)	Hyrax (n)	Mean (SD) (mm)	Weight %		Favors Hyrax	Favors Haas
Garib 2005	4	6.5 (1)	4	6.7 (0.4)	81.8	−0.20 (−1.26, 0.86)		
Oliviera 2004	9	8.49 (2.33)	10	3.73 (2.64)	18.2	4.76 (2.53, 6.99)		
Total	13		14		100	−0.25, 1.66		

Heterogeneity Chi^2 = 15.47, df = 1 (P = 0.00008); I^2 = 94%
Test for overall effect: Z = 1.45 (P = 0.15)

B, Comparison fixed slow (QH) versus removable slow EP – outcome molar expansion

				Mean difference, M-H, fixed 95%CI		
Authors	QH (n)	Expansion plate	Weight %	Risk Ratio	Favors EP	QH
Godoy 2011	33/33	30/33	74.4	1.1 (0.97, 1.24)		
Petr 2008	15/15	10/15	25.6	1.48 (1.02, 2.13)		
Total	48	48	100	1.20 (1.04, 1.37)		

Heterogeneity Chi^2 = 3.15, df = 1 (P = 0.08); I^2 = 68%
Test for overall effect Z = 2.58 (P = 0.0097)

Abbreviations: EP, expansion plate; QH, quad-helix.
Source: Adapted from Agostino *et al.* 2014.

Key Findings

- Greater molar expansion (medium-quality evidence) and more successful crossbite correction (low-quality evidence) was found using a fixed quad-helix appliance when compared to a slow maxillary expansion using a removable expansion plate.
- No difference in molar expansion was found between fixed Haas and Hyrax appliances at 3 months after completion of the expansion phase (low quality, high heterogeneity, I^2 = 94%).

Commentary

There is a very small amount of evidence (low to moderate) to suggest that fixed quad-helix appliances may be more successful than removable expansion plates at correcting posterior crossbites and expanding the inter-molar width in children with early mixed dentition (8 to 10 years of age). The remaining evidence (very low quality) was insufficient to conclude that any one intervention is better than another for any of the outcomes.

Additional references for Summary 23 can be found on page 205.

Acknowledgement

This Cochrane Review was published in the Cochrane Database of Systematic Reviews 2014, Issue 8. Cochrane Reviews are regularly updated as new evidence emerges and in response to feedback, and the Cochrane Database of Systematic Reviews should be consulted for the most recent version of the Cochrane Review.

S24

Long-term dental and skeletal changes in patients submitted to surgically assisted rapid maxillary expansion: a meta-analysis

Vilani GN, Mattos CT,* de Oliveira Ruellas AC, Maia LC. Oral Surg Oral Med Oral Pathol Oral Radiol 2012;114:689–697.

Background

The use of surgically assisted rapid maxillary expansion (SARME) to correct maxillary transverse dental and skeletal structures and its stability is controversial. This review aimed to summarize available evidence with a follow-up of at least 1 year.

Study Information

Population – individuals submitted to orthodontic and surgical treatment
Intervention – surgically assisted rapid maxillary expansion
Comparison – surgically assistant expansion compared with baseline measurements
Outcome – dental and skeletal measurements in dental casts or posteroanterior cephalometric radiographs for at least 1 year follow-up.

Search Parameters

Inclusion criteria – clinical trials; tooth-borne or bone-borne appliances
Databases searched – Scirus, Ovid, Web of Science, Cochrane Library, VHL, and PubMed
Dates searched – until June 2011
Other sources of evidence – hand searching of reference lists
Language restrictions – none.

Search Results

365 references were identified, seven of which met the inclusion criteria.

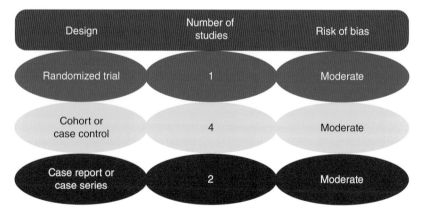

Design	Number of studies	Risk of bias
Randomized trial	1	Moderate
Cohort or case control	4	Moderate
Case report or case series	2	Moderate

Study Results

Three treatment outcomes at 1-year follow-up are shown in Table S24.1

Table S24.1 Comparison of three outcome measures for surgically assisted rapid maxillary expansion (SARME) for at least 1-year follow-up.

A, Follow-up outcome of alveolar width measured on posteroanterior radiographs Ma-Ma (mm)

Author	Mean	SD	Total	Mean	SD	Total	Weight	Mean difference Fixed, 95% CI	Favors decrease Favors increase
Berger *et al.* 1998	67.73	3.62	28	58.69	3.81	28	47.5	4.04 (2.09, 5.99)	
Koudstaal *et al.* 2009	61.4	3.8	23	58.8	4	23	35.4	2.60 (0.35, 4.85)	
Koudstaal *et al.* 2009	63.3	4.8	19	60.6	5.4	19	17.1	2.70 (−0.55, 5.95)	
Total			70			70	100	3.30 (1.96, 4.64)	

Heterogeneity: Chi^2 = 1.06, df = 2 (*P* = 0.59); I^2 = 0%
Test for overall effect: Z = 4.82 (*P* < 0.00001)

B, Follow-up outcome of intercanine width (cusp tips) measured on dental casts (mm)

Author	Mean	SD	Total	Mean	SD	Total	Weight	Mean difference Fixed, 95% CI
Berger *et al.* 1998	34.61	2.68	28	30.89	2.56	28	32.7	3.72 (2.35, 5.09)
Byloff and Mossaz, 2004	35.54	2.49	14	31.41	3.15	14	13.9	4.13 (2.03, 6.23)
Koudstaal *et al.* 2009	33.6	3.6	23	28.9	4.2	23	12.1	4.70 (2.44, 6.96)
Koudstaal *et al.* 2009	35.6	2.5	19	31.9	3.7	19	15.3	3.70 (1.69, 5.71)
Magnusson *et al.* 2009	32.85	3.08	31	30.45	3.11	31	26.0	2.40 (0.86, 3.94)
Total			115			115	100	3.55 (2.76, 4.33)

Heterogeneity: Chi^2 = 3.51, df = 4 (*P* = 0.48); I^2 = 0%
Test for overall effect: Z = 8.86 (*P* < 0.00001)

C, Follow-up outcome of intermolar width (mesiopalatal cusp tips) measured on dental casts (mm)

Author	Mean	SD	Total	Mean	SD	Total	Weight	Mean difference Fixed, 95% CI
Berger *et al.* 1998	41.79	2.86	28	37.02	3.45	28	44.3	4.77 (3.11, 6.43)
Sokucu *et al.* 2009	40.9	1.37	14	38.03	2.47	14	55.7	2.87 (1.39, 4,35)
Total			42			42	100	3.71 (2.61, 4.82)

Heterogeneity: Chi^2 = 2.80, df = 1 (*P* = 0.09); I^2 = 64%
Test for overall effect: Z = 6.59 (*P* < 0.00001)

Ma-Ma, maxillary alveolar width was assessed from the distance between the right and left intersection of the alveolar process and the maxillary molars on the posteroanterior cephalometric radiographs.
Source: Vilani *et al.* 2012. Reproduced with permission of Elsevier.

Key Findings

- There was an increase in maxillary alveolar, upper intercanine and intermolar widths at least 1 year after SARME compared to baseline.
- A significant relapse is expected in the upper intercanine width after expansion. No relapse was observed in the maxillary alveolar width.

Commentary

Additional randomized controlled trials have been published since this systematic review appeared and their evidence does not contradict the findings from this review (Kayalar *et al.* 2016; Prado *et al.* 2013; Zandi *et al.* 2014). However, none of them undertook a follow-up of more than 1 year.

Additional references for Summary 24 can be found on page 205.

S25

Long-term dental arch changes after rapid maxillary expansion treatment: a systematic review

Lagravere MO, Major PW, Flores Mir C.* Angle Orthod 2005;75:151–157.

Background

Maxillary expansion is among the most commonly used orthodontic procedures. Understanding long-term dentoalveolar impact of such appliance is crucial. This systematic review evaluated the long-term maxillary dental arch changes after nonsurgical rapid maxillary expansion (RME).

Study Information

Population – orthodontic patients with maxillary constricted arches
Intervention – nonsurgical RME
Comparison – untreated versus treated normal occlusions
Outcome – long-term dental arch measurements either through cephalometry or dental cast measurements (intercanine, intermolar, and arch perimeter).

Search Parameters

Inclusion criteria – randomized and nonrandomized clinical trials, and cohort studies that evaluated radiographically or through dental cast measurements the long-term changes in the maxillary dental arch
Databases searched – Medline, PubMed, LILACS, CDSR (Cochrane), and Web of Science
Dates searched – various initial dates, all up to March 2004
Other sources of evidence – reference lists of included studies
Language restrictions – none.

Search Results

Only four publications remained with long-term evaluations. Differences in the methodologies utilized made a meta-analysis questionable.

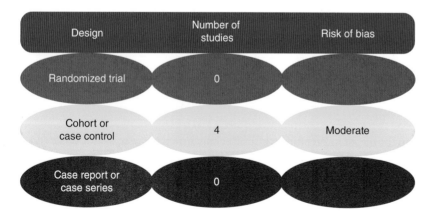

Design	Number of studies	Risk of bias
Randomized trial	0	
Cohort or case control	4	Moderate
Case report or case series	0	

Study Results

The outcomes of the four studies are shown in Table S25.1

Table S25.1 Long-term expansion based on rapid maxillary expansion versus control groups.

| | Test appliance Haas-type RME | | | Control/comparison group | | | Start and final evaluation (–/–) | |
| | | | | | | | Mean/median change in max/mand inter-canine distance compared to control (mm) | Mean/median change in max/mand intermolar distance compared to control (mm) |
Author	Sex	Start age	Final evaluation	Sex	Start age	Final evaluation		
McNamara *et al.* 2003	61 female 51 male	12 yr 2 mo ± 1 yr 4 mo	20 yr 5 mo ± 1 yr 7 mo	17 female 24 male,	11 yr 6 mo ± 1 yr	19 yr 7 mo	2.5/1.5	4/2.5
Handelman *et al.* 2000	Adult 28 female 19 male	29.9 yr ± 8 yr	2 ± 0.6 yr after start	31 female 21 male	32.27 ± 7.4 yr	2.1 ± 0.7 yr after start	2.8/1.1	4.8/0.9
	Child 29 female 18 male	9.5 yr ± 1.3 yr	N/K	–	–	–	4.2/0.6	5.9/0.6
Baccetti *et al.* 2001	Early 18 female 11 male	11 yr prepubertal (CVM)	19 yr 9 mo	2 female 9 male,	11 yr 3 mo	17 yr 5 mo	–	2.7/0.3
	Late 10 female 3 male	13 yr 7 mo post pubertal (CVM)	21 yr 9 mp	7 females 2 males	12 yr 4 mo	17 yr 7 mo	–	3.5/2.3
							Cephalometric measures	
Garib *et al.* 2001	14 female 11 male	13.5 yr, 11 to 17.3 yr	18.7 yr	13 female 13 male,	13.5 yr	18.7 yr	ANB -0.3dg SN to palatal plane 0.6dg	ANB -0.3dg SN to palatal plane 0.2dg

Source: Adapted from Lagravere *et al.* 2005.

- Based on direct dental cast measurements, long-term maxillary intermolar increases between 3.7 and 4.8 mm were attained.
- Based on direct dental cast measurements, long-term maxillary intercanine increases between 2.2 and 2.5 mm were attained.
- These transversal dental arch changes are more significant (>0.8 mm) in pubertal compared to prepubertal samples.
- Based on direct dental cast measurements, long-term maxillary arch perimeter increases of around 6 mm were attained.
- Based on direct dental cast measurements, long-term mandibular arch perimeter increases of around 4.5 mm were attained.
- Based on lateral cephalometric measurements, no long-term anteroposterior or vertical dental changes were observed.

Key Findings

- Long-term maxillary intermolar and intercanine increases could be considered clinically meaningful.
- Long-term maxillary and mandibular arch perimeter increases could be considered clinically meaningful.
- Differences between using the RME in pubertal versus prepubertal samples appears not to be of clinical significance.
- No long-term dental arch anteroposterior or vertical changes were observed.

Commentary

1) Only four retrospective cohorts studies were identified. They had moderate to high risk of bias.
2) The results included not only RME changes but also use of edgewise fixed appliances thereafter.
3) Because long-term changes were assessed the use of untreated control groups was considered indispensable.
4) These changes should not be extrapolated to SME procedures.

S26

Stability of deep-bite correction: a systematic review

Huang GJ,* Bates SB, Ehlert AA, Whiting DP, Chen SS, Bollen AM. J World Fed Orthod 2012;1:e89–e86.

Background

Deep bite occurs with a prevalence of about 15–20% in the US population. While correcting deep bites is a common goal of treatment, there are many methods that orthodontists employ. This review investigated the role of various parameters and treatments strategies on stability of deep bite correction.

Study Information

Population – orthodontic patients with deep bite malocclusion
Intervention – patient characteristics or treatment factors
Comparison – treated and untreated subjects or subjects with different initial characteristics or treatments
Outcome – overbite at end of treatment and at least 1 year after treatment.

Search Parameters

Inclusion criteria – clinical studies reporting on the stability of deep bite correction
Databases searched – PubMed, Web of Science, Embase, Cochrane
Dates searched – Jan 1966 to June 2012
Other sources of evidence – hand searching of reference lists
Language restrictions – none.

Search Results

1098 references were identified, with 23 meeting the inclusion criteria. Three additional studies were identified by hand searching, for a total of 26.

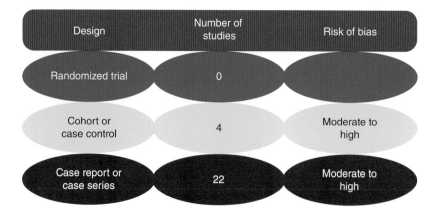

Design	Number of studies	Risk of bias
Randomized trial	0	
Cohort or case control	4	Moderate to high
Case report or case series	22	Moderate to high

Study Results

Weighted averages for overbite and follow-up time were calculated for each group: (A) Class I, (B) Class II Div 1, and (C) Class II Div 2, based on the sample size (Figure S26.1).

Figure S26.1 Weighted averages for overbite at various follow-up times from (a) Class I, (b) Class II Division I, and (c) Class II Division 2 studies. Abbreviations: NE, nonextraction, EXT, extraction; MIX, mixed. *Source:* Huang *et al.* 2012. Reproduced with permission of Sage Publications.

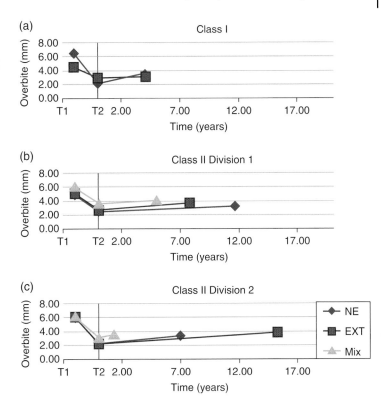

Deepbite

Key Findings

- Most studies were case series, and had significant risk for bias.
- Based on this relatively low-quality evidence, it appears that orthodontists have good success correcting deep bite cases, and that most of the correction is stable more than 1 year after treatment.

Commentary

There are two related articles, a systematic review from 2012 and a randomized controlled trial (RCT) from 2014. The systematic review reports on treatment and stability of Class II Div 2 malocclusion, and concludes that the existing evidence is at high risk for bias. The RCT stated that only 10% of deep bite patients relapsed to more than 50% overbite long term.

Additional References

Danz JC, Greuter C, Sifakakis I, *et al.,* 2014. Stability and relapse after orthodontic treatment of deep bite cases-a long-term follow-upstudy. *Eur J Orthod* 36, 522–530.

Millett DT, Cunningham SJ, O'Brien KD, *et al.,* 2012. Treatment and stability of Class II division 2 malocclusion in children and adolescents: a systematic review. *Am J Orthod Dentofacial Orthop* 142, 159–169.e9.

S27

Treatment and stability of Class II Division 2 malocclusion in children and adolescents: a systematic review

Millett DT, Cunningham SJ, O'Brien KD, Benson P, de Oliveira CM. Am J Orthod Dentofac Orthop 2012;142:159–169.e9.*

Background

Orthodontic treatment of Class II Division 2 malocclusion (Class II/2) is recognized as difficult to treat and prone to relapse. Randomized and controlled clinical trials were considered in a previous review, but as none were identified (Millett *et al.* 2006) this review has assessed all prospective and retrospective evidence regarding the effectiveness of orthodontic treatment and its stability for children and adolescents with Class II/2.

Study Information

Population – children and adolescents who had orthodontic treatment for Class II/2

Intervention – one or two arch full fixed appliances (with or without extractions), including cases with Class II elastics and no adjunctive appliances. Included also were cases treated by removable, functional, or headgear appliances, used on their own or in combination with fixed appliances.

Comparison – another treated Class II/2 group, untreated Class II/2 group, or neither

Outcome – primary: skeletal, soft-tissue, dental, occlusal, or gingival changes during treatment or observation period. Secondary: temporomandibular joint status or related muscular activity and quality of life.

Search Parameters

Inclusion criteria – clinical studies of Class II/2 treatment or stability of treatment.

Databases searched – the Cochrane Oral Health Trials Register, the Cochrane Central Register of Controlled Trials, MEDLINE, and EMBASE

Dates searched – various start dates to November 2011

Other sources of evidence – proceedings and abstracts of British and European Orthodontic and International Association for Dental Research Conferences. Reference lists of identified studies were screened. Contacted international researchers potentially involved in Class II/2 clinical trials to identify unpublished or ongoing randomized and controlled clinical trials.

Language restrictions – none.

Search Results

322 records identified; only 23 full-text articles (and one abstract) were retrieved. Three (plus the abstract) were subsequently excluded; 12 studies (four prospective, eight retrospective) dealt with treatment and eigth studies (all retrospective) dealt with stability (Table S27.1).

Table S27.1 Number of patients evaluated according to study types.

Study type	Test	Controls
Prospective treatment	122	74
Retrospective treatment	347	20
Retrospective stability	374	–

Source: Millett *et al.* 2012. Reproduced with permission of American Association of Orthodontists.

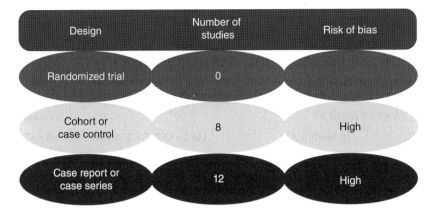

Design	Number of studies	Risk of bias
Randomized trial	0	
Cohort or case control	8	High
Case report or case series	12	High

Study Results

- Prospective but highly biased evidence exists regarding the effect of late mixed-dentition nonextraction treatment on facial growth in patients with Class II/2.
- Nonextraction treatment is favored and overbite correction is reasonably stable in the short term.
- International multicenter collaborative studies are required to gather appropriate epidemiologic evidence regarding this condition.

Key Findings

The evidence is highly biased in relation to the management and stability of Class II/2 in children and adolescents. Based on current evidence the following guidelines are suggested:

- Timely treatment to correct the overbite
- Nonextraction treatment is preferred
- Interincisal angle to be corrected and the upper incisors moved away from lower lip
- Long-term retention with an upper removable appliance incorporating a flat anterior bite plane and a bonded retainer to the upper labial segment.

Commentary

Stronger evidence is required on treatment and stability for Class II/2 in children and adolescents.

Additional Reference

Millett DT, Cunningham SJ, O'Brien KD, *et al.,* 2006. Orthodontic treatment for deep bite and retroclined upper front teeth in children. *Cochrane Database Syst Rev* (4), CD005972.

S28

Stability of Class II fixed functional appliance therapy – a systematic review and meta-analysis

Bock NC,* von Bremen J, Ruf S. Eur J Orthod. 2016;38:129–139.

Background

Many Herbst appliance derivatives have been introduced during the last 30 years. While the actual treatment effects have been analyzed, data on facial and dental changes after active treatment seem to be scarce. Therefore, the evidence on post-treatment changes was evaluated.

Study Information

Population – Class II patients
Intervention – fixed functional appliance treatment
Comparison – treatment changes
Outcome – ANB angle, overjet, overbite, Wits appraisal, molar relationship, soft tissue facial convexity.

Search Parameters

Inclusion criteria – fixed functional Class II treatment of ≥5 patients; numerical data on the post-treatment changes ≥ 1year (nonactive period)
Databases searched – PubMed, German Institute for Medical Documentation and Information (including Cochrane, Embase, Medline, and others), and the databases of 10 international orthodontic journals
Dates searched – up to December 2013
Other sources of evidence – hand searching of reference lists
Language restrictions – articles had to be in English or Danish, Finnish, French, German, Greek, Italian, Spanish, Swedish, Turkish.

Search Results

Of 2132 identified references, 20 articles finally met the inclusion criteria.

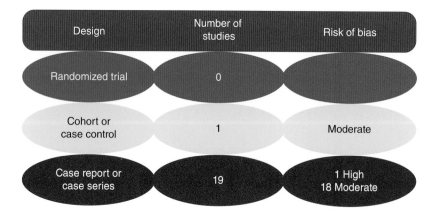

Design	Number of studies	Risk of bias
Randomized trial	0	
Cohort or case control	1	Moderate
Case report or case series	19	1 High 18 Moderate

Study Results

The outcomes for ANB angle are shown for fixed functional appliances (Table S28.1).

Table S28.1 Outcome of (A) ANB angle using a fixed functional appliance.

A, ANB angle (degrees) mean treatment changes 95% CI, random effects

	Treatment changes			Post-treatment changes		
	Effect (95% CI)	weights		Effect (95% CI)	weights	
Bock and Pancherz 2006	−1.3 (−1.72, −0.80)	1.0		0.2 (−0.22, 0.52)	1.1	
Bock and Ruf 2012	−0.8 (−1.29, −0.31)	1.0		0.2 (−0.21, 0.61)	1.0	
Bock and Ruf 2013	−1.5 (−1.83, −1.17)	1.1		0.2 (−0.19, 0.59)	1.1	
Bock *et al.* 2009	−1.2 (−1.71, −0.69)	1.0		0.0 (−0.30, 0.30)	1.3	
Chaiyonsirisern *et al.* 2009	−1.2 (−1.60, −0.80)	1.1		0.2 (−0.54, 0.98)	0.6	
Nelson *et al.* 2007	−1.6 (−2.07, −1.05)	1.0		−0.8 (−1.45, −0.19)	0.7	
Pancherz 1981	−2.0 (−2.31, −1.69)	1.1		0.1 (−0.27, 0.47)	1.1	
Pancherz 1991	−1.2 (−1.50, −0.80)	1.1				
Soytarhan and Isiksal 1990	−3.2 (−3.95, −2.35)	0.7		0.8 (0.38, 1.22)	1.0	
Summary	−1.48 (−1.81, −1.16)			0.14 (−0.11, 0.39)		
Heterogeneity: 0.2; *P* = 0				Heterogeneity: 0.079; *P* = 0.007		

Estimate heterogeneity variance 0.2; *P* = 0

Estimate heterogeneity variance 0.079; *P* = 0.007

Source: Bock *et al.* 2016. Reproduced with permission of Oxford University Press.

Key Findings

The main treatment relapses are highlighted below (% relates to relative treatment changes);

- ANB 0.2 degrees (12.4%);
- Overjet 1.8 mm (26.2%);
- Overbite Class II division 1 1.4 mm (44.7%) and Class II division 2 1 mm (22.2%);
- Wits appraisal 0.5 mm (19.5%);
- Sagittal molar relationship 1.2 mm/0.1 cusp width (21.8%/6.5%);
- Soft tissue facial convexity less than 0.1 degree (1%).

Commentary

- All 20 studies correspond to either Herbst appliance (n = 19) or twin force bite corrector (n = 1).
- The evidence on the stability of treatment results is nonexistent for most Class II fixed functional appliances except for Herbst treatment.
- Although most of the publications were of low quality (evidence level III), a meta-analysis revealed good dentoskeletal stability without clinically relevant changes for most variables.

S29

Treatment effects of fixed functional appliances in patients with Class II malocclusion: a systematic review and meta-analysis

Zymperdikas VF,* Koretsi V, Papageorgiou SN, Papadopoulos MA.* Eur J Orthod 2016;38:113–126.

Background

Class II malocclusion owing to mandibular retrognathism is a common condition. In growing patients, fixed functional appliances for mandibular advancement seem an appealing perspective, yet their clinical effects are much debated. The objective of this study is to assess the treatment effectiveness of fixed functional appliances in an evidence-based manner.

Study Information

Population – growing and nongrowing patients of any sex with Class II malocclusion
Intervention – orthodontic treatment with fixed functional appliances
Control group – untreated matched Class II subjects
Outcome – angular measurements from lateral cephalometric radiographs.

Search Parameters

Inclusion criteria – randomized and prospective controlled trials.
Databases searched – PubMed, Embase, Cochrane Library, Google Scholar, Web of Science, Evidence-Based
    Medicine, Scopus, LILACS, BBO, Ovid, Bandolier, Atypon Link, African Journals Online, ProQuest,
    Conference Paper Index, ZB MED, metaRegister of Controlled Trials
Dates searched – from inception to October 2014
Other sources of evidence – hand searching of reference lists and authors' communications
Language restrictions – none.

Search Results

9115 references were identified, nine unique datasets from 10 studies met the inclusion criteria.

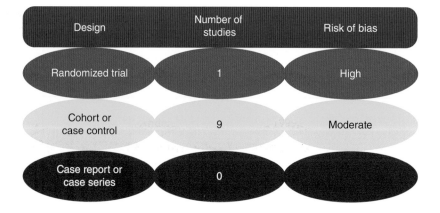

Design	Number of studies	Risk of bias
Randomized trial	1	High
Cohort or case control	9	Moderate
Case report or case series	0	

Study Results

The differences in the SNA and SNB angles for fixed functional appliances versus controls are shown in Table S29.1.

Table S29.1 Outcomes of fixed functional appliances versus controls (A) SNA, (B) SNB, and (C) ANB angles.

Study	Fixed functional appliances		Control				
	n	Mean (SD)	n	Mean (SD)	Weight	95% CI	Mean differences between fixed functional appliances and control groups
A, SNA angle change (degrees)							
Alali 2014	21	−0.60 (1.04)	17	0.30 (1.19)	15.44	−0.90 (−1.62, −0.18)	
Baysal 2011	20	−1.02 (0.84)	20	0.15 (0.53)	26.59	−1.17 (−1.61, −0.73)	
Gunay 2011	15	1.07 (1.80)	12	−0.08 (3.60)	2.31	1.15 (−1.08, 3.38)	
Karacay, 2006	32	−0.58 (8.16)	16	0.80 (8.00)	0.51	−1.38 (−6.21, 3.45)	
Latkauskiene 2012	40	−0.30 (0.90)	18	0.20 (1.10)	20.11	−0.50 (−1.08, 0.08)	
Oztoprak 2012	40	−0.55 (2.93)	19	−0.52 (3.10)	3.99	−0.03 (−1.69, 1.63)	
Phelan 2012	31	−0.80 (1.60)	30	0.50 (1.20)	15.77	−1.30 (−2.01, −0.59)	
Uyanlar 2014	15	−2.09 (3.33)	12	−0.16 (3.36)	1.80	−1.93 (−4.47, 0.61)	
De Almeida 2005	30	−0.80 (1.80)	30	−0.40 (1.30)	13.49	−0.40 (−1.19, 0.39)	
Total SNA ($I^2 = 27\%$; $P < 0.001$) with estimated predicted interval					100	−0.83 (−1.17, −0.48) (−1.58, −0.08)	
B, SNB angle (degrees)							
Alali 2014	21	2.54 (1.64)	17	−0.30 (1.04)	13.21	2.84 (1.98, 3.70)	
Baysal 2011	20	0.70 (0.89)	20	0.35 (0.73)	16.51	0.35 (−0.15, 0.85)	
Gunay 2011	15	1.07 (2.20)	12	1.16 (2.48)	6.52	−0.09 (−1.88, 1.70)	
Karacay 2006	32	3.90 (7.99)	16	0.40 (6.92)	1.53	3.50 (−0.88, 7.88)	
Latkauskiene 2012	40	0.80 (1.00)	18	0.10 (0.80)	16.70	0.70 (0.22, 1.18)	
Oztoprak 2012	40	1.20 (2.41)	19	0.52 (2.04)	10.36	0.68 (−0.50, 1.86)	
Phelan 2012	31	0.40 (1.50)	30	−0.20 (1.50)	14.21	0.60 (−0.15, 1.35)	
Uyanlar 2014	15	1.47 (2.86)	12	1.08 (2.28)	5.86	0.39 (−1.55, 2.33)	
De Almeida 2005	30	0.50 (1.30)	30	−0.10 (1.30)	15.11	0.60 (−0.06, 1.26)	
Total SNB ($I^2 = 72\%$; $P = 0.003$) with estimated predicted interval						0.87 (0.30, 1.43) (−0.84, 2.57)	

Source: Zymperdikas *et al.* 2016. Reproduced with permission of Oxford University Press.

Key Findings

The short-term effects of fixed functional appliances on the skeletal tissues of Class II patients were small and of minor clinical importance. In contrast, dentoalveolar and soft tissue changes were more pronounced, while the treatment results seem to be affected by patient- and appliance-related factors. The long-term effects of fixed functional appliances could not be assessed due to the lack of appropriate data.

Commentary

The skeletal short-term changes induced by Class II treatment with fixed functional appliances are not as evident as one would expect. Further studies with detailed reporting on patient and appliance data, as well as comparable cephalometric measures, are needed to examine the long-term stability of fixed functional appliance treatment.

Additional references for Summary 29 can be found on page 206.

Additional references for Summary 29 can be found on page 206.

S30

Effectiveness of orthodontic treatment with functional appliances on maxillary growth in the short term: a systematic review and meta-analysis

Nucera R, Lo Giudice A, Rustico L, Matarese G, Papadopoulos MA, Cordasco G. Am J Orthod Dentofacial Orthop 2016;149:600–611.e3.*

Background

This meta-analysis aimed to evaluate the best literature evidence from randomized controlled trials (RCTs) and prospective clinical controlled trials (pCCTs) in order to assess the short-term skeletal effects on maxillary growth of Class II patients of removable functional appliances that advance the mandible to a more forward position.

Study Information

Population – patients with skeletal Class II malocclusion
Intervention – removable functional protruding mandible appliances
Comparison/control group – untreated patients with skeletal Class II
Outcome – the following cephalometric parameters: SNA, anterior maxillary displacement (mm), maxillary plane rotation.

Search Parameters

Inclusion Criteria – RCTs, pCCTs, growing patients, no additional intervention
Databases searched – PubMed, Ovid, Embase, Cochrane Central Register of Controlled Trials, Web of Science, SCOPUS, LILACS, Google Scholar, Digital dissertation, Conference Paper Index, Clinicaltrials.gov, German Library of Med
Dates Searched – electronic searches were performed between 10th and 26th of April, 2015
Other sources of evidence – previously published systematic review performed on the same topic were hand searched
Language restrictions – none.

Search Results

2516 unique citations were identified. 191 trials remained after preliminary evaluation of title and abstract, 14 trials were considered after evaluation of full text. These 14 prospective clinical trials were used to perform qualitative evaluation and quantitative results synthesis.

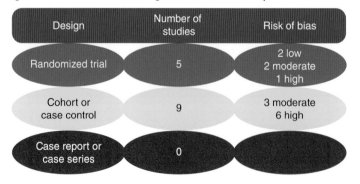

Design	Number of studies	Risk of bias
Randomized trial	5	2 low 2 moderate 1 high
Cohort or case control	9	3 moderate 6 high
Case report or case series	0	

Study Results

The outcomes for removable functional appliances versus controls in respect of: (1) SNA angle and (2) anterior maxillary displacement are shown in Table S30.1.

Table S30.1 Outcomes for removable functional appliances versus controls for (A) SNA angle and (B) anterior maxillary displacement.

A, SNA angle change (degrees)

Study	Functional n	Functional Mean (SD)	Control n	Control Mean (SD)	Weight (%)	Mean differences, Random, 95% CI (degrees) 95% CI	Favors functional / Favors control
Baysal *et al.* 2013	20	−0.56 (0.76)	20	0.15 (0.53)	12	−0.71 (−1.12, −0.30)	
Biligic *et al.* 2015	20	−1.6 (6.12)	20	0.8 (6.78)	0.8	−2.40 (−6.40, 1.60)	
Courtney *et al.* 1996	25	−0.11 (0.51)	17	0.23 (0.49)	12.8	−0.34 (−0.65, −0.03)	
Illing *et al.* 1998	34	−0.33 (2.73)	20	0.4 (2)	5.1	−0.73 (−2.00, 0.54)	
Kumar *et al.* 1996	16	−1.25 (2.69)	8	−0.22 (1.75)	3.1	−1.03 (−2.82, 0.76)	
Lund *et al.* 1998	36	0.08 (1.33)	27	0.25 (0.66)	11.1	−0.17 (−0.67, 0.33)	
Ozturk *et al.* 1994	17	0.13 (0.39)	19	0.55 (0.57)	12.7	−0.42 (−0.74, −0.10)	
Quintao *et al.* 2006	19	0.05 (1.07	19	0.95 (2.37)	5.7	−0.90 (−2.07, 0.27)	
Tulloch *et al.* 1997	53	0.11 (1.26)	61	0.26 (1.17)	11.6	−0.15 (−0.60, 0.33)	
Tumer *et al.* 1999	26	−0.08 (0.28)	13	0.18 (0.52)	12.9	−0.26 (−0.56, 0.04)	
Uner *et al.* 1989	11	−1.25 (0.49)	11	0.5 (0.4)	12.3	−1.75 (−2.12, −1.38)	
Total (95% CI)	277		235		100	−0.61 (−0.96, −0.25)	

Heterogeneity: Tau^2 = 0.24; Chi^2 = 52.95, df =10 (*P* < 0.00001); I^2 = 81%
Test for overall effect: Z = 3.30 (*P* = 0.001)

B, Anterior maxillary displacement (mm)

Study	Functional n	Functional Mean (SD)	Control n	Control Mean (SD)	Weight (%)	95% CI	
Baysal *et al.* 2013	20	0.35 (0.9)	20	1.05 (0.81)	14.0	−0.7 (−1.23, −0.17)	
Biligic *et al.* 2015	20	0.6 (11.28)	20	0.5 (14.86)	0.1	0.10 (−8.08, 9.28)	
Courtney *et al.* 1996	25	0.24 (0.7)	17	0.56 (0.57)	18.0	−0.32 (−0.71, 0.07)	
Illing *et al.* 1998	34	−0.24 (1.87)	20	1.07 (1.47)	7.4	−1.31 (−2.21, −0.41)	
Jacobbson *et al.* 1967	16	−0.53 (0.87)	17	0.47 (0.95)	12.0	−1.00 (−1.62, −0.38)	
Martina *et al.* 2012	23	1.47 (1.27)	23	2.5 (2.5)	5.1	−1.03 (−2.18, 0.12)	
O'Brien *et al.* 2003	89	0.46 (0.45)	85	1.16 (1.16)	21.7	−0.70 (−0.96, 0.44)	
Tulloch *et al.* 1997	53	0.04 (1)	61	0.17 (0.14)	21.5	−0.13 (−0.40, 0.14)	
Total (95% CI)	280		263		100	−0.61 (−0.90, −0.32)	

Heterogeneity: Tau^2 = 0.08; Chi^2 = 17.17, df =7 (*P* < 0.02); I^2 = 59%
Test for overall effect: Z = 4.10 (*P* < 0.0001)

Source: Nucera *et al.* 2016. Reproduced with permission of Elsevier.

Key Findings

Evidence suggests that removal functional treatment in growing Class II patients causes, in the short term, the following significant annual changes:

- maxillary growth inhibition (ANB = −0.61°);
- A-point anterior projection reduction (A-reference line = −0.61 mm).

Commentary

Removable functional protruding mandible appliances in Class II growing patients appear to slightly inhibit sagittal maxillary growth in the short term.

These conclusions should be considered with caution because of the high level of heterogeneity and the low quality of evidence found amongst the original studies.

Additional references for Summary 30 can be found on page 206.

S31

The effectiveness of the Herbst appliance for patients with Class II malocclusion: a meta-analysis

Yang X, Zhu Y, Long H, Zhou Y, Jian F, Ye N, Gao M, Lai W.* Eur J Orthod 2016;38:324–333.

Background

Of all the functional appliances used for Class II malocclusion correction, the Herbst appliance is one of the most commonly used. We present an up-to-date meta-analysis to investigate the effectiveness of Herbst appliance.

Study Information

Population – Class II division I malocclusion patients treated with any kind of Herbst appliance
Intervention – Herbst appliance
Comparison – patients treated with and without the Herbst appliance
Outcome – the net changes of cephalometrically derived skeletal angular and linear measurements before and immediately after Herbst treatment.

Search Parameters

Inclusion criteria – randomized controlled trials (RCTs) or clinical controlled trials; using Herbst appliances to correct Class II division 1 malocclusions; skeletal and/or dental changes evaluated through lateral cephalograms
Databases searched – PubMed, Web of Science, Embase, CENTRAL, SIGLE and ClinicalTrial.gov
Dates searched – up to December 2014
Other sources of evidence – none
Language restrictions – none.

Search Results

57 references were identified, 12 of which met the inclusion criteria.

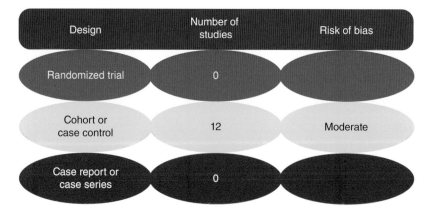

Study Results

The mean differences for the 11 outcome measures are shown in Table S31.1.

Table S31.1 Sensitivity analysis for Herbst appliance versus control.

Outcome measure	Original estimates	Exclusion of studies	Exclusion of low-quality studies	Effect model, mean difference, Random, 95% CI		Direction of forest plot summary
				Fixed	Random	
SNA	−0.56 (−0.99, −0.14)	−0.52 (−0.99, −0.06)	−0.30 (−0.87, 0.26)	−0.62 (−0.88, −0.37)	−0.56 (−0.99, −0.14)	Favors Herbst
SNB	1.06 (0.53, 1.60)	1.08 (0.49, 1.66)	1.85 (1.05, 2.64)	0.89 (0.66, 1.13)	1.06 (0.53, 1.60)	Favors Herbst
ANB	−1.08 (−2.16, −0.00)	−0.96 (−2.12, 0.20)	−0.99 (−3.70, 1.73)	−0.60 (−0.81, −0.38)	−1.08 (−2.16, −0.00)	Favors Herbst
Mandibular plane angle	0.17 (−0.09, 0.42)		0.08 (0.24, 0.39)	0.17 (−0.09, 0.42)	0.17 (−0.09, 0.42)	Favors Herbst
Overjet	−4.82 (−5.83, −3.80)	−4.51 (·5.51, −3.51)	−5.09 (−5.82, −4.36)	4.40 (4.75, −4.05)	−4.82 (−5.83, −3.80)	Favors Herbst
Overbite	−1.69 (·3.18, −0.21)	1.57 (−3.23, 0.08)	3.01 (·3.47, −0.55)	2.40 (·2.69, −2.11)	1.69 (−3.18, −0.21)	Favors Herbst
Co-Go	1.76 (1.27, 2.26)		1.73 (0.90,2.56)	1.76 (1.27, 2.26)	1.76 (1.27, 2.26)	Favors Herbst
Co-Gn	1.74 (0.95,2.53)	2.03 (1.30,2.76)	1.67 (0.41, 2.93)	1.94 (1.41, 2.48)	1.74 (0.95, 2.53)	Favors Herbst
Molar relationship	−5.70 (−6.71, −4.69)	−5.50 (−6.74–, −4.26)	−6.12 (−7.05, −5.18)	−5.75 (−6.15, −5.34)	−5.70 (−6.71, −4.69)	Favors Herbst
A point-OIp.	−0.52 (−0.73, −0.30)	−0.53 (−0.75, −0.30)	−0.37 (−0.71, −0.03)	−0.52 (−0.73. −0.30)	−0.52 (−0.73, -0.30)	Favors Herbst
Pg OIp	1.45 (0.43, 2.47)	2.00 (0.27, 2.50)	2.46 (1.95, 2.97)	1.23 (0.89, 1.56)	1. 45 (0.43, 2.47)	Favors Control

Abbreviation: OLp, occlusal plane perpendicular.
Source: Yang *et al.* 2016. Reproduced with permission of Oxford University Press.

Key Findings

- The Herbst appliance can improve sagittal intermaxillary relationship, probably by a combination restricting the maxilla and allowing mandibular growth. The Herbst appliance has minimal effect on the mandibular angle.
- The Herbst appliance can improve the sagittal dental discrepancy.
- The results based on 12 nonrandomised controlled suggests that the Herbst appliance is effective for patients with Class II malocclusion.

Commentary

The limitations of this analysis are: the paucity high quality studies, preferably RCTs, lack of long-term outcomes, and unknown cephalometric magnifications. Due to low quality of evidence and publication bias, the results should be interpreted with caution.

Additional Reference

Manni A,Mutinelli S,Pasini M,*et al.,* 2016. Herbst appliance anchored to miniscrews with 2 types of ligation: effectiveness in skeletal Class II treatment. *Am J Orthod Dentofacial Orthop* 149, 871–880.

S32

Enamel roughness and incidence of caries after interproximal enamel reduction: a systematic review

Koretsi V, Chatzigianni A, Sidiropoulou S. Orthod Craniofac Res 2014;17:1–13.*

Background

Interproximal enamel reduction (IER) has become a widespread clinical procedure in orthodontics. The aim of this study was to investigate (i) enamel roughness and (ii) caries incidence after different IER methods on tooth surfaces as compared with untreated tooth surfaces.

Study Information

Population – tooth surfaces
Intervention – Any method or system of IER
Control group – untreated and healthy tooth surfaces
Outcome – (i) enamel roughness and (ii) incidence of caries after IER

Search Parameters

Inclusion criteria – (i) enamel roughness: *in vitro*/*in vivo* controlled studies, IER performed by one operator, control group of untreated enamel, scanning electron microscopy (SEM) and/or quantitative evaluation of enamel roughness; (ii) caries incidence: controlled clinical studies with or without randomization, treated and untreated teeth derived from the same patient, follow-up time of at least 1 year, clinical and/or radiographic examinations

Databases searched – PubMed, Scopus, the Cochrane Library, ProQuest, Web of Science, LILACS and the Brazilian bibliography of dentistry

Dates searched – up to March 2012, without limitations for date of publication

Other sources of evidence – hand searching of reference lists

Language restrictions – none

Search Results

After removal of duplicates, a total of 1740 records remained for assessing eligibility. Finally, 18 studies were included: (i) 14 assessing enamel roughness and (ii) four investigating caries incidence after IER. One of the latter studies evaluated teeth instead of tooth surfaces and thus was excluded.

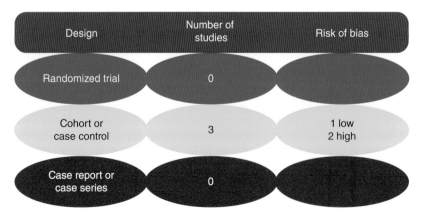

Design	Number of studies	Risk of bias
Randomized trial	0	
Cohort or case control	3	1 low 2 high
Case report or case series	0	

Study Results

The results for interproximal enamel reduction versus controls are shown in Table S32.1.

(i) Enamel roughness: due to high heterogeneity among included studies, namely various IER methods and systems and/or assessment methods, no quantitative synthesis of the data was possible.
(ii) Caries incidence: three studies were suitable for meta-analysis. Detailed results are presented in Table S32.1.

Table S32.1 Forest plot and confidence intervals (CI) for the incidence of caries after interproximal enamel reduction (IER) on tooth surfaces compared with untreated tooth surfaces (clinical and radiographic assessments).

		IER		Control			Odds ratio (95% CI)		
Study	Patients	Tooth surfaces	Carious lesions	Tooth surfaces	Carious lesions	Follow-up after IER		Favors IER	Favors control
Crain and Sheridan 1990	20	151	7	512	21	2 to 5 yr	1.137 (0.474, 2.727)		
Jarjoura *et al.* 2006	40	376	3	376	6	1 to 6.5 yr	0.496 (0.123, 1.998)		
Zachrisson *et al.* 2011	43	278	7	84	2	3.5 to 7 yr	1.059 (0.216, 5.197)		
Point estimate and 95% CI							0.926 (0.473, 1.812)		

Based on fixed effects: Heterogeneity Q = 1.01; df (Q) = 2, *P* = 0.603

Source: Koretsi *et al.* 2014. Reproduced with permission of John Wiley & Sons.

Key Findings

- Enamel roughness: it was not possible to draw firm conclusions on enamel roughness after IER owing to heterogeneity among studies.
- The incidence of caries on tooth surfaces previously treated with IER was statistically equivalent to that of untreated surfaces. IER did not increase the risk of caries on treated teeth.

Commentary

Even though no meta-analysis on enamel roughness after IER could be conducted, qualitative analysis was suggestive of the importance of polishing after any IER method or system used. Furthermore, more studies are needed with respect to caries incidence after IER to enable strong clinical conclusions.

S33

Prevalence of peg-shaped maxillary permanent lateral incisors: a meta-analysis

Hua F,* He H,* Ngan P,* Bouzid W. Am J Orthod Dentofacial Orthop 2013;144:97–109.

Background

Peg-shaped maxillary permanent lateral incisors (peg-laterals) can lead to esthetic, orthodontic, and periodontal problems for affected persons. The aims of this systematic review were to provide insight into the prevalence of peg-laterals and its association with races, sexes, population types, and continents of origin.

Study Information

Population – general population / dental patients / orthodontic patients
Intervention – not applicable (observational studies in epidemiology)
Comparison – not applicable (observational studies in epidemiology)
Outcome – prevalence of peg-laterals (number of people affected with peg-laterals divided by the number of people studied).

Search Parameters

Inclusion criteria – cross-sectional or retrospective studies using a diagnostic standard the same as or similar to "the incisal mesiodistal width of the tooth crown is shorter than the cervical width" with each participant as a study unit
Databases searched – PubMed, EMBASE, Google Scholar, Cochrane Central Register of Controlled Trials, metaRegister of Controlled Trials, OpenGrey
Dates searched – from inception to October 2011
Other sources of evidence – hand searching of reference lists
Language restrictions – none.

Search Results

3337 records were identified, of which 30 (36 studies / substudies, 17 countries, 87 172 subjects) remained after the application of eligibility criteria.

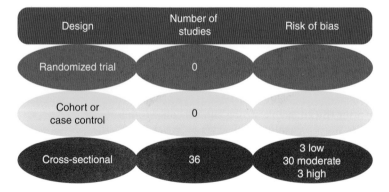

Design	Number of studies	Risk of bias
Randomized trial	0	
Cohort or case control	0	
Cross-sectional	36	3 low 30 moderate 3 high

Study Results

The prevalence of peg-shaped lateral incisors in different population groups are shown in Tables S33.1 and S33.2.

Table S33.1 Prevalence of peg-shaped lateral in differenta populations.

Study	Sample size	Prevalence in % (95% CI)	Weight (%)	
A, General population 22 studies				
Subtotal (I^2=94.4%, P=0.000)	65728	1.6 (1.2, 2.0)	66.87	
B, Dental patients 6 studies				
Subtotal (I^2=93.4%, P =0.000)		1.9 (0.9, 2.8)	16.23	
C, Orthodontic patients 8 studies				
Subtotal (I^2=81.7%, P=0.000)	12269	2.7 (1.9, 3.5)	16.90	
Overall (I^2=94.5%, P=0.000)	9175	1.8 (1.5, 2.1)	100	
Weights – random effects analysis				0 ——— 15.5%

Source: Hua *et al*. 2013. Reproduced with permission of Elsevier.

Tables S33.2 Prevalence of peg-shaped laterals by gender in different ethnic groups.

Study	Female		Male		Risk ratio, 95% CI	Weight (%)	Favors Female	Favors Male
	Events	Total	Events	Total				
A, Black (2 studies)	24	1300	15	1264	1.56 (0.82, 2.96)	7.2		
Heterogeneity: Chi^2 = 0.65 df = 1 (P = 0.42), I^2 = 0% Test for overall effect: Z = 1.36 (p = 0.18)								
B, White (3 studies)	50	4090	50	6054	1.42 (0.95, 2.12)	19.0		
Heterogeneity: Chi^2 = 2.89 df = 2 (P = 0.24), I^2 = 31% Test for overall effect: Z = 1.69 (P = 0.09)								
C, Mongoloid (3 studies)	213	3951	146	3700	1.31 (1.07, 1.61)	73.4		
Heterogeneity: Chi^2 = 0.76 df = 2 (P = 0.68), I^2 = 0% Test for overall effect: Z = 2.59 (P = 0.010)								
D, Indian (1 study)	1	210	1	290	1.38 (0.09, 21.95)	0.4		
Heterogeneity: Not applicable Test for overall effect: Z = 0.23 (P = 0.82)								
Total (95% CI)	228	9551	212	11308	1.35 (1.13, 1.61)	100		
Heterogeneity: Chi^2 = 4.51 df = 8 (P = 0.81), I^2 = 0% Test for overall effect: Z = 3.35 (P = 0.0008) Test for subgroup differences: Chi^2 = 0.32 df = 3 (P = 0.96), I^2 = 0%							0.02 0.1 1 10 50	

Source: Hua *et al*. 2013. Reproduced with permission of Elsevier.

Key Findings

- About 1 in every 55 people (1.8%) is affected with peg-laterals.
- Women are 35% more likely than men to have peg-laterals.
- The prevalence of peg-laterals is higher in Mongoloid people (3.1%) than in black (1.5%) and white (1.3%) people.
- Although unilateral and bilateral peg-laterals seem equally common, the left side is twice as common as the right side among unilateral cases.
- Subjects with unilateral peg-laterals have a 55% chance of having lateral incisor hypodontia on the contralateral side.

Commentary

The epidemiological features summarized in this review are helpful for orthodontists, especially those working in multiethnic communities, in their examination and treatment of patients with peg-laterals. Findings of several recent studies are similar to those reported in this review (Karatas *et al.* 2014; Kim *et al.* 2014).

Additional references for Summary 33 can be found on page 206.

S34

Craniofacial and upper airway morphology in adult obstructive sleep apnea patients: a systematic review and meta-analysis of cephalometric studies

Neelapu BC, Kharbanda OP,* Sardana HK, Balachandran R, Sardana V, Kapoor P, Gupta A, Vasamsetti S. Sleep Med Rev 2017;31:79–90.

Background

The objective of the systematic review is to determine any altered craniofacial anatomy on lateral cephalograms in adult subjects with established obstructive sleep apnea (OSA).

Study Information

Population – nonsyndrome adult subjects >18 years of age with a diagnosis of OSA by overnight polysomnography (PSG)

Interventions – studies evaluating craniofacial and neck regions in adult OSA subjects using lateral cephalograms (including cone beam computed tomography derived)

Comparators – healthy non-OSA individuals versus OSA patients

Outcome – studies providing craniofacial and upper airway morphology in terms of linear and angular measurements.

Search Parameters

Inclusion criteria – randomized controlled trials assessing DBP and SBP
Databases searched – PUBMED, SCOPUS, and Google Scholar
Dates searched – up to Dec 2014
Other sources of evidence – hand searching of reference lists.
Language restrictions – only English.

Search Results

Initial search revealed 646 articles of which 241 were duplicates, 328 articles excluded based on abstracts, and 51 excluded based on full text. Finally, only 26 articles fulfilled inclusion criteria of this study and were analyzed for systematic review.

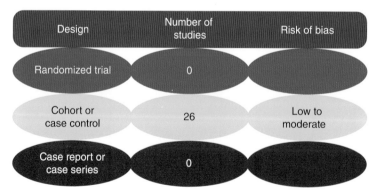

Design	Number of studies	Risk of bias
Randomized trial	0	
Cohort or case control	26	Low to moderate
Case report or case series	0	

Study Results

Out of the 27 craniofacial parameters originally evaluated only two are shown: (A) posterior nasal spine to pharyngeal wall and (B) anterior nasal spine to gnathion (Table S34.1).

Table S34.1 Effect of obstructive sleep apnea on two craniofacial measurements.

A, Pooled results for posterior nasal spine to pharyngeal wall (PNS to Phw)

Authors	OSA Mean	SD	Total	Control Mean	SD	Total	Weight %	Mean difference, Random, 95% CI
Kukaw 1988	27	4	30	30	4	12	9.6	−3.00 (−5.68 to −0.32)
Blanks 1988	29	4	90	29	4	12	11.5	0.00 (−2.41 to 2.41)
Seto 2001	23.4	0.8	29	24.85	0.59	21	72.1	−1.45 (−1.84 to −1.06)
Vidovic 2103	24.34	5.36	20	27.49	5.1	20	6.8	−3.15 (−6.39 to 0.09)
Summary			169			65	100	−1.5 (−2.43 to −0.67)

Favors OSA patient | Favors controls

Heterogeneity: Tau^2 = 0.24; Chi^2 = 3.73, df = 3; P = 0.29; I^2 = 19%
Test for overall effect Z = 3.44 (P = 0.0006)

B, Pooled results for anterior lower face height (ANS to Gn)

Andersson 1991	70.4	6.8	23	69.8	5.2	28	20.9	0.60 (−2.78 to 3.98)
Hui 2003	71.9	5.9	69	69.9	5.2	25	33.8	2.00 (−0.47 to 4.47)
Tangugsorn 1995	75.93	6.34	100	72.22	4.7	36	45.3	3.71 (1.73 to 5.69)
Summary			192			89	100	2.48 (0.78 to 4.19)

Heterogeneity: Tau^2 = 0.66; Chi^2 = 2.78, df = 2; P = 0.25; I^2 = 29%
Test for overall effect Z = 2.85 (P = 0.004)

Source: Neelapu *et al.* 2017. Reproduced with permission of Elsevier.

Key Findings

- 2.48 mm increase in lower anterior facial height;
- 5.45 mm inferior position of hyoid bone;
- 6.89 mm increase sella to hyoid bone;
- 495.74 mm^2 decreased pharyngeal airway space and 151.14 mm^2 decrease in oropharyngeal airway.

Caution should be given to the following parameters due to significant heterogeneity between primary studies:

- 2.25 mm decrease in S-N and 1.45 degree decrease in cranial base angle N-S-Ba;
- 1.49 degrees SNB, less prominent mandible;
- 5.66 mm decreased mandibular length;
- 1.76 mm decrease in maxillary length;
- 366.5 mm^2 increase in tongue area;
- 125 mm^2 increase in soft palate area;
- 5.39 mm increase in upper airway length.

Commentary

Further assessments could have been made on three-dimensional volumetric analysis of craniofacial and pharyngeal structures (Kecik 2017).

Additional Reference

Kecik D, 2017. Three-dimensional analyses of palatal morphology and its relation to upper airway area in obstructive sleep apnea. *Angle Orthod* 87, 300–306.

S35

Myofunctional therapy to treat obstructive sleep apnea: a systematic review and meta-analysis

Camacho M,* Certal V, Abdullatif J, Zaghi S, Ruoff CM, Capasso R, Kushida CA. Sleep 2015; 38:669–675. (Additional summary authors: Fernandez-Salvador C and Reckley L)

Background

One of the major causes for obstructive sleep apnea (OSA) is due to the laxity of the dilator muscles of the upper airway, which fail to maintain a patent airway during sleep. As a result, researchers have focused a tremendous effort at treatment modalities that target oral and oropharyngeal muscular structures for OSA. This systematic review is aimed at evaluating myofunctional therapy (MT) as treatment for OSA in children and adults and to perform a meta-analysis on the polysomnographic, snoring, and sleepiness data.

Study Information

Population – children and adults with OSA
Intervention – myofunctional therapy treatment
Comparison – myofunctional therapy versus patients never trained to perform the exercises
Outcome – Apnea-Hypopnea Index (AHI), lowest oxygen saturations (low O_2), snoring and Epworth Sleepiness Scale (ESS).

Search Parameters

Inclusion criteria – evaluating oral or oropharyngeal MT as an isolated treatment for either adult or pediatric OSA
Databases searched – PubMed, Medline, Web of Science, Scopus, and Cochrane
Dates searched – the searches were performed through June 18, 2014
Other sources of evidence – nonelectronic journals were hand searched
Language restrictions – none.

Search Results

A total of 226 citations were identified. After further review, a total of 11 studies met criteria and were included in this review.

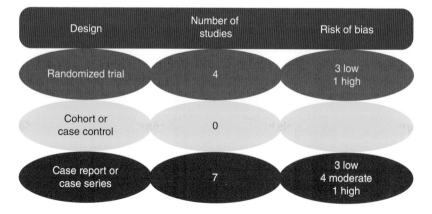

Design	Number of studies	Risk of bias
Randomized trial	4	3 low 1 high
Cohort or case control	0	
Case report or case series	7	3 low 4 moderate 1 high

Study Results

The outcomes for Apnea-Hypoapnea Index, low oxygen saturations, and Epworth Sleepiness Scale are shown in Table S35.1

Table S35.1 Outcomes for pre- and postmyofunctional therapies in terms of Apnea-Hypopnea Index (AHI), low oxygen levels, and Epworth sleepiness scale (ESS) (9 studies).

Study design Includes PCS, RCT, RCR, RCS, ABS	n	Age (yr)	BMI (kg/m^2)	AHI (event/h) Pre-MT	AHI (event/h) Post-MT	Low O$_2$ (%) Pre-MT	Low O$_2$ (%) Post-MT	ESS Pre-MT	ESS Post-MT
Total	120	44.5 ± 11.6	28.9 ± 6.2	24.5 ± 14.3	12.3 ± 11.8	83.9 ± 6.0	86.6 ± 7.3	14.8 ± 3.5	8.2 ± 4.1

Nine studies: Suzuki *et al.* 2013, Kronbauer *et al.* 2013, Diaferia *et al.* 2013, Baz *et al.* 2012, Guimaraes *et al.* 2009, de Paula Silva *et al.* 2007, Berreto *et al.* 2007, Guimaraes *et al.* 2003, Guimaraes *et al.* 1999.
Abbreviations: BMI, body mass index; MT, myofunctional therapy; PCS, prospective case series; RCR, retrospective case report; RCS, retrospective case series; RCT, randomized controlled trial.
Source: Adapted from Camacho *et al.* 2015.

Key Findings

- Evidence demonstrates that myofunctional therapy decreases Apnea-Hypopnea Index by approximately 50% in adults and 62% in children.
- Lowest oxygen saturations, snoring, and sleepiness outcomes are shown to improve in adults after proper myofunctional therapy.
- Myofunctional therapy was not shown to be curative, but could serve as an adjunct to other obstructive sleep apnea treatments.

Commentary

Since the publication of this systematic review and meta-analysis, there has been additional published literature validating the efficiency and effectiveness of myofunctional therapy for obstructive sleep apnea (Chuang *et al.* 2017; Corrêa Cde and Berretin-Felix 2015; Guilleminault and Akhtar 2015; Morgan 2016).

Additional References

Chuang L, Yun-Chia L, Hervy-Auboiron M, *et al.*, 2017. Passive myofunctional therapy applied on children with obstructive sleep apnea: A 6-month follow-up. *J Formos Med Assoc* 116, 536–541.

Corrêa Cde C, Berretin-Felix G, 2015. Myofunctional therapy applied to upper airway resistance syndrome: A case report. *Codas* 27, 604–609.

Guilleminault C, Akhtar F, 2015. Pediatric sleep-disordered breathing: New evidence on its development. *Sleep Med Rev* 24, 46–56.

Morgan T, 2016. Novel approaches to the management of sleep-disordered breathing. *Sleep Med Clin* 11, 173–187.

Disclaimer

The views expressed in this abstract/manuscript are those of the author(s) and do not reflect the official policy or position of the Department of the Army, Department of Defense, or the US Government.

S36

CPAP vs mandibular advancement devices and blood pressure in patients with obstructive sleep apnea: a systematic review and meta-analysis

Bratton DJ, Gaisl T, Wons AM, Kohler M.* JAMA 2015;314:2280–2293.

Background

Obstructive sleep apnea (OSA) is associated with higher levels of blood pressure, which can lead to increased cardiovascular risk.

Study Information

Population – subjects 18+ years of age with a diagnosis of obstructive sleep apnea (defined as a apnea-hypopnea index of ≥5 per hour)

Interventions – continuous positive air pressure (CPAP) or mandibular advancement devices (MADs)

Comparison – different devices or inactive devices

Outcome – reduction in diastolic (DBP) and systolic (SBP) blood pressure

Search Parameters

Inclusion criteria – randomized controlled trials (RCTs) assessing DBP and SBP

Databases searched – MEDLINE, EMBASE, and the Cochrane Library

Dates searched – up to August 2015

Other sources of evidence – hand searching of reference lists

Language restrictions – none.

Search Results

Inclusion was restricted to trials reported in English. 872 studies were identified, of which 51 RCTs (4888 participants) met the inclusion criteria. 44 RCTs compared CPAP with an inactive control, three compared MADs with an inactive control, one compared CPAP with an MAD, three compared CPAP, MADs, and an inactive control. No more than 10% of the included trials were deemed to be at high risk of bias.

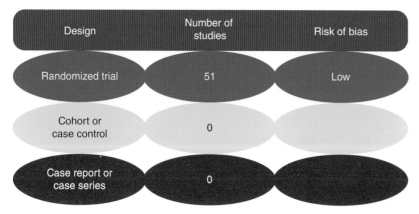

Design	Number of studies	Risk of bias
Randomized trial	51	Low
Cohort or case control	0	
Case report or case series	0	

Study Results

The study outcomes for systolic blood pressure using MAD and CPAP versus controls are shown in Tables S36.1 and S36.2.

Table S36.1 Treatment effect for change in Systolic Blood Pressure (SBP) in the included trial of continuous airway pressure (CPAP) versus Inactive control.

CPAP versus Inactive control	Change in SBP Treatment Difference (95%CI), mmHg	Weight %	Favors CPAP	Favors inactive control
2-Group trials				
44 RCTs CPAP versus inactive control (summarized)	−2.5 (−3.4 to 1.5)	92.6		
3-Group trials				
Barnes *et al.* 2004	−0.9 (−3.3 to 1.5)	3.9		
Dal-Fabbro *et al.* 2014	−1.4 (−7.2 to 4.4)	1.9		
Lam *et al.* 2007	−6.1 (−12.8 to 0.6)	1.6		
Pairwise meta-analysis	**−2.6 (−3.6 to −1.6)**			
Network meta-analysis	**−2.5 (−3.5 to −1.5)**			

The size of each data marker is proportional to the weight carried by the corresponding study in the random-effects pairwise meta-analysis.
Source: Adapted from Bratton *et al.* 2015.

Table S36.2 Treatment effect for change in systolic blood pressure (SBP) in the included trials of mandibular advancement device (MAD) versus continuous positive airway pressure (CPAP) and versus inactive controls.

MAD versus inactive control	Change in SBP treatment difference (95%CI), mmHg	Favors MAD	Favors inactive controls
2 and 3 group trials			
Pairwise meta-analysis	−1.9 (−3.2 to −0.6)		
Network meta-analysis	−2.1 (−3.4 to −0.8)		

Change in SBP treatment difference (95% CI), mmHg

2 group trails: Andrén *et al.* 2013, Gotsopoulos *et al.* 2004, Quinnell *et al.* 2014
3 group trials: Barnes *et al.* 2004, Dal-Fabbro *et al.* 2014, Lam *et al.* 2007

CPAP versus MAD		Favors CPAP	Favors MAD
2 and 3 group trials			
Pairwise meta-analysis	0.3 (−1.0 to 1.5)		
Network meta-analysis	−0.5 (−2.0 to 1.0)		

Change in SBP treatment difference (95% CI), mmHg

2 group trial: Phillips *et al.* 2013
3 group trials: Barnes *et al.* 2004, Dal-Fabbro *et al.* 2014, Lam *et al.* 2007

Source: Adapted from Bratton *et al.* 2015.

Key Findings

- Both CPAP and MADs were associated with a significant reduction in blood pressure (2 mmHg).
- Network meta-analysis did not identify a statistically significant difference between the BP outcomes with these two therapies.

Commentary

A recent network meta-analysis comparing CPAP versus MADs indicates that CPAP devices are more effective than MADs at reducing daytime sleepiness (although both are effective) (Bratton *et al.* 2015). A 2 mmHg reduction in blood pressure can reduce by 10% the societal burden of blood pressure-related chronic heart disease, stroke, and heart failure (Hardy *et al.* 2015).

Additional references for Summary 36 can be found on page 206.

S37

Orthodontic and orthopaedic treatment for anterior open bite in children

Lentini-Oliveira DA,* Carvalho FR, Rodrigues CG, Ye Q, Hu R, Minami-Sugaya H, Carvalho LBC, Prado LBF, Prado GF. Cochrane Database Syst Rev 2014;(9):CD005515.

Background

Anterior open bite (AOB) is a lack of vertical overlap or contact of the upper and lower incisors. Etiological factors include inherited features, environmental factors, digit sucking, and breathing disorders. Although there is extensive literature written on anterior open bite, the various interventions are not supported by any strong scientific evidence. The aim of this systematic review was to evaluate orthodontic and orthopedic treatments to correct anterior open bite in children.

Study Information

Population – children and adolescents with anterior open bite
Intervention – orthodontic or orthopedic interventions (nonsurgical)
Comparison – orthopedic treatment versus no intervention, or another technique
Outcome – correction of AOB; stability; impact on atypical swallowing or respiratory diseases.

Search Parameters

Inclusion criteria – randomized controlled trials (RCTs) or quasi RCTs
Databases searched – Cochrane Library, MEDLINE, EMBASE, LILACS, Brazilian Bibliography of Odontology, SciELO, and ClinicalTrials.gov
Dates searched – up to 14th February 2014
Other sources of evidence – hand searching reference lists. Chinese publications were also searched
Language restrictions – none.

Search Results

576 studies were identified, three studies met the inclusion criteria.

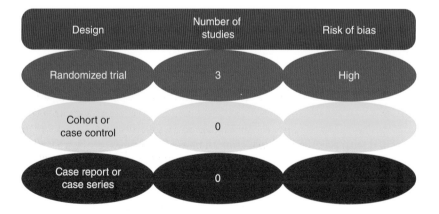

Design	Number of studies	Risk of bias
Randomized trial	3	High
Cohort or case control	0	
Case report or case series	0	

Study Results

The effect of the interventions to correct open bite are shown in Table S37.1.

Table S37.1 Treatment effects of two interventions on open bite (mm) versus no treatment.

Author	Study	Control	Intervention	Weight %	Mean difference, Risk ratio (fixed) 95%CI		
						Favors intervention	Favors control
Almeida 2005	Removable appliance with palatal crib associated with high-pull chin cup versus no treatment controls	4	24	100	0.23 (0.11 to 0.48)		
Total	Test for overall effect Z = 3.94 (*P* < 0.0001)	4	24	100	0.23 (0.11 to 0.48)		
Erbay 1995	Frankel functional regulator FR-4) and lip sealing treatment versus no treatment controls	0	20	100	0.02 (0.00, 0.38)		
Total	Test for overall effect Z = 2.66 (*P* = 0.008)	0	20	100	0.02 (0.00, 0.38)		

The study using repelling magnetic splints versus bite blocks was terminated early due to side effects (Kiliaridis 1990).
Source: Adapted from Lentini-Oliveira *et al.* 2014.

Key Findings

- The studies on AOB lack standardization. Therefore, there is no clear evidence on which to make a clinical decision for the type of intervention to use in AOB patients.
- The evidence is weak for two interventions: Frankel's function regulator-4 with lip-seal training and removable palatal crib with high-pull chin cup.

Commentary

Studies on the correction of AOB require sample sizes based on power calculation, adequate and detailed sequence of randomization with allocation concealment, blind outcome assessment, and completeness of follow up. If there are drop outs, an intention-to-treat analysis should be done and all data described. In addition, the possible association among open bite, respiratory pattern, sleep respiratory disturbance, and snoring should be considered by researchers (Pacheco *et al.* 2015).

Additional Reference

Pacheco MC, Fiorott BS, Finck NS, *et al.*, 2015. Craniofacial changes and symptoms of sleep-disordered breathing in healthy children. *Dental Press J Orthod* 20, 80–87.

Acknowledgement

This Cochrane Review was published in the Cochrane Database of Systematic Reviews 2014, Issue 9. Cochrane Reviews are regularly updated as new evidence emerges and in response to feedback, and the Cochrane Database of Systematic Reviews should be consulted for the most recent version of the Cochrane Review.

S38

Stability of treatment for anterior open-bite malocclusion: a meta-analysis

Greenlee GM,* Huang GJ,* Chen SS, Chen J, Koepsell T, Hujoel P. Am J Orthod Dentofacial Orthop 2011;139:154–169.

Background

Historically, anterior open-bite malocclusions have been challenging to correct, and perhaps even more challenging to retain. In this review, we aimed to investigate the stability of open-bite correction based on the best available literature.

Study Information

Population – orthodontic patients with anterior open-bite
Intervention – conventional dentoalveolar correction
Comparison – treatment follow-up in nonsurgical and surgical corrections of open bites
Outcome – stability 12 or more months after treatment.

Search Parameters

Inclusion criteria – clinical studies reporting on stability of open-bite correction longer than 1 year
Databases searched – PubMed, Embase, Cochrane Library
Dates searched – 1949 to May 2009
Other sources of evidence – hand searching of reference lists
Language restrictions – none.

Search Results

105 references were identified, 21 of which met the inclusion criteria. Overbite means from 16 studies were analyzed in forest plots, and 15 used in a dichotomous stability analysis (presence of positive overbite).

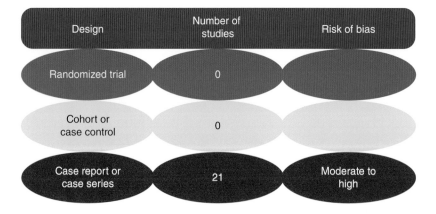

Design	Number of studies	Risk of bias
Randomized trial	0	
Cohort or case control	0	
Case report or case series	21	Moderate to high

Study Results

The long-term follow-up for open bite correction in surgical and nonsurgical patients are shown in Tables S38.1 and S38.2.

Table S38.1 Long-term overbite status in surgical studies.

Authors	Class/type	Follow-up years	Overbite (mm) Random effects model, 95% CI
Lawry 1990	–	1.5	
McNance 1992	Class II	1	
McNance 1992	Class III	1	
Kahnberg 1994	–	1.5	
Hoppenreijs 1997	–	5.7	
Arpornmaeklong 2000	–	2	
Fischer 2000	–	2	
Moldez 2000	Max. impaction	5	
Moldez 2000	Rotation	5	
Ding 2007	–	15	
Espeland 2008	–	3	
Total 95% CI			1.27

Source: Greenlee *et al.* 2011. Reproduced with permission of Elsevier.

Table S38.2 Long-term overbite status in nonsurgical studies.

Authors	Class/type	Follow-up years	Overbite (mm) Random effects model, 95% CI
Nelson 1991	–	2	
Katsaros 1993	–	2	
Küçükkeles 1999	–	1	
Kim 2000	Growing	2	
Kim 2000	Nongrowing	2	
Suguwara 2002	–	1	
Janson 2006	Nonextraction	5.2	
Janson 2006	Extraction	8.4	
Remmers 2008	–	5	
Total 95% CI			0.76

Source: Greenlee *et al.* 2011. Reproduced with permission of Elsevier.

Key Findings

- The surgical studies reported on adults, while the nonsurgical studies largely reported on adolescents.
- The success rates based on dichotomous presence of overbite at the latest follow-up time were 82% and 75%, respectively.
- The included evidence consists of lower level studies, and these results should be viewed with caution.

Commentary

Due to the differences in age between the two study populations, it is difficult to draw direct comparisons. However, the initial mean open-bite values were similar in the surgical and nonsurgical populations, while the mandibular plane angles in the surgical patients were slightly steeper. Since the time of this review, more literature has been published utilizing temporary anchorage devices (TADs) to intrude molars, thereby assisting with bite closure. This mechanism is similar to that accomplished with maxillary impaction surgery, but the long-term stability of intrusion with TADs has not been well documented to date. Additionally, some are advocating mandibular surgery to correct anterior open-bites. Finally, there have been reports that aligners with occlusal coverage may be a useful strategy to close open-bites, as they may create a posterior bite block effect. Inclusion of six new studies in the dichotomous analysis indicates similar long-term stability of closure at 82% for surgical treatment and 80% for nonsurgical treatment. More evidence is needed for all of these newer techniques.

Additional references for Summary 38 can be found on page 206.

S39

Pharmacological interventions for pain relief during orthodontic treatment

Monk AB, Harrison JE,* Worthington HV, Teague A. Cochrane Database Syst Rev 2017;(11):CD003976.

Background

Studies suggest that up to 95% of orthodontic patients report pain during their treatment. Pain during orthodontic treatment is the most common reason for patients wanting to discontinue treatment and ranked as the worst aspect of treatment (Oliver and Knapman 1985). The objective of this review was to determine the most effective drug intervention for pain relief during orthodontic treatment.

Study Information

Population – participants of any age receiving any type of orthodontic treatment
Intervention – any pharmacological pain relief, taken by any route, dose, form, or combination, at any time during treatment
Comparison – placebo or the same intervention at a different dose, intensity, or time interval
Outcome – self-reported pain intensity/relief measured by any scale.

Search Parameters

Inclusion criteria – randomized controlled trials (RCTs) relating to pain control during orthodontic treatment measured on a visual analogue scale (VAS), numerical rating scale (NRS), or any categorical scale
Databases searched – OHG Trials Register, Cochrane Pain, Palliative and Supportive Care Group Trials Register, Cochrane Central Register of Controlled Trials, MEDLINE, EMBASE, CINAHL
Dates searched – 1966 to June 19, 2017
Other sources of evidence – hand searching of reference lists
Language restrictions – none.

Search Results

The search identified 32 relevant RCTs, which included 3110 participants aged 9 to 34 years, 2348 of whom were included in the analyses.

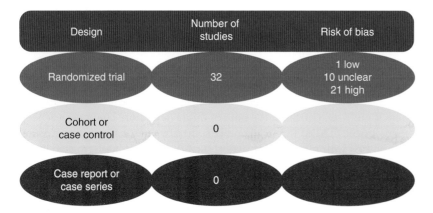

Design	Number of studies	Risk of bias
Randomized trial	32	1 low 10 unclear 21 high
Cohort or case control	0	
Case report or case series	0	

Pain

Study Results

Table S39.1 Pain measured using visual analogue scales (VAS) during orthodontic treatment: analgesic versus controls.

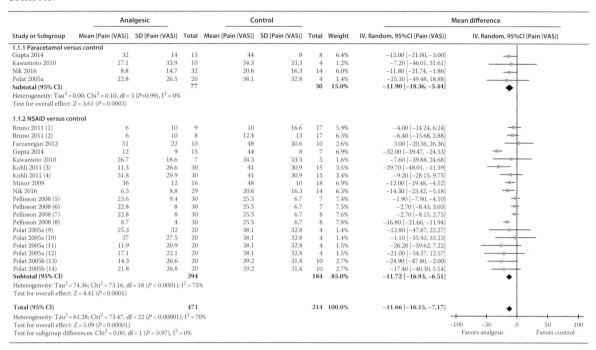

Study or Subgroup	Analgesic Mean [Pain (VAS)]	SD [Pain (VAS)]	Total	Control Mean [Pain (VAS)]	SD [Pain (VAS)]	Total	Weight	Mean difference IV, Random, 95%CI [Pain (VAS)]
1.1.1 Paracetamol versus control								
Gupta 2014	32	14	15	44	8	8	6.4%	−12.00 [−21.00, −3.00]
Kawamoto 2010	27.1	33.9	10	34.3	33.3	4	1.2%	−7.20 [−46.01, 31.61]
Nik 2016	8.8	14.7	32	20.6	16.3	14	6.0%	−11.80 [−21.74, −1.86]
Polat 2005a	22.8	26.5	20	38.1	32.8	4	1.4%	−15.30 [−49.48, 18.88]
Subtotal (95% CI)			**77**			**30**	**15.0%**	**−11.90 [−18.36, −5.44]**
Heterogeneity: Tau² = 0.00; Chi² = 0.10, df = 3 (P=0.99), I² = 0%								
Test for overall effect: Z = 3.61 (P = 0.0003)								
1.1.2 NSAID versus control								
Bruno 2011 (1)	6	10	9	10	16.6	17	5.9%	−4.00 [−14.24, 6.24]
Bruno 2011 (2)	6	10	8	12.4	13	17	6.3%	−6.40 [−15.68, 2.88]
Farzanegan 2012	51	22	10	48	30.6	10	2.6%	3.00 [−20.36, 26.36]
Gupta 2014	12	9	15	44	8	7	6.9%	−32.00 [−39.47, −24.53]
Kawamoto 2010	26.7	18.6	7	34.3	33.3	5	1.6%	−7.60 [−39.88, 24.68]
Kohli 2011 (3)	11.3	26.6	30	41	30.9	15	3.5%	−29.70 [−48.01, −11.39]
Kohli 2011 (4)	31.8	29.9	30	41	30.9	15	3.4%	−9.20 [−28.15, 9.75]
Minor 2009	36	12	16	48	10	18	6.9%	−12.00 [−19.48, −4.52]
Nik 2016	6.3	8.8	29	20.6	16.3	14	6.3%	−14.30 [−23.42, −5.18]
Pellisson 2008 (5)	23.6	9.4	30	25.5	6.7	7	7.4%	−1.90 [−7.90, −4.10]
Pellisson 2008 (6)	22.8	8	30	25.5	6.7	7	7.5%	−2.70 [−8.43, 3.03]
Pellisson 2008 (7)	22.8	8	30	25.5	6.7	8	7.6%	−2.70 [−8.15, 2.75]
Pellisson 2008 (8)	8.7	4	30	25.5	6.7	8	7.8%	−16.80 [−21.66, −11.94]
Polat 2005a (9)	25.3	32	20	38.1	32.8	4	1.4%	−12.80 [−47.87, 22.27]
Polat 2005a (10)	37	27.5	20	38.1	32.8	4	1.4%	−1.10 [−35.43, 33.23]
Polat 2005a (11)	11.9	20.9	20	38.1	32.8	4	1.5%	−26.20 [−59.62, 7.22]
Polat 2005a (12)	17.1	22.1	20	38.1	32.8	4	1.5%	−21.00 [−54.57, 12.57]
Polat 2005b (13)	14.3	26.6	20	39.2	31.8	10	2.7%	−24.90 [−47.80, −2.00]
Polat 2005b (14)	21.8	26.8	20	39.2	31.8	10	2.7%	−17.40 [−40.30, 5.54]
Subtotal (95% CI)			**394**			**184**	**85.0%**	**−11.72 [−16.93, −6.51]**
Heterogeneity: Tau² = 74.36; Chi² = 73.16, df = 18 (P < 0.0001); I² = 75%								
Test for overall effect: Z = 4.41 (P < 0.0001)								
Total (95% CI)			**471**			**214**	**100.0%**	**−11.66 [−16.15, −7.17]**
Heterogeneity: Tau² = 61.28; Chi² = 73.47, df = 22 (P < 0.00001); I² = 70%								
Test for overall effect: Z = 5.09 (P < 0.00001)								
Test for subgroup differences: Chi² = 0.00, df = 1 (P = 0.97), I² = 0%								

Favors analgesic   Favors control

Source: Monk *et al.* 2017. Reproduced with permission of John Wiley & Sons.

Key Findings

- Paracetamol and nonsteriodal anti-inflammatory drugs (NSAIDs) were effective at reducing pain intensity when compared to control at 2, 6, and 24 hours.
- There was no difference between NSAIDs and paracetamol at 2, 6, or 24 hours.
- Pre-emptive ibuprofen gave better pain relief at 2 hours than ibuprofen taken post-treatment.

Commentary

There is moderate to low quality evidence that the use of paracetamol or NSAIDs reduces the pain associated with orthodontic treatment. We found no clear evidence of a difference between the effect of ibuprofen and paracetamol at reducing pain associated with orthodontic treatment.

Additional Reference

Oliver R, Knapman Y, 1985. Attitudes to orthodontic treatment. *Br J Orthod* 12, 179–188.

Acknowledgement

This Cochrane Review was published in the Cochrane Database of Systematic Reviews 2017, Issue 11. Cochrane Reviews are regularly updated as new evidence emerges and in response to feedback, and the Cochrane Database of Systematic Reviews should be consulted for the most recent version of the Cochrane Review.

S40

Pharmacological management of pain during orthodontic treatment: a meta-analysis

Angelopoulou MV, Vlachou V, Halazonetis DJ. Orthod Craniofac Res 2012;15:71–83.*

Background

Pain during orthodontic treatment is a frequent complaint. Nonsteroidal anti-inflammatory drugs (NSAIDs) are the most common pain management method, but their effectiveness is debatable. The aim of this meta-analysis was to evaluate the effectiveness of NSAIDs in managing pain arising from orthodontic interventions.

Study Information

Population – orthodontic patients treated with fixed appliances
Intervention – nonsteroidal anti-inflammatory drugs
Comparison - NSAIDs versus placebo
Outcome – experience of pain evaluated with visual analogue scale (VAS).

Search Parameters

Inclusion criteria – randomized clinical trials comparing the efficacy of NSAIDs to placebo assessed by VAS in patients with fixed orthodontic appliances
Databases searched – PubMed, Google Scholar, Clinical Trials Cochrane
Dates searched – up to July 2010
Other sources of evidence – hand searching of reference lists
Language restrictions – none.

Search Results

1127 references were identified, seven of which met the inclusion criteria.

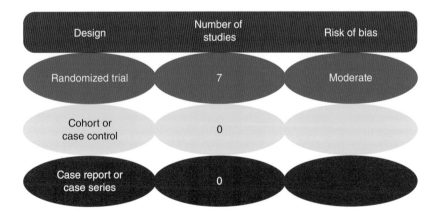

Design	Number of studies	Risk of bias
Randomized trial	7	Moderate
Cohort or case control	0	
Case report or case series	0	

Study Results

The pain reduction for chewing and biting activities for ibruprofen versus placebo and ibuprofen versus acetaminophen is shown in Table S40.1.

Table S40.1 Meta-analysis results: standardized treatment effect, calculated as Hedges' g, 95% confidence interval (CI) using random effects model, and I^2 values.

Activity	Time (hr)	Ibruprofen versus placebo (6 studies)			Ibuprofen versus acetaminophen (3 studies)		
		Treatment effect	95% CI	I^2	Treatment effect	95% CI	I^2
Chewing	2	−0.206	−0.550 to 0.138	0.456	0.049	−0.507 to 0.606	0.711*
	6	−0.386	−0.638 to −0.133	0.000	−0.076	−0.600 to 0.447	0.679*
		−0.270	−0.642 to 0.102	0.532	−0.003	−0.266 to 0.261	0.000
Biting	2	−0.560	−1.065 to −0.056	0.691*	−0.106	−0.488 to 0.276	0.421
	6	−0.513	−0.847 to −0.179	0.313	0.054	−0.617 to 0.725	0.801*
	24	−0.395	−0.828 to 0.037	0.592*	−0.072	−0.335 to 0.191	0.000

*$P < 0.05$

6 studies (Ngan *et al.* 1994; Steen Law *et al.* 2000; Polat *et al.* 2005; Polat and Karaman 2005; Salmassian *et al.* 2009; Minor *et al.* 2009).
3 studies (Arias and Marquez-Orozco 2006; Bird *et al.* 2007; Salmassian *et al.* 2009).
Source: Angelopoulou *et al.* 2012. Reproduced with permission of John Wiley & Sons.

Key Findings

- The results of this meta-analysis showed that NSAIDs reduced pain 2 and 6 hours after orthodontic intervention, but do not have a significant effect at 24 hours, when maximum pain occurs.
- Ibuprofen and acetaminophen were found equally effective, at all time points and activities, but the evidence is weak.
- Based on these findings NSAIDs can only achieve moderate pain reduction during orthodontic treatment.

Commentary

Additional RCTs have been published since this systematic review appeared, and according to a recent meta-analysis NSAIDs can be effective in reducing pain at its peak (Sandhu *et al.* 2016). In addition, more studies have tested the effect of laser therapy on pain management during orthodontic treatment, which can be an alternative option to comfort orthodontic patients (Ren *et al.* 2015).

Additional References

Sandhu SS, Cheema MS, Khehra HS, 2016. Comparative effectiveness of pharmacologic and nonpharmacologic interventions for orthodontic pain relief at peak pain intensity: a Bayesian network meta-analysis. *Am J Orthod Dentofacial Orthop* 150,13–32.
Ren C, McGrath C, Yang Y, 2015. The effectiveness of low-level diode laser therapy on orthodontic pain management: a systematic review and meta-analysis. *Lasers Med Sci* 30,1881–1893.

S41

Factors associated with patient and parent satisfaction after orthodontic treatment: a systematic review

Pachêco-Pereira C, Pereira JR, Dick BD, Perez A, Flores Mir C.* Am J Orthod Dentofacial Orthop 2015;148:652–659.

Background

Because of the different reasons for seeking orthodontic treatment, patients, parents, and orthodontists may assess treatment outcomes differently. Perceived satisfaction results from a combination of several factors. This systematic review aimed to identify factors associated with orthodontic treatment satisfaction among patients and their parents after orthodontic treatment.

Study Information

Population – patients or their legal representatives
Intervention – orthodontic treatment
Comparison – observational study
Outcome – satisfaction with orthodontic results.

Search Parameters

Inclusion criteria – patients, parents, or caregivers opinion about treatment results after orthodontic treatment
Databases searched – Medline, PubMed, Embase, EMB reviews, LILACS, Web of Science and Google Scholar
Dates searched – various initial dates, all up to March 2014
Other sources of evidence – partial gray literature and reference lists of included studies
Language restrictions – none.

Search Results

1149 unique citations were identified. 18 publications remained after inclusion criteria applied, but differences in their methodologies to assess treatment satisfaction made a meta-analysis questionable.

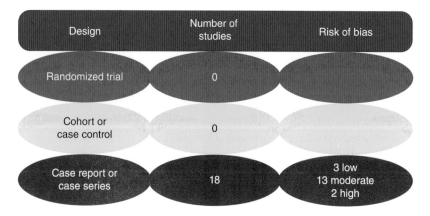

Design	Number of studies	Risk of bias
Randomized trial	0	
Cohort or case control	0	
Case report or case series	18	3 low 13 moderate 2 high

Study Results

The timing of data collection, surveying methods, response rate, and risk of bias are shown in Table S41.1.

Table S41.1 Summary of timing of data collection, surveying methods, response rate and risk of bias for the included studies.

Authors	Timing	Method of application of survey / response rate	RoB
Feldman 2014	At the first rescheduled visit (6 weeks) of retention	During retainer recall. Response rate 90–100%	4
Oliveira *et al.* 2013	Completed orthodontic treatment	Questionnaire applied in a recall consultation (timing not declared). Response rate 100%	3
Keles and Bos 2013	3 years of postorthodontics	Questionnaire applied 6 weeks after debonding. Response rate 55%	4
Maia *et al.* 2010	Postorthodontic treatment (mean 8.5 years)	Randomly selected by phone calls and invited to new records and questionnaire. Response rate 100%	4
Mollov *et al.* 2010	Retention stage average 5.3 years	Students surveyed during class time and finished patients were mailed. Response rate 77,11%	3
Anderson *et al.* 2009	Maximum 3.5 years postorthodontics	Questionnaire mailed. Response rate 96%	5
Uslu and Akcam 2007	Post-retention stage (5–22.5 years)	Mailed questionnaire. Response rate 15.8%	3
Al-Omiri and Abu Alhaija 2006	Retention stage (6–12 months)	Questionnaire mailed. 10 patients retested. Response rate 84%	6
Barker *et al.* 2005	Not specified. Patients at age 26	Questioned if treatment was either: excellent, pretty good, fair, or poor. Response rate 95.6%	5
Bos *et al.* 2005	3 years postorthodontic treatment	Questionnaire mailed to patients. Response rate 70%	4
Mascarenhas *et al.* 2005	At least 6 months of completion of treatment	Self-administered parental questionnaire at the end of orthodontic treatment. Response rate N/D	3
Bennett *et al.* 2001	Within 2 years after debonding	Phone interview and 18 month by a focus group. Final questionnaire mailed. Response rate 65% and 49%	7
Eberting *et al.* 2001	Not specified	Mailed questionnaire with 9 questions. Response rate 46.5%	2
Birkeland *et al.* 2000 2000	Children T1 and T2 + parents	Questionnaires filled by children on the day of examination. Parents mailed questionnaire. Response rate parents 83.3%, children 81.6%	5
Fernandes *et al.* 1999	Children and parents T1 and T2	Questionnaire at the examination follow up. Response rate child: 94.9%, parents 93.9%	5
Rieldmann *et al.* 1999	Adult patients >30 years, 42% wearing long-term retention	Mailed questionnaire. Response rate 80%	6
Bergstrom *et al.* 1998	8 years after the first consultation	Mailed questionnaire. Response rate 81%	6
Espeland and Stenvik 1993	Completed orthodontic treatment	During their annual visit. Response rate N/D	5

Abbreviation: RoB, risk of bias. The higher the number the higher the quality.
Source: Pachêco-Pereira *et al.* 2015. Reproduced with permission of Elsevier.

Key Findings

- Patients' and their parents' satisfaction levels with orthodontic treatment were generally high.
- Overall satisfaction was associated with pleasing perceived esthetic outcomes, perceived psychological benefits of treatment, positive patients' personality traits.
- Satisfaction also correlated to good quality of care linked to dentist–staff–patient.

Commentary

1) This systematic review reflects studies with limited evidence.
2) Dissatisfaction was associated with longer treatment duration, increased pain or discomfort levels, and problems with retention appliance usage.
3) The timing between treatment completion and assessment of patient treatment outcome satisfaction could affect answers.

S42

The effects of orthodontic therapy on periodontal health: a systematic review of controlled evidence

Bollen AM,* Cunha-Cruz J, Bakko DW, Huang GJ, Hujoel PP. J Am Dent Assoc 2008;139:413–422.

Background

It has been suggested that orthodontic treatment leads to improved periodontal health. The objective of this systematic review was to compare periodontal status between individuals who had received contemporary orthodontic treatment and those who had not by means of periodontal measures after end of treatment.

Study Information

Population – human (excluded studies on patients with periodontal disease or craniofacial anomalies)
Intervention – orthodontic treatment (excluded studies of treatment with fully banded appliances)
Comparison – no orthodontic treatment
Outcome – periodontal status
Length of follow-up – excluded studies that assessed periodontal outcomes only during treatment or at time of appliance removal.

Search Parameters

Inclusion Criteria – randomized controlled trials, cohort, case–control, and cross-sectional studies
Databases searched – Electronic search of eight databases: PubMed, Medline, Web of Science, Cochrane Library, Cochrane Central, Cochrane CDSR, DARE, HTA
Dates searched – 1980 to 2006
Other sources of evidence – search of bibliographic reference listings of published primary and review studies; contacted authors of relevant studies for additional information; electronic search of gray literature (Clinical Trials.gov, National Research Register UK, Pro-Quest Dissertation Abstracts, and Thesis Database); hand search of six dental journals
Language restrictions – none.

Search Results

The electronic search identified 3552 unique citations; the hand search identified 214 unique citations. After the inclusion criteria were applied, 12 publications remained. Differences in outcome measures (periodontal status) limited the possible statistical comparisons.

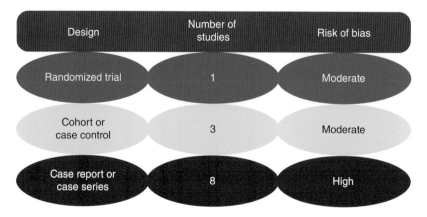

Design	Number of studies	Risk of bias
Randomized trial	1	Moderate
Cohort or case control	3	Moderate
Case report or case series	8	High

Study Results

The summary estimates for the three outcome measures (A) alveolar bone loss, (B) periodontal pocket depth, and (C) gingival recession are shown in Table S42.1.

Table S42.1 Summary estimate and individual results of cohort and cross-sectional studies reporting on the effect of orthodontic therapy on periodontal health: (A) alveolar bone loss, (B) periodontal pocket depth, and (C) gingival recession.

Study	Years after treatment	Mean difference, 95% CI	Favors orthodontic treatment	Favours control
A, Alveolar bone loss				
Ogaard 1988	5.7	0.13 (0.02, 0.24)		
Bondemark 1988	2.2	0.11 (−0.03, 0.25)		
Janson *et al.* 2003	2.7	0.16 (0.04, 0.28)		
Total		0.13 (0.07, 0.20)		

Heterogeneity: $Chi^2 = 0.31$, df = 2, $P = 0.86$, $I^2 = 0\%$
Test for overall effect: z = 3.88, $P = 0.0001$

B, Periodontal pocket depth				
Janson 1984	2.7	0.12 (−0.02, 0.26)		
Ribeiral *et al.* 1999	6.5	0.26 (0.18, 0.34)		
Total		0.23 (0.15, 0.30)		

Heterogeneity: $Chi^2 = 2.70$, df = 1, $P = 0.10$, $I^2 = 63\%$
Test for overall effect: z = 6.10, $P = 0.00001$

C, Gingival recession				
Ribeiral *et al.* 1999	6.5	0.03 (0.01, 0.05)		
Thomson 2002	8+	0.02 (−0.00, 0.04)		
Allais and Melsen 2003	NR	0.11 (−0.07, 0.29)		
Total		0.03 (0.01, 0.04)		

Heterogeneity: $Chi^2 = 1.27$, df = 2, $P = 0.53$, $I^2 = 0\%$
Test for overall effect: z = 4.08, $P = 0.0001$

(Forest plot axis: −0.5 −0.25 0 0.25 0.5)

Key Findings

- There is an absence of reliable evidence on the positive effects of orthodontic treatment on periodontal health.
- The existing limited evidence suggests a small overall worsening of periodontal status after orthodontic treatment.
- Claims that orthodontic treatment results in improved overall periodontal health cannot be supported with existing controlled evidence.

Commentary

1) The main limitation of the included studies is the lack of measurement of periodontal status prior to orthodontic treatment.
2) The limited data analyses indicated that orthodontic treatment slightly increased alveolar bone loss, periodontial pocket depth, and gingival recession.
3) Recent evidence supports the findings of the systematic review.

Additional references for Summary 42 can be found on page 207.

S43

Retention procedures for stabilizing tooth position after treatment with orthodontic braces

Littlewood SJ,* Millett DT, Doubleday B, Bearn DR, Worthington HV. Cochrane Database Syst Rev 2016;(1):CD002283.

Background

Retention is the phase of orthodontic treatment that attempts to keep teeth in the corrected positions after treatment. To reduce relapse, almost every orthodontic patient will require some type of retention after treatment. This Cochrane review evaluates the effects of different retention strategies used to stabilize tooth position after orthodontic braces.

Study Information

Population – orthodontic patients
Intervention – retainers or adjunctive procedures to reduce relapse
Comparison – different types of retainers or adjunctive procedures or no retainers
Outcome – stability, failures of retainers, adverse effects on health, patient satisfaction.

Search Parameters

Inclusion criteria – randomized controlled trials (RCTs) of retainers or adjunctive techniques
Databases searched – Cochrane Oral Health Groups Trial Register, Cochrane Central Register of Controlled Trials, MEDLINE, EMBASE
Dates searched – 1946 to Jan 2016
Other sources of evidence – ongoing trials registers, conference proceedings and abstracts, reference lists
Language restrictions – none.

Search Results

487 references were identified. 15 RCT studies met the inclusion criteria.

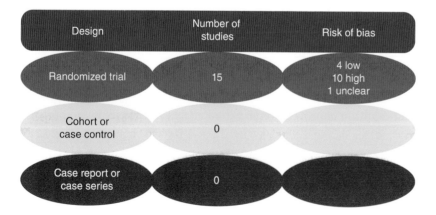

Design	Number of studies	Risk of bias
Randomized trial	15	4 low 10 high 1 unclear
Cohort or case control	0	
Case report or case series	0	

Study Results

Comparison of four different retention regimes after orthodontic tooth movement are shown in Table S43.1.

Table S43.1 Comparison of different retention regimes after orthodontic tooth movement (based on Little's Irregularity index for the lower labial segment).

Authors	Retention A n	Mean (SD)	Retention B n	Mean (SD)	Weight %	Odds ratio, Random, 95% CI
1, (A) Night wear Hawley 1 year versus						
(B) 24-hour wear for 6 months followed by night-time wear for 6 months						
Shawesh 2010	24	2 (1)	28	1.8 (0.7)	100	0.20 (−0.28, 0.68)
Subtotal	24		28			0.20 (−0.28, 0.68)
Test for overall effect: Z = 0.82 (P = 0.41)						
2, (A) Hawley 24-hour wear for 3 months followed by 12-hour wear versus						
(B) Thermoplastic for 12-hour wear for 1 week followed by night-time wear						
Rowland 2007	155	1.2 (0.98)	155	0.78 (0.72)	100	0.42 (0.23, 0.61)
Subtotal	155		155			0.42 (0.23, 0.61)
Test for overall effect: Z = 4.30 (P = 0.000017)						
3, (A) Upper and lower Begg 24-hour wear versus						
(B) Upper and lower thermoplastic retainers 24-hour wear						
Kumar 2011	112	0.37 (0.29)	112	0.12 (0.12)	100	0.25 (0.19, 0.31)
Subtotal	112		112			0.25 (0.19, 0.31)
Test for overall effect: Z = 8.43 (P = 0.00001)						
4, (A) Part-time 8 hours per day thermoplastic versus						
(B) 24 hours per day thermoplastic						
Gill 2007	29	0.31 (0.79)	28	0.29 (0.57)	100	0.02 (−0.34, 0.38)
Subtotal						0.02 (−0.34, 0.38)
Test for overall effect: Z = 0.11 (P = 0.91)						

Source: Littlewood *et al.* 2016. Reproduced with permission of John Wiley & Sons.

Key Findings

- There is no evidence that wearing thermoplastic retainers full time provides greater stability than wearing part time, but this was assessed in only a small number of participants.
- Patients who were judged to need a fixed retainer were excluded from the study.
- Overall there is insufficient high-quality evidence to make recommendations on retention procedures for stabilizing tooth position after orthodontic treatment.

Commentary

Retention studies are not easy to undertake, but several randomized controlled clinical trials have now been completed, showing that this research is feasible (Edman *et al.* 2013, Gill *et al.* 2007, O'Rouke *et al.* 2016, Thickett and Power 2010). Ideally, trials with longer-term follow-up of patients would be beneficial, looking at stability, survival of retainers, adverse effects on oral health, and patient satisfaction.

Additional references for Summary 43 can be found on page 207.

Acknowledgement

This Cochrane Review was published in the Cochrane Database of Systematic Reviews 2016, Issue 1. Cochrane Reviews are regularly updated as new evidence emerges and in response to feedback, and the Cochrane Database of Systematic Reviews should be consulted for the most recent version of the Cochrane Review.

S44

Performance of clear vacuum-formed thermoplastic retainers depending on retention protocol: a systematic review

Kaklamanos EG,* Kourakou M, Kloukos D, Doulis I, Kavvadia S. Odontology 2017;105:237–247.

Background

There still remains some uncertainty regarding the parameters of definitive retention protocols after orthodontic treatment. This review sought to investigate whether different vacuum-formed retainers (VFRs) wearing protocols perform differently in maintaining the therapeutic result.

Study Information

Population – patients in retention after orthodontic treatment of any type
Intervention – protocols including VFRs of any type and wearing schedule
Comparison – different VFR wearing schedules
Outcome – primarily, teeth alignment, arch form, and occlusion. Secondarily, patient reported outcomes, compliance, data on retainer condition and longevity, hard and soft oral tissue health, and possible adverse effects.

Search Parameters

Inclusion criteria – randomized and prospective controlled clinical trials comparing "full time" and "part time" VFRs wearing protocols
Databases searched – MEDLINE, EMBASE, Cochrane Oral Health Group's Trials Register, CENTRAL, ClinicalTrials.gov, the National Research Register, ProQuest Dissertation, and Theses Global
Dates searched – inception to August 2014
Other sources of evidence – hand searching of reference lists
Language restrictions – none.

Search Results

184 references were identified, three of which met the inclusion criteria.

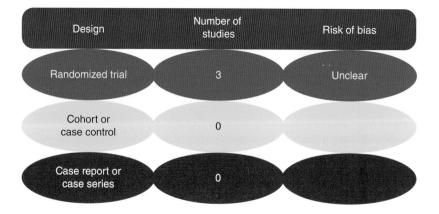

Design	Number of studies	Risk of bias
Randomized trial	3	Unclear
Cohort or case control	0	
Case report or case series	0	

Study Results

The various outcome measures for Little's Index, intercanine/molar widths, arch length, overjet, overbite, and PAR score are shown in Table S44.1.

Table S44.1 Comparisons between various clear vacuum-formed thermoplastic retainers based of wear regime (*p* values).

	Observation period (months)	Little's Index		Intercanine width		Intermolar width		Arch length		Overjet	Overbite	PAR score
		Max	Mand	Max	Mand	Max	Mand	Max	Mand			
Gill *et al.* 2007[a]	6	0.60	0.93	0.89	0.56	0.81	0.74	–		0.80	0.11	–
Thickett and Power 2010[b]	6	0.67	0.08	0.34	0.31	0.62	0.69	0.40	0.14	0.55	0.02 (P/T > F/T)	>0.05
Jäderberg *et al.* 2012[b]	6	>0.05	>0.05	–	–	–	–	–	–	>0.05	>0.05	–
Thickett and Power 2010[b]	12	0.80	0.50	0.52	0.65	0.68	0.61	0.97	0.06	0.37	0.05 (P/T > F/T)	>0.05

Abbreviations: P/T, part-time; F/T, full-time; Max, Maxilla; Mand, Mandible.
[a] *t* test.
[b] Mann–Whitney.
Source: Adapted from Kaklamanos *et al.* 2017.

Key Findings

Overall, no statistically significant differences were observed between the compared VFRs wear regimes, regarding Little's Irregularity Index (Gill *et al.* 2007; Thickett and Power 2010; Jäderberg *et al.* 2012), intermolar and intercanine width (Gill *et al.* 2007; Thickett and Power 2010), arch length (Thickett and Power 2010), overjet (Gill *et al.* 2007; Thickett and Power 2010; Jäderberg *et al.* 2012), and PAR score (Thickett and Power 2010). The overall level of certainty in the evidence was judged to be moderate (ADA 2013). For overbite a statistically significant greater measurement in the "part-time" wearing group was noted compared to "full-time" wear (Thickett and Power 2010). The overall level of certainty in the evidence was judged to be low (ADA 2013). No specific data on secondary outcomes could be evaluated.

Commentary

In general, there exists a moderate level of certainty that "part-time" VFR use could possibly be sufficient in maintaining the orthodontic treatment result. Practically, potential advantages could accrue regarding the health of the hard and soft tissues, retainer longevity, cost-effectiveness, as well as, patient satisfaction and overall compliance.

Additional References

American Dental Association (ADA), 2013. *ADA Clinical Practice Guideline Handbook: 2013 Update.* Chicago: American Dental Association.
Gill DS, Naini FB, Jones A, Tredwin CJ, 2007. Part-time versus fulltime retainer wear following fixed appliance therapy: a randomized prospective controlled trial. *World J Orthod* 8, 300–306.
Jäderberg S, Feldmann I, Engström C, 2012. Removable thermoplastic appliances as orthodontic retainers – a prospective study of different wear regimens. *Eur J Orthod* 34, 475–479.
Thickett E, Power S, 2010. A randomized clinical trial of thermoplastic retainer wear. *Eur J Orthod* 32,1–5.

S45

A meta-analysis of mandibular intercanine width in treatment and postretention

Burke S, Silveira AM,* Goldsmith LJ, Yancey J, Van Stewart A, Scarfe W. Angle Orthod 1998;68:53–60.

Background

This meta-analysis summarizes the influence of Angle classification and extraction on post-treatment stability using intercanine dimensional change as an index of mandibular dental arch form without retaining devices.

Study Information

Population – nonsurgical orthodontic patients
Intervention – fixed appliance orthodontic therapy
Comparison – pretreatment status, Angle classification, extraction or nonextraction
Outcome – mean treatment change (T1–T2) and postretention (T2–T3) intercanine dimensional change (mm).

Search Parameters

Inclusion Criteria – clinical studies comparing intercanine width pretreatment (T1), immediately post-treatment (T2) and postretention (T3)
Databases searched – PubMed
Dates searched – prior to 1997
Other sources of evidence – hand searching of reference lists unpublished Master's thesis, personal communications
Language restrictions – none.

Search Results

1233 patients identified from 26 studies which met the inclusion criteria.

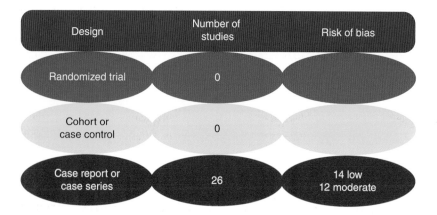

Design	Number of studies	Risk of bias
Randomized trial	0	
Cohort or case control	0	
Case report or case series	26	14 low 12 moderate

Study Results

The change in intercanine widths for the different malocclusions and interventions are shown in Table S45.1

Table S45.1 Comparison of mean intercanine widths pre- and post-treatment for various types of malocclusion and interventions.

	n	Mean treatment change (mm) T1–T2	Mean postretention change (mm) T2–T3	Samples+/ No change/ Samples –	Mean net change (mm) T1–T3	SD T1–T3	Degrees of freedom T1–T3	95% CI	P value
All patients	1233	1.57	−1.24	34+/3'0'/21−	0.33	1.77	391	(0.23, 0.43)	0*
Nonextraction	616	1.45	−1.17	18+/2'0'/9−	0.28	1.79	237	(0.14, 0.41)	0.0001*
Extraction	510	1.78	−1.41	15+/1'0'/11−	0.39	1.67	153	(0.26, 0.55)	0*
Class I	194	1.86	−1.48	7+/1'0'/5−	0.36	2.15	94	(0.55, 0.66)	0.0228
Class II	413	1.40	−1.32	13+/2'0'/10−	0.09	1.61	151	(−0.06, 0.24)	0.2762
Class II div 1	166	1.13	−1.31	2+/5−	−0.18	1.61	94	(−0.42, 0.68)	0.1601
Class II div 2	34	1.91	−1.44	4+/1−	0.49	1.68	16	(−0.12, 1.09)	0.1122
Nonextraction Class I	73	1.80	−1.60	4+/1'0'/1−	0.13	2.79	41	(−0.53, 0.70)	0.6843
Extraction Class I	121	1.90	−1.41	3+/4−	0.49	1.43	52	(0.23, 0.76)	0.0003*
Nonextraction Class II	223	1.19	−1.26	1+/1'0'/5−	−0.07	1.41	108	(−0.25, 0.11)	0.4457
Extraction Class II	190	1.64	−1.39	6+/1'0'/5−	0.27	1.81	42	(0.00, 0.53)	0.0444*
Nonextraction Class II div 1	92	0.81	−1.20	1+/3−	−0.40	1.42	69	(0.07, 0.66)	0.0155*
Extraction Class II div 1	74	1.50	−1.50	1+/2−	0.10	1.68	24	(−0.34, 0.46)	0.7632
Nonextraction Class II div 2	24	2.02	−1.60	3+	0.41	1.68	16	(−0.32, 1.13)	0.2558
Extraction Class II div 2	10	1.66	−1.00	1+/1−	0.68	–	–	–	–

*$P < 0.05$

Source: Burke *et al.* 1998. Reproduced with permission of Allen Press, Inc.

Key Findings

Regardless of Angle classification or orthodontic technique, mandibular intercanine width:

- tends to expand during treatment by 0.8 mm to 2.0 mm;
- tends to constrict postretention by 1.2 mm to 1.9 mm;
- ranges postretention from 0.5 mm expansion to 0.6 mm constriction.

Commentary

This meta-analysis and more recent publications (Basciftci *et al.* 2014; Shirazi *et al.* 2016) confirm that without retaining devices, mandibular intercanine dimensions relapse postorthodontic therapy.

Additional References

Basciftci FA, Akin M, Ileri Z, *et al.,* 2014. Long-term stability of dentoalveolar, skeletal, and soft tissue changes after non-extraction treatment with a self-ligating system. *Korean J Orthod* 44, 119–127.

Shirazi S, Kachoei M, Shahvaghar-Asl N, *et al.,* 2016. Arch width changes in patients with Class II division 1 malocclusion treated with maxillary first premolar extraction and non-extraction method. *J Clin Exp Dent* 8, e403–e408.

S46

Radiologically determined orthodontically induced external apical root resorption in incisors after non-surgical orthodontic treatment of Class II division 1 malocclusion: a systematic review

Tieu LD, Saltaji H, Normando D, Flores Mir C.* Prog Orthod 2014;15:48.

Background

Nonsurgical correction of Class II malocclusions with a significant skeletal involvement require meaningful incisor root apical movements. Such movements are known to be a factor that facilitates orthodontically induced external apical root resorption (OIEARR). This systematic review aimed to evaluate OIEARR among incisors from patients that underwent nonsurgical orthodontic treatment of their Class II division 1 malocclusion.

Study Information

Population – Class II division 1 malocclusion individuals with a significant skeletal involvement of any age that underwent orthodontic treatment

Intervention – nonsurgical orthodontic treatment

Comparison – other type of treatments or nontreated control sample

Outcome – OIEARR as quantified through radiographic evaluation.

Search Parameters

Inclusion criteria – randomized and nonrandomized clinical trials, and cohort studies that compared radiographically OIARR during nonsurgical orthodontic management of Class II division 1 malocclusions

Databases searched – Medline, and PubMed

Dates searched – various initial dates, all up to July 2013

Other sources of evidence – reference lists of included studies

Language restrictions – none.

Search Results

A total of 1831 unique citations were initially identified, but only eight publications remained. Methodological and clinical heterogeneity precluded a meta-analysis.

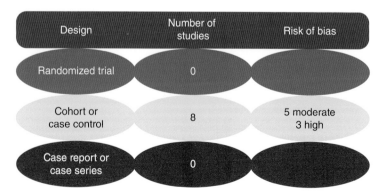

Design	Number of studies	Risk of bias
Randomized trial	0	
Cohort or case control	8	5 moderate 3 high
Case report or case series	0	

Study Results

The findings of the various studies are shown in Table S46.1.

Table S46.1 Root resorption related to treatment duration, sex, appliance type, and incisors affected.

Article	Treatment duration (months)	Radiograph	Results
DeShields 1969	M: 20.5 F: 22.5 M + F: 21.6 ± 5.2	PA	51/52 cases had resorption in at least 1 maxillary incisor
Hollender *et al.* 1980	Mean 18	PA	Maxillary anterior teeth most affected 48/60 Lateral incisor 22/24 No mild apical blunting (<3 mm) resorption
Eisel *et al.* 1994	38 ± 20	PA	Only 29 patients had periapicals to quantify RR. No explanation why only these ones. RR dx through Linge and Linge (1991) method
Reukers *et al.* 1998	Overall 20.4 ± 6.0 Straight wire 21.6 ± 4.8 Edgewise 19.2 ± 6.0	PA	Statistical test showed no difference in root resorption between straight wire and edgewise Study only focused on root resorption of maxillary central incisors
Taner *et al.* 1999	28.1 ± 9.0	Cephalogram	Mean root resorption 2.1 ± 1.6 mm
Mavragani *et al.* 2000	N/K	PA	Same data as 2002
Mavragani *et al.* 2002	N/K	PA	Root elongation was noted for 50/280 teeth Age at treatment start was significantly higher among patients showing root shortening of lateral incisors than those showing root elongation ($P < 0.05$) Roots that were incompletely developed before treatment reached a significantly greater length than those that were fully developed at the treatment start
Liou and Chang 2010	En-masse (Group I) 28.3 ± 7.3 FFA (Group II) 22.7 ± 5.0	PA	Group I (ANB 7.1° ± 1.9°) Group II (ANB 3.2° ± 2.9°) Apical root resorption of maxillary central incisor was significantly correlated to the duration of treatment ($P = 0.026$) but not to the amount of en-masse retraction, intrusion, or palatal tipping of maxillary Incisors Maxillary lateral incisors were significantly greater in Group I than in Group 2
Martins *et al.* 2012	28.0 ± 9.4	PA	All cases had resorption in at least 1 maxillary incisor

Source: Adapted from Tieu *et al.* 2014.

Commentary

1) Only seven retrospective and one prospective cohort studies were identified. They had moderate to high risk of bias. Only radiographic assessment methods were considered.
2) The reported OIEARR prevalence in this systematic review varied between 66 and 100%. Reasons could be related to different used definitions. Additionally, no distinction between OIEARR that will have clinical implications was made.
3) Diverse methodologies and orthodontic mechanics prevent any strong conclusions.
4) Some important factors to consider are the use of only two-dimensional radiography to quantify OIEARR, diverse Class II management mechanics, diverse amounts of incisor apical displacement, and distinct treatment times.

S47

Root resorption of endodontically treated teeth following orthodontic treatment: a meta-analysis

Ioannidou-Marathiotou I, Zafeiriadis AA,* Papadopoulos MA.* Clin Oral Investig 2013;17:1733–1744.

Background

The aim of this meta-analysis was to investigate the effect of orthodontic treatment on root resorption of endodontically treated teeth compared to vital teeth.

Study Information

Population – patients with endodontically treated incisors
Intervention – orthodontic treatment
Comparison – contralateral incisors root filled versus vital teeth
Outcome – external apical root resorption.

Search Parameters

Inclusion criteria – human controlled clinical studies investigating apical root resorption of endodontically treated teeth compared to vital teeth subjected to orthodontic treatment
Databases searched – PubMed, Medline, Embase, Cochrane, Google Scholar, Web of Science, Evidence-based medicine, Scopus, Lilacs, Bibliografia Brasileira de Odontologia, Ovid, Bandolier, Atypon Link, African Journals Online, Digital dissertations (UMI ProQuest), Conference Paper Index, ZB MED, metaRegister of Controlled Trials
Dates searched – up to January 2012
Other sources of evidence – manual searching
Language restrictions – none.

Search Results

1942 unique citations were identified. 11 publications remained after inclusion criteria applied. Five studies were excluded (not accessible or use of an improper control group), leaving only six studies for qualitative evaluation. Furthermore, two studies used data of the same subgroup, while another used a different methodology. In total, four studies were included in the meta-analysis.

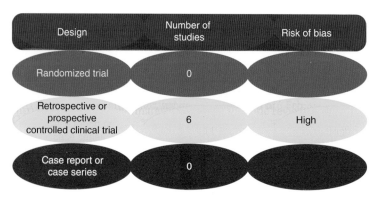

Design	Number of studies	Risk of bias
Randomized trial	0	
Retrospective or prospective controlled clinical trial	6	High
Case report or case series	0	

Study Results

The results comparing root resorption in root treated versus vital teeth are shown in Table S47.1.

Table S47.1 Comparison of root resorption during orthodontic treatment: endodontically treated teeth versus teeth with vital pulps.

	Endodontic teeth		Vital teeth			Mean difference, Fixed, 95% CI		
Study	Total	Mean (SD)	n	Mean (SD)	Weight		Favors endodontic teeth (less resorption)	Favors vital teeth
Esteves *et al.* 2007	16	0.81 (1.19)	16	1.04 (1)	19.2%	−0.23 (−0.99, 0.53)		
Kreia *et al.* 2005	20	1.14 (1.02)	20	1.34 (1.34)	20.4%	−0.20 (−0.94, 0.54)		
Mirabella and Artun 1995	28	0.91 (1.03)	28	1.38 (1.53)	23.8%	−0.47 (−1.15, 0.21)		
Spurrier *et al.* 1990	43	1.28 (1.09)	43	2.05 (1.49)	36.5%	−0.77 (−1.32, −0.22)		
Subtotal	107		107		100%	−0.48 (−0.81, −0.14)		

Heterogeneity: $Chi^2 = 2.03$, df = 3 ($P = 0.57$), $I^2 = 0\%$
Test for overall effect: $Z = 2.81$ ($P = 0.005$)

Source: Ioannidou-Marathiotou *et al.* 2013. Reproduced with permission of Springer.

Key Findings

- Following orthodontic treatment, endodontically treated teeth exhibit relatively less root resorption than teeth with vital pulps, although the overall amount of this resorption (0.48 mm) might be of little clinical importance.
- There was no indication of publication bias, while heterogeneity of the source data was low ($I^2 = 0\%$). The overall quality of the included studies was considered as "low."
- Clinicians should consider orthodontic movement of endodontically treated teeth as a relatively safe clinical procedure.

Commentary

1) The results of this meta-analysis should be interpreted with some caution, due to the small number and the low quality of included studies.
2) More high-quality studies could produce strong evidence to further support the current findings, as well as to answer the questions that remained unanswered in this meta-analysis due to lack of appropriate data, such as the effect of appliances used in orthodontic treatment, the orthodontic treatment duration, the timing of endodontic therapy, and the materials used in endodontic therapy.

Additional references for Summary 47 can be found on page 207.

S48

Radiographic comparison of the extent of orthodontically induced external apical root resorption in vital and root-filled teeth: a systematic review

Walker SL, Tieu LD, Flores Mir C. Eur J Orthod 2013;35:796–802.*

Background

There is some controversy in the literature regarding orthodontically induced external apical root resorption (OIEARR) in endodontically treated teeth. This systematic review critically analyzes the available scientific literature comparing radiographically OIEARR in human in vivo root-filled versus vital teeth.

Study Information

Population – individuals of any age that underwent fixed appliance orthodontic tooth movement
Intervention – orthodontic movement of asymptomatic root-filled teeth
Comparison – orthodontic movement of nonvital versus contralateral vital teeth
Outcome – OIEARR as quantified through radiographic evaluation.

Search Parameters

Inclusion criteria – randomized and nonrandomized clinical trials, cohort and case–control studies that compared radiographically OIEARR between vital and root-filled teeth
Databases searched – Medline, PubMed, EMBASE, Scopus, CDSR (Cochrane), CINAHL, and Web of Science
Dates searched – up to July 2012
Other sources of evidence – partial Google Scholar search and reference lists of included studies
Language restrictions – none.

Search Results

165 unique citations were initially identified but only four publications satisfied the entry criteria. Due to differences in methodologies a meta-analysis was not possible.

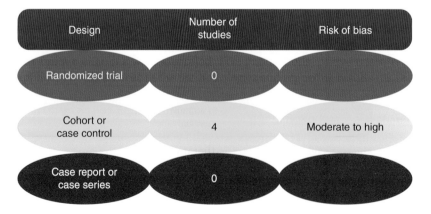

Design	Number of studies	Risk of bias
Randomized trial	0	
Cohort or case control	4	Moderate to high
Case report or case series	0	

Study Results

The outcomes for four studies comparing OIEARR in nonvital and vital teeth are detailed in Table S48.1.

Table S48.1 Outcome of radiographic assessment of root resorption.

Authors	Assessment method	Results
Llamas-Carreras *et al.* 2010	Sample size = 77 (73% female). Mean age 32.7 + 10.7. Mean treatment time 26.8 months. Pre- and postorthodontic radiographs were standardized by measurement of the greatest distance from incisal/occlusal edge to the cementoenamel junction (CEJ). Differences were calculated as shortening/lengthening factors. Root lengths were calculated by measuring the distance from CEJ to a line between root apices. Root resorption was calculated as the proportion of root resorption. That is root resorption in root-filled teeth/root resorption in vital contralateral teeth.	No statistically significant difference between amount of root resorption in root-filled teeth compared with contralateral vital teeth following orthodontic treatment (proportion of root resorption = 1.00 + 0.13). Greater root resorption in root-filled teeth compared to contralateral vital teeth following orthodontic treatment in women ($P = 0.0255$; OR = 4.2; 95% CI = 1.2–14.6), and incisors ($P = 0.0014$; OR = 6.3; 95% CI = 2.0–19.4).
Esteves *et al.* 2007	Sample size = 16. Age not stated. Treatment time greater than 20 months. Pre- and postorthodontic treatment radiographs were standardized by measuring the greatest distance from the incisal edge to the CEJ junction, differences were calculated as shortening/lengthening factors. All teeth were measured from incisal edge to apex of the root in pre- and postorthodontic treatment radiographs.	No statistically significant difference between amount of root resorption in root-filled teeth and contralateral vital teeth following orthodontic treatment ($P > 0.05$). Vital teeth showed slightly greater mean apical root resorption (0.22 mm). Statistically significant root resorption following orthodontic treatment occurred in root-filled teeth ($P = 0.007$) and vital teeth ($P = 0.0004$).
Mirabella and Artun 1995	Sample size = 39 (51% female). Mean age greater than 20. Treatment time range 6 to 62 months. Total tooth length was measured from incisal edge to root apex along the long axis of the tooth. Root resorption was calculated by subtracting the total tooth length following orthodontic treatment from total tooth length prior to orthodontic treatment (no standardization).	The teeth with root canal fillings resorbed less than vital contralateral teeth following orthodontic treatment (mean difference = 0.45 mm; SD = 1.21, $P < 0.05$).
Spurrier *et al.* 1990	Sample size = 43. Mean age 13.9. Treatment time mean 25 months. Pre- and post-treatment radiographs were standardized by measurement of the greatest distance from incisal edge to CEJ; differences were calculated as shortening/lengthening factors. All teeth were measured from greatest incisor-apical dimension on pre-and post-treatment radiographs.	Teeth with root canal fillings resorbed significantly less than vital contralateral teeth (mean difference = 0.77 mm, $P = 0.006$). Statistically significant root resorption occurred in root-filled teeth ($P = 0.003$) and vital contralateral teeth ($P = 0.0008$). No significant difference existed in root resorption of root-filled teeth following orthodontic treatment in males and females. Males exhibited significantly more resorption in control teeth following orthodontic treatment than females ($P < 0.02$).

Source: Walker *et al.* 2013. Reproduced with permission of Oxford University Press.

Key Findings

- Although the included studies were not directly comparable there was agreement that root-filled teeth do not appear to be more susceptible to OIEARR when compared to vital teeth.
- Furthermore, there is some evidence to suggest that root-filled teeth may exhibit less OIEARR than vital teeth.

Commentary

1) Only radiographic assessment methods were considered.
2) The reason for why the teeth were root filled are not reported and this may have an influence on root resorption as well as other factors such as, age, timing and severity of trauma or pathology, presence of external root resorption prior to treatment, the degree of tooth movement, and the different orthodontic mechanics undertaken.

S49

Root resorption associated with orthodontic tooth movement: a systematic review

Weltman B,* Vig KW,* Fields HW, Shanker S, Kaizar EE. Am J Orthod Dentofacial Orthop 2010;137:462–466.

Background

Apical root resorption results from a combination of individual biological variability, genetic predisposition, and the effect of mechanical factors. This systematic review aimed to evaluate root resorption as an outcome for patients undergoing orthodontic tooth movement, in order provide the best available evidence for clinical decisions to minimize the risks and severity of root resorption.

Study Information

Population – patients with no history of root resorption
Intervention – orthodontic treatment
Comparison/control group – teeth that were not moved orthodontically
Outcome – external apical root resorption.

Search Parameters

Inclusion criteria – human randomized controlled trials (RCTs) recording root resorption during and/or after orthodontic treatment
Databases searched – PubMed, Medline, Web of Science, Embase, Cochrane, Lilacs, DARE
Dates searched – various initial dates, all up to 2008
Other sources of evidence – nonelectronic journals were hand searched and experts in the field consulted
Language restrictions – none.

Search Results

921 unique citations were identified. 13 publications, of 11 trials, remained after inclusion criteria applied, but differences in the methodologies and reporting results made statistical comparisons impossible.

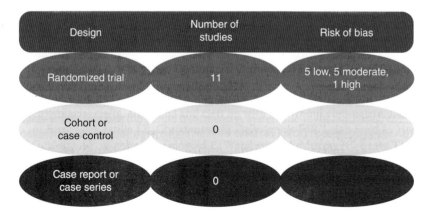

Design	Number of studies	Risk of bias
Randomized trial	11	5 low, 5 moderate, 1 high
Cohort or case control	0	
Case report or case series	0	

Study Results

The outcomes for root resorption are shown in Table S49.1

Table S49.1 Orthodontic tooth movement and associated root resorption.

Study	Random-ization	Allocation concealed	Assessor blinding	Dropouts described	Risk of bias	Study outcome
Acar *et al.* 1999	No	Unclear	Unclear	Yes	High	Teeth experiencing orthodontic tooth movement had significantly more root resorption than control teeth. Continuous forces produced significantly more resorption than discontinuous force application.
Barbagallo *et al.* 2008	Yes	No	No	Yes	Moderate	Heavy forces produced significantly more resorption than light forces or thermoplastic appliance force application.
Brin *et al.* 2003	Yes	Yes	Yes	Yes	Low–retrospective	As treatment time increased, the odds of orthodontically induced inflammatory root (OIIRR) resorption also increased. Teeth with roots with unusual morphology before treatment were not statistically more likely to have moderate to severe root resorption than those with normal root form.
Chan and Darendeliler 2004	Yes	No	No	Yes	Moderate	Heavy forces produced significantly more root resorption than light forces or control.
Chan and Darendeliler 2006	Yes	No	No	Yes	Moderate	The mean volume of the resorption crater in the light force group was 3.49 times greater than in the control group (not significant).
Han *et al.* 2005	Yes	Yes	Yes	Yes	Low	Intrusive forces significantly increased the percentage of resorbed root area.
Harris *et al.* 2006	Yes	No	No	Yes	Moderate	Heavy force application produced significantly more root resorption than light forces or control.
Levander *et al.* 1994	Yes	Unclear	Unclear	Yes	Moderate	Root resorption was significantly less in patients treated with a pause than those treated with continuous forces without a pause.
Mandall *et al.* 2006	Yes	Yes	Yes	Yes	Low	History of incisor trauma was not associated with increased root resorption. No statistically significant differences between archwire sequences were found between the proportion of patients with/without root resorption.
Reukers *et al.* 1998	Yes	Yes	Yes	Yes	Low	No statistically significant differences in the amount of tooth root loss or prevalence of root resorption between straightwire and standard edgewise groups.
Scott *et al.* 2008	Yes	Unclear	Yes	Yes	Low	Mandibular incisor root resorption was not statistically different between self-ligating Damon 3 and conventional Synthesis systems.

Source: Weltman *et al.* 2010. Reproduced with permission of Elsevier.

Key Findings

- Evidence suggests that comprehensive orthodontic treatment causes an increase in the incidence and severity of root resorption, and heavy forces are particularly harmful.
- Orthodontically induced inflammatory root resorption (OIIRR) appears to be unaffected by archwire sequencing, bracket prescription, or self-ligation.
- There is some evidence that a 2 to 3-month treatment pause may decrease total root resorption.

Commentary

1) More recent evidence from RCTs does not contradict original findings.
2) Other trends could not be substantiated because of small subject numbers and short treatment times.
3) Standard reporting methods of future clinical trials are recommended so data can be pooled and stronger clinical recommendations made as meta-analysis is still not possible.

Additional References

Eross E, Turk T, Elekdag-Turk S, *et al.*, 2015. Physical properties of root cementum: Part 25. Extent of root resorption after the application of light and heavy buccopalatal jiggling forces for 12 weeks: A microcomputed tomography study. *Am J Orthod Dentofacial Orthop* 147, 738–746.

Leite V, Conti AC, Navarro R, *et al.*, 2012. Comparison of root resorption between self-ligating and conventional preadjusted brackets using cone beam computed tomography. *Angle Orthod* 82, 1078–1082.

S50

Influence of orthodontic treatment, midline position, buccal corridor and smile arc on smile attractiveness

Janson G,* Branco NC, Fernandes TMF, Sathler R, Garib D, Lauris JRP. Angle Orthod 2011;81:155–163.

Background

Some studies have suggested that orthodontic treatment, midline position, axial midline angulation, buccal corridor, and smile arc may affect smile attractiveness. Therefore, the aim of this systematic review was to analyze the scientific evidence on the influence of these variables in smile attractiveness.

Study Information

Population – untreated subjects and orthodontic patients
Intervention – digitally altered images and orthodontic treatment
Comparison – normal occlusion
Outcome – smile attractiveness.

Search Parameters

Inclusion criteria – studies on the influence of at least one of these variables: orthodontic treatment, midline position, axial midline angulation, buccal corridor, and smile arc on smile esthetics
Databases searched – PubMed, Web of Science, Embase, and All Evidence-Based Medicine Reviews (EBM Reviews)
Dates searched – 1979 to 2009
Other sources of evidence – hand search of reference lists
Language restrictions – English only.

Search Results

203 articles were identified and 20 met the inclusion criteria.

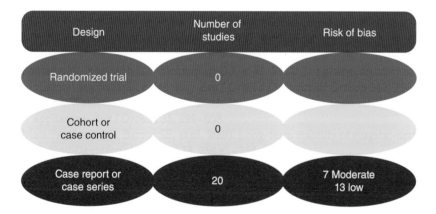

Design	Number of studies	Risk of bias
Randomized trial	0	
Cohort or case control	0	
Case report or case series	20	7 Moderate 13 low

Study Results

The conclusion for the 20 studies are shown in Table S50.1

Table S50.1 The conclusions of the 20 studies regarding midline position, buccal corridor and smile arc on smile attractiveness.

Authors	Conclusions
Ioi *et al.* 2009	Both the orthodontists and dental students preferred broader smiles to medium or narrow smiles.
Rodrigues *et al.* 2009	Variations from beauty norms of a smile do not necessarily result in reduced attractiveness.
Gul-e-Erum and Fida 2008	A broad and a flat smile in the male are preferred; a medium-broad and a flat/consonant smile in the female are preferred; midline deviation was considered unattractive in the male subjects by only orthodontic residents, while in the female subject it was considered unattractive by all groups, except operative residents.
McNamara *et al.* 2008	No correlation was found between the size or ratio value of the buccal corridors distal to the most posterior teeth visible on smile. No correlation was found between smile arc and smile esthetics.
Shyagali *et al.* 2008	Discrepancies of 2 mm or more are likely to be noticed by both orthodontic and laypeople.
Ker *et al.* 2008	The ideal buccal corridor size was 16%, and the acceptability range was 8 to 22%; raters preferred a consonant smile but accepted a smile with minimal curvature as well; maxillary to mandibular midline deviation was acceptable until it exceeded 2.1 mm and one-third of the respondents accepted the maxillary to face maximal deviation of 2.9 mm.
Martin *et al.* 2007	Large buccal corridors are considered less attractive than those with small buccal corridors.
Parekh *et al.* 2007	Large buccal corridors and flat smile arcs are rated as less acceptable.
Pinho *et al.* 2007	Midline shifts were perceived at 1 mm by orthodontists and 3 mm by prosthodontists; layperson did not notice midline shifts of 4 mm.
Gracco *et al.* 2006	A minimal buccal corridor was considered more attractive.
Isiksal *et al.* 2006	Treatment modality alone has no predictable effect on the overall esthetic assessment of a smile; transverse characteristics of the smile appeared to be of little significance to an attractive smile.
Parekh *et al.* 2006	Large buccal corridors and flat smile arcs are considered less attractive.
Moore *et al.* 2005	Large buccal corridors are considered less attractive than those with small buccal corridors.
Roden-Johnson *et al.* 2005	Buccal corridors do not influence smile esthetics.
Kim and Gianelly 2003	There is no predictable relationship between extraction and nonextraction treatment and the esthetics of the smile.
Thomas *et al.* 2003	Mean acceptable midline angulation for the male subject was 6.6 ± 4.5° for orthodontists and 10.7 ± 6.2° for laypeople. For the female subject, the mean acceptable threshold was 6.4 ± 4.0° for orthodontists and 10.0 ± 6.1° for laypeople. Discrepancies of 10° were unacceptable by 68% of orthodontists and 41% of laypeople.
Johnston *et al.* 1999	Dental to facial midline discrepancies of 2 mm are likely to be noticed by 83% of orthodontists and more than 56% of young laypeople.
Kokich *et al.* 1999	A maxillary midline deviation of 4 mm was necessary before orthodontists rated is significantly less esthetic than the others; dentists and laypeople were unable to detect a 4 mm midline deviation.
Beyer and Lindauer 1998	The mean threshold for acceptable dental midline deviation was 2.2 ± 1.5 mm.
Johnson and Smith 1995	There is no predictable relationship between extraction and nonextraction treatment and the esthetics of the smile.

Source: Adapted from Janson *et al.* 2011.

Key Findings

- Nonextraction or four-premolar extraction treatments seem to have no predictable effects on smile attractiveness.
- The dental midline can be deviated up to 2.2 mm without any detrimental effect on smile esthetics. However, an axial midline angulation of 10 degrees is very apparent.
- The buccal corridor size or the smile arc alone do not seem to affect smile attractiveness in investigations with actual subjects.

Commentary

1) Recent investigations confirm the conclusions obtained (Ghaffar and Fida 2011; Meyer *et al.* 2014; Yang *et al.* 2015).
2) More studies with actual subjects are recommended to provide more valid conclusions.

Additional references for Summary 50 can be found on page 208.

S51

Systematic review and meta-analysis of randomized controlled trials evaluating intraoral orthopedic appliances for temporomandibular disorders

Fricton J,* Look JO, Wright E, Alencar FG Jr, Chen H, Lang M, Ouyang W, Velly AM. J Orofac Pain 2010;24:237–254.

Background

Intraoral appliances have been advocated for managing temporomandibular disorders (TMJD). The most common types of appliances are the hard and soft acrylic stabilization type, anterior positioning appliances, and anterior bite appliances. Despite their widespread use, there is still controversy regarding their efficacy in clinical trials. Therefore the purpose of this review is to ascertain whether TMJD treatments effectively reduce TMJD pain compared to placebo/control or no treatment?

Study Information

Population – patients with reported TMJD pain

Interventions – hard and soft stabilization appliances, anterior positioning appliances, anterior bite planes, as well as appliances compared to other treatments, such as self-care, acupuncture, cognitive behavioral therapy, physical medicine, pharmacological treatments, and occlusal therapies

Comparison – different appliances against inactive controls

Outcome – successful outcome reported as approximately 50% reduction in a self-report measure of pain.

Search Parameters

Inclusion criteria – randomized controlled trials (RCTs)

Databases searched – MEDLINE, EMBASE, and the Cochrane Library

Dates searched – up to September 2013

Other sources of evidence – hand searching of reference lists

Language restrictions – none.

Search Results

47 publications citing 44 RCTs with 2218 subjects were included.

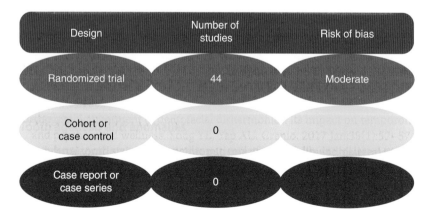

Design	Number of studies	Risk of bias
Randomized trial	44	Moderate
Cohort or case control	0	
Case report or case series	0	

Study Results

The outcome for (A) hard stabilization appliances versus palatal nonoccluding appliances and (B) stabilization appliances versus no treatment to reduce TMJD pain are shown in Table S51.1.

Table S51.1 Comparison of intervention outcomes (A) two appliances and (B) stabilization appliance versus control.

Study	OR	Lower limit	Upper limit	Z value	P	OR and 95% CI
A, Forest plot based on 7 randomized clinical trials totaling 385 subjects and evaluating the efficacy of hard stabilization appliances compared to palatal nonoccluding appliances as a control treatment						
Summary	2.45	1.56	3.86	3.89	0.00	
Ekberg et al. 1998–1999, Raphael et al. 2001, Ekberg et al. 2003, Dao et al. 1994, Rubinoff et al. 1987, Wassell et al. 2004, Conti et al. 2006						
B, Forest plot based on 3 randomized clinical trials including 216 subjects and evaluating the efficacy of stabilization appliances compared to no treatment as the control.						
Summary	2.14	0.80	5.75	1.51	.12	
List et al. 1992, part I, List et al. 1992, part II, Lundh et al. 1992						

The size of the squares suggests the size of the effect for each study. A position to the right of "1" suggests more efficacy is demonstrated by the stabilization appliance over the control appliance and is plotted along a log scale.
Source: Adapted from Fricton *et al.* 2010.

Key Findings

Sufficient evidence from this study supports;

- full coverage well adjusted part-time use of intraoral orthopedic appliances that do not change the occlusion

Other systematic reviews support the following therapeutic or preventive measures to treat TMJD pain:

- self-management treatments including exercise to restore normal jaw function and oral habit change to reduce jaw strain
- physical medicine treatments including ultrasound, laser therapy, and transcutaneous nerve simulation (TENS)
- non-opioid pharmacologic therapies
- cognitive-behavioral and psychological therapy
- temporomandibular joint (TMJ) surgery in selected cases with significant dysfunction.

Insufficient evidence to support therapeutic or preventive treatment to treat TMJD pain:

- partial coverage or fulltime use of intraoral orthopedic appliances that change the occlusion
- occlusal therapy including occlusal adjustment, orthodontics, restorative dentistry, and orthognathic surgery but may be indicated for occlusal dysfunction.

S52

The role of mandibular third molars on lower anterior teeth crowding and relapse after orthodontic treatment: a systematic review

Zawawi KH,* Melis M.* ScientificWorldJournal 2014;2014:615429.

Background

Mandibular third molars have been historically implicated as a causative factor in anterior crowding of the teeth, particularly after orthodontic treatment. This systematic review aimed to clarify the role of mandibular third molars on lower anterior crowding and relapse after orthodontic treatment.

Study Information

Population – orthodontic patients, as well as treated and untreated individuals
Interventions – extraction of mandibular third molars
Comparison – nonextraction or agenesis of third molars
Outcome – crowding of mandibular anterior teeth.

Search Parameters

Inclusion criteria – controlled trials
Databases searched – Pubmed
Dates searched – up to December 2013
Other sources of evidence – hand searching of reference lists
Language restrictions – English.

Search Results

96 articles were initially identified. After examining the titles and the abstracts, 26 studies remained, and five additional publications were added after the manual search of their references. Seven articles could not be acquired because the year of publication was very old. In the end, 12 studies were included.

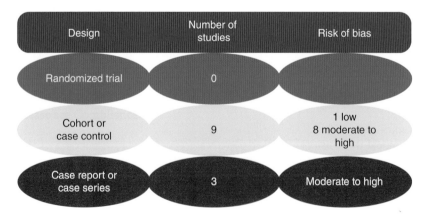

Design	Number of studies	Risk of bias
Randomized trial	0	
Cohort or case control	9	1 low 8 moderate to high
Case report or case series	3	Moderate to high

Study Results

The influence of the presence of third molars on anterior crowding is shown in Table S52.1.

Table S52.1 The influence of third molars on lower anterior crowding.

Authors	Study groups	n	Type of study	Results
Shanley 1962	Untreated subjects (1) bilaterally impacted (2) bilaterally erupted (3) bilaterally congenitally absent	44	Cross-sectional	No differences between the groups
Sheneman 1969	Treated subjects, (1) in occlusion, (2) unerupted (3) missing	49	Retrospective/ longitudinal	More stability in patients with congenital missing 3rd molars compared with 3rd molars present
Kaplan 1974	Treated subjects (1) bilaterally erupted into function (2) bilaterally impacted, (3) bilateral agenesis	75	Retrospective/ longitudinal	No differences between the groups
Lindqvist and Thilander 1982	Untreated subjects (1) extracted on one side, (2) retained on the contralateral side	52	Prospective/ longitudinal	Extraction side had a more favorable development than the control side
Richardson 1982	Untreated subjects (1) bilaterally impacted, (2) bilaterally nonimpacted	51	Retrospective/ longitudinal	3rd molars that become impacted tend to be associated with crowding
Ades *et al.* 1990	Treated subjects (1) impacted (2) erupted into function (3) congenitally absent (4) extracted at least 10 years earlier	97	Retrospective/ longitudinal	No differences among the groups
van der Schoot *et al.* 1997	Treated subjects (1) erupted, (2) nonerupted, (3) extracted, (4) congenitally absent	99	Retrospective/ longitudinal	No differences among the groups
Harradine *et al.* 1998	Treated subjects (1) extracted, (2) nonextracted	164	Prospective/ longitudinal	No differences between the groups
Little 1999	Treated subjects (1) impacted, (2) erupted, (3) extracted (4) agenesis	97	Retrospective/ longitudinal	No differences between the groups
Buschang and Shulman 2003	Random sample of untreated subjects as part of the Third National Health and Nutrition Examination Survey	9044	Cross-sectional	Erupted 3rd molars not associated with increased crowding
Niedzielska 2005	Untreated subjects (1) bilaterally extracted (2) unilaterally extracted, (3) bilaterally retained (4) unilaterally retained	47	Prospective/ longitudinal	Retained 3rd molars associated with increased crowding in relation to Ganss ratio (the ratio between the third molar width and the retromolar space)
Sidlauskas and Trakiniene 2006	Untreated subjects with mandibular 3rd molars: (1) erupted, (2) nonerupted, (3) agenesis	91	Cross-sectional	No differences between the groups

Source: Zawawi and Melis 2014. Available at: https://www.hindawi.com/journals/tswj/2014/615429/abs/. Licensed under CC-BY 3.0.

Key Findings

- There is no definitive conclusion on the role of the third molars in the development of anterior tooth crowding.
- A high risk of bias was found in most of the studies.
- A cause-and-effect relationship between mandibular third molars and anterior tooth crowding or postorthodontic relapse was not found.

Commentary

A recent review and two studies have been published since this systematic review; however, there is still no definitive conclusion (Esan and Schepartz 2016; Selmani *et al.* 2016; Stanaitytė *et al.* 2014).

Additional references for Summary 52 can be found on page 208.

S53

Coronectomy vs. total removal for third molar extraction: a systematic review

Long H, Zhou Y, Liao L, Pyakurel U, Wang Y, Lai W.* J Dent Res 2012;91:659–665.

Background

Coronectomy, partial odontectomy, or root retention is claimed to reduce the incidence of many surgical complications, especially nerve injury. However, its effectiveness in reducing surgical complications has yet to be concluded. This systematic review aimed to critically appraise the efficacy of coronectomy versus conventional total removal in reducing extraction complications.

Study Information

Population – patients requiring the extractions of third molars with high risk of nerve injury
Intervention – coronectomy
Comparison – conventional total removal
Outcome – nerve injury, postoperative infection, dry socket, and pain.

Search Parameters

Inclusion criteria – clinical studies comparing coronectomy and conventional total removal
Databases searched – PubMed, Web of Science, Embase, Cochrane, and SIGLE
Dates searched – 1990 to November 2011
Other sources of evidence – none
Language restrictions – none.

Search Results

38 references were identified, four of which met the inclusion criteria.

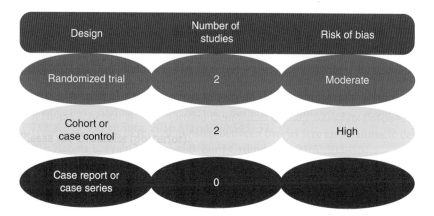

Design	Number of studies	Risk of bias
Randomized trial	2	Moderate
Cohort or case control	2	High
Case report or case series	0	

Study Results

The risk ratios for (A) coronectomy versus total removal and (B) infection are shown in Table S53.1.

Third molars

Table S53.1 Risk ratios for (A) coronectomy versus total removal and (B) postoperative infections.

Authors	Coronectomy		Total removal		Weight (%)	Risks ratio, M-H Fixed, 95% CI	
	Events	Total	Events	Total		Favors coronectomy	Favors total removal
A, Risk ratio for coronectomy versus total removal of 3rd molars							
Renton 2005	0	58	24	138	46.3	0.05 (0.00, 0.78)	
Leung 2009	1	155	10	194	28.2	0.13 (0.02, 0.97)	
Hatano 2009	1	102	6	118	17.7	0.19 (0.02, 1.58)	
Cilasun 2011	0	86	2	89	7.8	0.21 (0.01, 4.25)	
Total	2	401	42	539	100	0.11 (0.01, 4.25)	

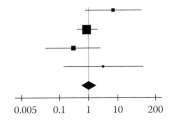

Heterogeneity: Chi^2 = 0.82, df = 3, P = 0.85, I^2 = 0%,
Test for overall effect: Z = 3.59, P = 0.0003

B, Risk ratio regarding postoperative infections for coronectomy vs. total removal							
Renton 2005	3	58	1	138	3.6	7.14 (0.76, 67.20)	
Leung 2009	9	155	13	194	70.7	0.87 (0.38, 1.97)	
Hatano 2009	1	102	4	118	22.7	0.29 (0.03, 2.55)	
Cilasun 2011	1	86	0	89	3.0	3.10 (0.13, 75.15)	
Total	14	401	18	539	100	1.03 (0.54, 1.98)	

Heterogeneity: Chi^2 = 4.80, df = 3, P = 0.19, I^2 = 38%,
Test for overall effect: Z = 0.09, P = 0.93

Source: Long *et al.* 2012. Reproduced with permission of Sage Publications.

Key Findings

- Coronectomy is superior to conventional total removal in protecting inferior alveolar nerves in the extractions of third molars with high risk of nerve injury.
- The incidence of postoperative infections, dry socket, and pain were similar between the two techniques.

Commentary

This systematic review is a pioneer study investigating the effectiveness of coronectomy in reducing nerve injury among patients requiring the extractions of third molars with high risk of nerve injury. Subsequently, several additional studies and systematic reviews have reported similar findings.

Additional References

Cervera-Espert J, Perez-Martinez S, Cervera-Ballester J, *et al.*, 2016. Coronectomy of impacted mandibular third molars: A meta-analysis and systematic review of the literature. *Med Oral Patol Oral Cir Bucal* 21, e505–513.
Martin A, Perinetti G, Costantinides F, *et al.*, 2015. Coronectomy as a surgical approach to impacted mandibular third molars: a systematic review. *Head Face Med* 11, 9.

S54

How long does treatment with fixed appliances last? A systematic review

Tsichlaki A, Chin SY, Pandis N, Fleming PS.* Am J Orthod Dentofacial Orthop 2016;149:308–318.

Background

There is little agreement on the duration of a course of orthodontic treatment; however, a consensus appears to have emerged that fixed appliance treatment is excessive. This has led to the development and marketing of novel approaches directed to reduce treatment times, occasionally with an acceptance that occlusal outcomes may be compromised. The aim of this study was to determine the mean duration and the number of visits required for comprehensive orthodontic treatment involving fixed appliances.

Study Information

Population – orthodontic patients treated with fixed appliances
Intervention – any patient undergoing fixed appliances without adjunctive use of functional or removable appliances or adjunctive surgical interventions
Comparison – observational in respect to treatment time
Outcomes – treatment duration and visits.

Search Parameters

Inclusion criteria – randomized and controlled clinical trials, prospective cohort studies
Databases searched – MEDLINE, Cochrane
Dates searched – to November 2014
Other sources of evidence – gray literature and reference lists
Language restrictions – none.

Search Results

1750 references were identified, 24 of which were considered for meta-analysis.

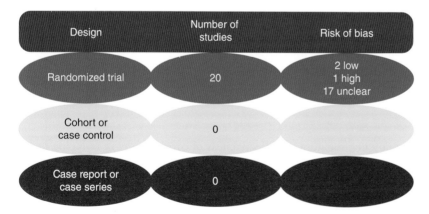

Design	Number of studies	Risk of bias
Randomized trial	20	2 low 1 high 17 unclear
Cohort or case control	0	
Case report or case series	0	

Study Results

The treatment times for the 24 studies are shown in Table S54.1.

Table S54.1 Treatment times for orthodontic treatment.

Authors	Weight %	Effect size, mean difference
Al Maaitah 2013	6.47	14.42 (13.17, 15.67)
Banks 2000 (F)	5.11	19.20 (17.79, 20.61)
Banks 2000 (non-F)	1.90	20.40 (18.09, 20.61)
Boros 2012 (PI)	0.40	28.66 (23.62, 33.70)
Boros 2000 (TPA)	0.54	33.33 (28.98, 37.68)
Cattaneo 2011 (SLB-A)	1.52	21.10 (18.51, 23.69)
Catteneo 2011 (SLB-P)	2.41	22.40 (20.35, 24.45)
DiBiase 2011	3.58	23.83 (22.14, 25.52)
Fleming 2010	4.25	19.92 (18.37, 21.47)
Jenatschke 2001 (CHX)	1.34	21.06 (18.30, 23.82)
Jenatschke 2001 (Placebo)	0.78	21.73 (18.13, 25.33)
Jiang 2013 (APF)	11.00	18.40 (17.44, 19.36)
Jiang 2013 (Placebo)	14.81	17.50 (16.67, 18.33)
Johansson 2012 (SLB-A)	3.27	20.40 (18.64, 22.16)
Johansson 2012 (CB)	2.83	18.20 (16.30, 20.10)
Liu 2009 (TAD)	1.76	25.65 (23.24, 28.06)
Liu 2009 (TPA)	1.05	26.88 (23.77, 29.99)
Magnius 2014	2.71	22.80 (20.86, 24.74)
Manning 2006	1.52	21.70 (19.11, 24.29)
Miller 1996	0.54	30.10 (25.77, 34.43)
Millett 1999	10.35	15.30 (14.31, 16.29)
Millett 2000	2.74	21.30 (19.37, 23.23)
Noreval 1996	3.07	21.48 (19.66, 23.30)
Polat 2008 (SLB-A)	0.67	23.30 (19.40, 27.20)
Polat 2008 (CB)	0.51	21.40 (16.94, 25.86)
Reukers 1998	4.49	20.40 (18.89, 21.91)
Sandler 2008 (PI)	1.37	25.80 (23.08, 28.52)
Sandler 2008 (EOT)	1.20	26.76 (23.84, 29.68)
Sander 2014	3.73	27.42 (25.77, 29.07)
Van der Veen 2010	2.45	18.10 (16.06, 20.14)
Xu 2010 (En masse)	0.73	30.00 (26.26, 33.74)
Xu 2010 (2-step)	0.89	31.20 (27.82, 34.58)
Overall $I^2 = 94.4\%$, $P = 0.000$	100	19.90 (19.58, 20.22)

X-axis: 0 10 20 30 35

Source: Tsichlaki *et al.* 2016. Reproduced with permission of Elsevier.

Key Findings

- On the basis of this review orthodontic treatment with fixed appliances requires considerably less than 2 years (19.9 months) on average.
- However, a wide range of treatment durations (14–33 months) were reported. This variation may relate to baseline and treatment-related differences, although important potential confounders were minimized by omitting studies involving adjunctive appliances, additional treatment phases, and combined orthodontic–surgical treatment.

Commentary

It now seems reasonable to assume that the average duration of comprehensive treatment is less than 2 years. If adjuncts or alternatives to reduce the treatment time are suggested, it would be sensible that these interventions are recommended with an awareness of this yardstick.

Additional references for Summary 54 can be found on page 208.

S55

Surgically facilitated orthodontic treatment: a systematic review

Hoogeveen EJ, Jansma J, Ren Y.* Am J Orthod Dentofacial Orthop 2014;145: S51–S64. (Additional summary author: Ong SH).

Background

Corticotomy and dental distraction have been proposed as effective and safe methods to shorten orthodontic treatment duration in adolescent and adult patients. A systematic review was performed to evaluate the evidence supporting these claims.

Study Information

Population – adolescent and adult orthodontic patients
Intervention – surgical orthodontics (corticotomy-facilitated/ dental distraction)
Comparison – conventional orthodontics
Outcome – tooth movement velocity and shortening of treatment time.

Search Parameters

Inclusion criteria – human randomized controlled trials (RCTs), clinical controlled trials (CCTs), and case series with >5 patients recording tooth movement velocity or treatment time shortening with surgical orthodontics
Databases searched – PubMed, Embase, Cochrane
Dates searched – various initial dates, all up to April 2013
Other sources of evidence – hand searching of reference lists
Language restrictions – none.

Search Results

510 unique citations were identified of which 45 full-text articles were assessed for eligibility. 18 studies were included after application of the inclusion criteria, exclusion of one Chinese study based on language and one for overlap of data with another study. Together, these 18 studies included 286 surgical-orthodontically treated patients (203 distraction procedures; 83 corticotomy procedures).

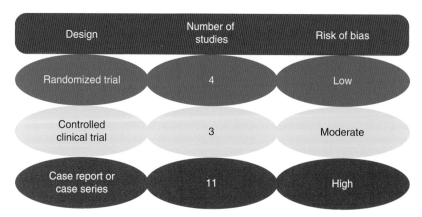

Design	Number of studies	Risk of bias
Randomized trial	4	Low
Controlled clinical trial	3	Moderate
Case report or case series	11	High

Study Results

The rate of tooth movements for distraction and corticotomy versus controls are shown in Table S55.1.

Table S55.1 Outcomes for tooth movements in respect of (A) distraction and (B) corticotomy.

Authors	Study design	n	Rate of tooth movement	
			Intervention	Control group
A) Dental distraction				
Mowafy and Zaher 2012	RCT	30	Upper canine: 5.9 ± 1.4 mm in 37 ± 10 days	Upper canine: 4.7 ± 1.6 mm in 195 ± 47 days
Kharkar *et al.* 2010	CCT	6	Full canine retraction in 12.5 days	Full canine retraction in 19.5 days[a]
B) Corticotomy				
Aboul-Ela *et al.* 2011	RCT	10	Upper canine: 5.7 mm in 120 days	Upper canine: 3.4 mm in 120 days
Fischer 2007	RCT	6	Upper canine: 10–14 mm in 266–378 days	Upper canine: 11–15 mm in 406–546 days
Shoreiba *et al.* 2012	RCT	10	Lower canine retraction: 17 weeks (14–20)	Lower canine retraction: in 16.7 weeks (14–20)[a]
Shoreiba *et al.* 2012	CCT	10	Lower canine retraction: 17.5 weeks	Lower canine retraction: 49 weeks
Gantes *et al.* 1990	CCT	9	Full arch closure: 14.8 months (11–20)	Full arch closure: 28.3 months (24–35)
3 other studies	CS	29		

[a] Other corticotomy/distraction procedure.
Source: Hoogeveen *et al.* 2014. Reproduced with permission of Elsevier.

Key Findings

- Corticotomy was found to double the rate of tooth movement in two RCTs with a split-mouth control group (Aboul-Ela *et al.* 2011; Fischer 2007). After 3 months, the acceleratory effect ceased.
- The treatment time reduction was evaluated in two other corticotomy studies and found to be 30–70%, based on controls with similar crowding (Shoreiba *et al.* 2012) or malocclusion (Gantes *et al.* 1990).
- Dentoalveolar distraction can lead to full canine retraction in 2–5 weeks, dependent on the exact surgical technique and subsequent activation regime (Mowafy and Zaher 2012; Kharkar *et al.* 2010).
- Limited evidence shows nonincreased risks for periodontal problems and root resorption. Tooth nonvitality after surgical orthodontics was not observed in any study. However, this was based on poor diagnostics and provides no evidence.
- Concluding, surgical orthodontics causes temporarily accelerated tooth movement in cases where careful treatment planning, early activation, and short check-up intervals are employed.

Commentary

The heterogeneity of clinical indications, treatment plans, surgical techniques, and force systems does not permit a meta-analysis. Most of the included studies had small samples. Only four of the 18 studies used a control group treated with conventional orthodontics. Due to a lack of comparative data, it is unclear which surgical protocol is preferable regarding treatment efficiency and safety. Further research is needed to elaborate on patient comfort, long-term stability, the underlying mechanism, and efficiency with different surgical approaches and clinical indications.

Additional references for Summary 55 can be found on page 208.

S56

Fluorides for the prevention of early tooth decay (demineralised white lesions) during fixed brace treatment

Benson PE,* Parkin NA, Dyer FM, Millett DT, Furness S, Germain P. Cochrane Database Syst Rev 2013;(12):CD003809.

Background

A study has found that 32% of participants had white lesions on their teeth before treatment with fixed orthodontic appliances and this increased to 74% after treatment (Enaia *et al.* 2011). Fluoride is effective in reducing decay in susceptible individuals in the general population. Individuals receiving orthodontic treatment may be prescribed various forms of fluoride treatment. This review compares the effects of various forms of fluoride used during orthodontic treatment on the development of demineralized lesions. This review is an update of a Cochrane review first published in 2004, updated in 2013 and is currently being updated again. Additional information from this planned update has been included.

Study Information

Population – orthodontic patients undergoing treatment with fixed appliances
Interventions – any type of topical fluoride or fluoride-releasing material
Comparison – no fluoride or alternative fluoride intervention
Outcome – presence/ absence of new demineralized lesions by participant.

Search Parameters

Inclusion criteria – randomized controlled trials (RCTs) (not intraindividual) recording demineralized lesions preferably before and/or after treatment
Databases searched – Cochrane Oral Health Group's Trials Register and Central Register of Controlled Trials (CENTRAL), MEDLINE via OVID, EMBASE via OVID
Dates searched – various initial dates, all up to 2013
Other sources of evidence – bibliographies of identified RCTs and review articles. US National Institutes of Health Trials Register
Language restrictions – none.

Search Results

191 unique citations were identified. Five publications, of five trials, remained after inclusion criteria were applied, but differences in the methodologies and reporting results made statistical comparisons impossible.

Design	Number of studies	Risk of bias
Randomized trial	5	3 low 1 high 1 unclear
Cohort or case control	0	
Case report or case series	0	

Study Results

The outcomes for five studies are shown in Table S56.1.

Table S56.1 Relative risk ratios for intervention and control/comparison groups.

Study	Intervention	Control/comparison group	n	Relative effect, RR – Risk Ratio (95% CI)	Risk of bias
Stecksen-Blicks 2007	Difluorsilane varnish (1000 ppm F$^-$)	No fluoride varnish	243	0.31 (0.21, 0.44)	Low
Jiang 2013	Acidulated phosphate fluoride foam (12,300 ppm F$^-$)	No fluoride foam	95	0.26 (0.11, 0.57)	Low
Sonesson 2014	Sodium fluoride toothpaste (5000 ppm F$^-$)	Sodium fluoride toothpaste (1450 ppm F$^-$)	380	0.68 (0.46, 1.00)	Low
Luther 2005	Sodium fluoride glass bead (133,000 ppm F$^-$)	Sodium fluoride mouth rinse (225 ppm F$^-$)	37	1.41 (0.61, 3.26)	High
Van der Kaaij 2015	Amine/sodium fluoride mouth rinse (250 ppm F$^-$)	No fluoride mouth rinse	81	0.65 (0.37, 1.77)	Unclear

Source: Adapted from Benson *et al.* 2013.

Key Findings

- Moderate evidence that regular professionally applied fluoride varnish/foam or home use of high concentration fluoride toothpaste (one trial for each intervention) reduces the incidence of demineralized lesions during orthodontic treatment with fixed appliances (Stecksen-Blicks *et al.* 2007; Jiang *et al.* 2013; Sonesson *et al.* 2014).
- Low evidence for other fluoride interventions (Luther *et al.* 2005; van der Kaaij *et al.* 2015).

Commentary

1) Further well-designed studies are required to confirm these findings.
2) Standard reporting methods of future clinical trials are recommended so data can be pooled and stronger clinical recommendations made as meta-analysis is still not possible.

Additional References

Enaia M, Bock N, Ruf S, 2011. White-spot lesions during multibracket appliance treatment: A challenge for clinical excellence. *Am J Orthod Dentofacial Orthop* 140, e17–24.

Jiang H, Hua F, Yao L, *et al.*, 2013. Effect of 1.23% acidulated phosphate fluoride foam on white spot lesions in orthodontic patients: a randomized trial. *Pediatr Dent* 35, 275–278.

Luther F, Tobin M, Robertson AJ, *et al.*, 2005. Fluoride-releasing glass beads in orthodontic treatment to reduce decay: a randomized, controlled clinical trial. *WorldJournalOrthodontics* 6 (Suppl.), 166–167.

Sonesson M, Twetman S, Bondemark L, 2014. Effectiveness of high-fluoride toothpaste on enamel demineralization during orthodontic treatment-a multicenter randomized controlled trial. *Eur J Orthod* 36, 678–682.

Stecksen-Blicks C, Renfors G, Oscarson ND, *et al.*, 2007. Caries-preventive effectiveness of a fluoride varnish: a randomized controlled trial in adolescents with fixed orthodontic appliances. *Caries Res* 41, 455–459.

van der Kaaij NC, van der Veen MH, van der Kaaij MA, *et al.*, 2015. A prospective, randomized placebo-controlled clinical trial on the effects of a fluoride rinse on white spot lesion development and bleeding in orthodontic patients. *Eur J Oral Sci* 123, 186–193.

Acknowledgement

This Cochrane Review was published in the Cochrane Database of Systematic Reviews 2013, Issue 12. Cochrane Reviews are regularly updated as new evidence emerges and in response to feedback, and the Cochrane Database of Systematic Reviews should be consulted for the most recent version of the Cochrane Review.

Summary 3 Additional References

Banks P, Macfarlane TV, 2007. Bonded versus banded first molar attachments: a randomized controlled clinical trial. *J Orthod* 34, 128–136.

Nazir M, Walsh T, Mandall NA, *et al.* 2011. Banding versus bonding of first permanent molars: a multi-centre randomized controlled trial. *J Orthod* 38, 81–89.

Summary 7 Additional References

Ioannidis JP, 2016. The mass production of redundant, misleading, and conflicted systematic reviews and meta-analyses. *Milbank Q* 94, 485–514.

Meursinge Reynders RA, 2016. *Evidence-based knowledge creation on orthodontic mini-implants: 'Why we know so little'.* PhD thesis October 26 2016. Department of Oral and Maxillofacial Surgery, Academic Medical Center, University of Amsterdam. Available at: http://dare.uva.nl/document/2/177074 (accessed November 2016).

Sterne JA, Hernán MA, Reeves BC, *et al.*, 2016. ROBINS-I: a tool for assessing risk of bias in non-randomised studies of interventions. *BMJ* 355, i4919.

Summary 19 Additional References

Letra A, Menezes R, Granjeiro JM, *et al.*, 2007. Defining cleft subphenotypes based on dental development. *J Dent Res* 86, 986–991.

Menezes R, Vieira AR, 2008. Dental anomalies as part of the cleft spectrum. *Cleft Palate Craniofac J* 45, 414–419.

Vieira AR, 2008. Unraveling human cleft lip and palate research. *J Dent Res* 87, 119–125.

Vieira AR, 2012. Genetic and environmental factors in human cleft lip and palate. In: Cobourne MT (ed). *Cleft Lip and Palate. Epidemiology, Aetiology and Treatment. Frontiers of Oral Biology*, Vol. 16. Basel, Karger, 19–31.

Summary 20 Additional References

Clark L, Teichgraeber JF, Fleshman RG, *et al.,* 2011. long-term treatment outcome of presurgical nasoalveolar molding in patients with unilateral cleft lip and palate. *J Craniofac Surg* 22, 333–336.

Noverraz RLM, Disse MA, Ongkosuwito EM, *et al.,* 2015. Transverse dental arch relationship at 9 and 12 years in children with unilateral cleft lip and palate treated with infant orthopedics: a randomized clinical trial (DUTCHCLEFT). *Clin Oral Investig* 19, 2255–2265.

Summary 23 Additional References

Garib DG, Henriques JF, Janson G, *et al.,* 2005. Rapid maxillary expansion - tooth tissue-borne versus tooth-borne expanders: a computed tomography evaluation of dentoskeletal effects. *Angle Orthod* 75, 548–557.

Godoy F, Godoy-Bezerra J, Rosenblatt A, 2011. Treatment of posterior crossbite comparing 2 appliances: a community based trial. *Am J Orthod Dentofacial Orthop* 139, e45–52.

Oliveira NL, Da Silveira AC, Kusnoto B, *et al.,* 2004. Three dimensional assessment of morphologic changes of the maxilla: a comparison of 2 kinds of palatal expanders. *Am J Orthod Dentofacial Orthop* 126, 354–362.

Petrén S, Bondemark L, 2008. Correction of unilateral posterior crossbite in the mixed dentition: a randomized controlled trial. *Am J Orthod Dentofacial Orthop* 133, 790.e7–13.3.

Summary 24 Additional References

Kayalar E, Schauseil M, Kuvat SV, *et al.*, 2016. Comparison of tooth-borne and hybrid devices in surgically assisted rapid maxillary expansion: A randomized clinical cone-beam computed tomography study. *J Craniomaxillofac Surg* 44, 285–293.

Prado GP, Pereira MD, Bilo JP, *et al.*, 2013. Stability of surgically assisted rapid palatal expansion: a randomized trial. *J Dent Res* 92 (7 Suppl.), 49S–54S.

Zandi M, Miresmaeili A, Heidari A, 2014. Short-term skeletal and dental changes following bone-borne versus tooth-borne surgically assisted rapid maxillary expansion: a randomized clinical trial study. *J Craniomaxillofac Surg* 42, 1190–1195.

Summary 29 Additional Reference

Koretsi V, Zymperdikas VF, Papageorgiou SN, Papadopoulos MA, 2015. Treatment effects of removable functional appliances in patients with Class II malocclusion: a systematic review and meta-analysis. *Eur J Orthod* 37, 418–434.

Summary 30 Additional References

Higgins JPT, Green S (eds), 2011. *Cochrane Handbook for Systematic Reviews of Interventions*, version 5.1.0, updated March 2011. Cochrane Collaboration. Available at: www.handbook.cochrane.org (accessed November 2017).

Martina R, Cioffi I, Galeotti A, *et al.*, 2013. Efficacy of the Sander bite-jumping appliance in growing patients with mandibular retrusion: a randomized controlled trial. *Orthod Craniofac Res* 16,116–126.

O'Brien K, Wright J, Conboy F, *et al.*, 2003. Effectiveness of early orthodontic treatment with the twin-block appliance: a multicenter, randomized, controlled trial. Part 1: dental and skeletal effects. *Am J Orthod Dentofacial Orthop* 124, 234–243.

Tulloch JF, Phillips C, Koch G, *et al.*, 1997. The effect of early intervention on skeletal pattern in Class II malocclusion: a randomized clinical trial. *Am J Orthod Dentofacial Orthop* 111, 391–400.

Summary 33 Additional References

Karatas M, Akdag MS, Celikoglu M, 2014. Investigation of the peg-shaped maxillary lateral incisors in a Turkish orthodontic subpopulation. *J Orthod Res* 2, 125.

Kim J, Ko Y, Kim H, *et al.*, 2014. Distribution of the peg-laterals and associated dental anomalies in Korean children: a radiological study. *J Korean Acad Pediatr Dent* 41, 241–246.

Summary 36 Additional References

Bratton DJ, Gaisl T, Schlatzer C, *et al.*, 2015. Comparison of the effects of continuous positive airway pressure and mandibular advancement devices on sleepiness in patients with obstructive sleep apnoea: a network meta-analysis. *Lancet Respir Med* 3, 869–878.

Hardy ST, Loehr LR, Butler KR, *et al.*, 2015. Reducing the blood pressure-related burden of cardiovascular disease: impact of achievable improvements in blood pressure prevention and control. *J Am Heart Assoc* 4, e002276.

Summary 38 Additional References

Fontes AM, Joondeph DR, Bloomquist DS, *et al.*, 2012. Long-term stability of anterior open-bite closure with bilateral sagittal split osteotomy. *Am J Orthod Dentofacial Orthop* 142, 792–800.

Geron S, Wasserstein A, Geron Z, 2013. Stability of anterior open bite correction of adults treated with lingual appliances. *Eur J Orthod* 35, 599–603.

Maia FA, Janson G, Barros SE, *et al.*, 2010. Long-term stability of surgical-orthodontic open-bite correction. *Am J Orthod Dentofacial Orthop* 138, 254.e1–254.e10.

Mucedero M, Franchi L, Giuntini V, *et al.*, 2013. Stability of quad-helix/crib therapy in dentoskeletal open bite: a long-term controlled study. *Am J Orthod Dentofacial Orthop* 143, 695–703.

Teittinen M, Tuovinen V, Tammela L, *et al.*, 2012. Long-term stability of anterior open bite closure corrected by surgical-orthodontic treatment. *Eur J Orthod* 34, 238–243.

Zuroff JP, Chen SH, Shapiro PA, *et al.*, 2010. Orthodontic treatment of anterior open-bite malocclusion: stability 10 years postretention. *Am J Orthod Dentofacial Orthop* 137, 302.e1–302.e8.

Summary 42 Additional References

Allais D, Melsen B, 2003. Does labial movement of lower incisors influence the level of the gingival margin? A case-control study of adult orthodontic patients. *Eur J Orthod* 25, 343–352.

Bondemark L, 1998. Interdental bone changes after orthodontic treatment: a 5-year longitudinal study. *Am J Orthod Dentofacial Orthop* 114, 25–31.

Davies TM, Shaw WC, Worthington HV, *et al.*, 1991. The effect of orthodontic treatment on plaque and gingivitis. *Am J Orthod Dentofacial Orthop* 99, 155–161.

Feliu JL, 1982. Long-term benefits of orthodontic treatment on oral hygiene. *Am J Orthod* 82, 473–477.

Jager A, Polley J, Mausberg R, 1990. [Effects of orthodontic expansion of the mandibular arch on the periodontal condition of the posterior teeth]. *Dtsch Zahnarztl Z* 45, 113–115.

Janson G, Bombonatti R, Brandao AG, *et al.*, 2003. Comparative radiographic evaluation of the alveolar bone crest after orthodontic treatment. *Am J Orthod Dentofacial Orthop* 124, 157–164.

Janson M, 1984. [Gingival and periodontal relationships after orthodontic therapy. A study of class-II patients]. *Dtsch Zahnarztl Z* 39, 254–256.

Motegi E, Nomura M, Miyazaki H, *et al.*, 2002. Gingival recession in long-term post-orthodontic patients. *J Dent Res* 81, A372–A372.

Ogaard B, 1988. Marginal bone support and tooth lengths in 19-year-olds following orthodontic treatment. *Eur J Orthod* 10, 180–186.

Paolantonio M, Festa F, di Placido G, *et al.*, 1999. Site-specific subgingival colonization by *Actinobacillus actinomycetemcomitans* in orthodontic patients. *Am J Orthod Dentofacial Orthop* 115, 423–428.

Ribeiral MBC, Bolognese AM, Feres EJ, 1999. Periodontal evaluation after orthodontic treatment. *J Dent Res* 78, 979–979.

Thomson WM, 2002. Orthodontic treatment outcomes in the long term: findings from a longitudinal study of New Zealanders. *Angle Orthod* 72, 449–455.

Summary 43 Additional References

Edman Tynelius G, Bondemark L, 2013. A randomized controlled trial of three orthodontic retention methods in Class I four premolar extraction cases - stability after 2 years in retention. *Orthod Craniofacial Res* 16,105–115.

Gill DS, Naini FB, Jones A, *et al.*, 2007. Part-time versus full-time retainer wear following fixed appliance therapy: a randomized prospective controlled trial. *World J Orthod* 8, 300–306.

O'Rourke N, Albeedh H, Sharma P, *et al.*, 2016. Effectiveness of bonded and vacuum-formed retainers: A prospective randomized controlled clinical trial. *Am J Orthod Dentofacial Orthop* 150, 406–415.

Thickett E, Power S, 2010. A randomized clinical trial of thermoplastic retainer wear. *Eur J Orthod* 32, 1–5.

Summary 47 Additional References

Esteves T, Ramos AL, Pereira CM, *et al.*, 2007. Orthodontic root resorption of endodontically treated teeth. *J Endod* 33, 119–122.

Kreia TB, Tanaka O, Lara F, *et al.*, 2005. Avaliação da reabsorção radicular após a movimentação ortodôntica em dentes tratados endodonticamente/Evaluation of root resorption after orthodontic treatment in endodontically treated teeth. *Rev Odonto Ciênc* 20, 50–56.

Llamas-Carreras JM, Amarilla A, Solano E, *et al.*, 2010. Study of external root resorption during orthodontic treatment in root filled teeth compared with their contralateral teeth with vital pulps. *Int Endod J* 43, 654–662.

Mirabella AD, Årtun J, 1995. Risk factors for apical root resorption of maxillary anterior teeth in adult orthodontic patients. *Am J Orthod Dentofacial Orthop* 108, 48–55.

Spurrier SW, Hall SH, Joondeph DR, *et al.*, 1990. A comparison of apical root resorption during orthodontic treatment in endodontically treated and vital teeth. *Am J Orthod Dentofacial Orthop* 97, 130–134.

Summary 50 Additional References

Ghaffar F, Fida M, 2011. Effect of extraction of first four premolars on smile aesthetics. *Eur J Orthod* 33, 679–683.

Meyer AH, Woods MG, Manton DJ, 2014. Maxillary arch width and buccal corridor changes with orthodontic treatment. Part 2: attractiveness of the frontal facial smile in extraction and nonextraction outcomes. *Am J Orthod Dentofacial Orthop* 145, 296–304.

Yang S, Guo Y, Yang X, *et al.*, 2015. Effect of mesiodistal angulation of the maxillary central incisors on esthetic perceptions of the smile in the frontal view. *Am J Orthod Dentofacial Orthop* 148, 396–404.

Summary 52 Additional References

Esan T, Schepartz LA, 2016. Third molar impaction and agenesis: influence on anterior crowding. *Ann Hum Biol* 9, 1–7.

Selmani ME, Gjorgova J, Selmani ME, *et al.*, 2016. Effects of lower third molar angulation and position on lower arch crowding. *Int J Orthod* 27, 45–49.

Stanaitytė R, Trakinienė G, Gervickas A, 2014. Do wisdom teeth induce lower anterior teeth crowding? A systematic literature review. *Stomatologija* 16, 15–18.

Summary 54 References

Fleming PS, Fedorowicz Z, Johal A, *et al.*, 2015. Surgical adjunctive procedures for accelerating orthodontic treatment. *Cochrane Database Syst Rev* (6), CD010572.

Woodhouse NR, DiBiase AT, Johnson N, *et al.*, 2015. Supplemental vibrational force during orthodontic alignment a randomized trial. *J Dent Res* 94, 682–689.

Summary 55 Additional References

Aboul-Ela SM, El-Beialy AR, El-Sayed KM, *et al.*, 2011. Miniscrew implant-supported maxillary canine retraction with and without corticotomy-facilitated orthodontics. *Am J Orthod Dentofacial Orthop* 139, 252–259.

Fischer TJ, 2007. Orthodontic treatment acceleration with corticotomy-assisted exposure of palatally impacted canines. *Angle Orthod* 77, 417–420.

Gantes B, Rathbun E, Anholm M, 1990. Effects on the periodontium following corticotomy-facilitated orthodontics. Case reports. *J Periodontol* 61, 234–238.

Kharkar VR, Kotrashetti SM, 2010.Transport dentoalveolar distraction osteogenesis-assisted rapid orthodontic canine retraction. *Oral Surg Oral Med Oral Pathol Oral Radiol Endod* 109, 687–693.

Liem AML, Hoogeveen EJ, Jansma J, *et al.*, 2015. Surgically facilitated experimental movement of teeth: systematic review. *Br J Oral Maxillofac Surg* 53, 491–506.

Mowafy MI, Zaher AR, 2012. Anchorage loss during canine retraction using intermittent versus continuous force distractions; a split mouth randomized clinical trial. *Prog Orthod* 13, 117–125.

Shoreiba EA, Salama AE, Attia MS, *et al.*, 2012. Corticotomy-facilitated orthodontics in adults using a further modified technique. *J Int Acad Periodontol* 14, 97–104.

Systematic Reviews in Orthodontics

Systematic Reviews in Orthodontics searched in PubMed through June 30, 2017.

Accelerated tooth movement

Corticotomy

Effectiveness of minimally invasive surgical procedures in the acceleration of tooth movement: a systematic review and meta-analysis. Alfawal AM, Hajeer MY, Ajaj MA, Hamadah O, Brad B. Prog Orthod. 2016 Dec;17(1):33.

Corticotomies as a surgical procedure to accelerate tooth movement during orthodontic treatment: A systematic review. Fernández-Ferrer L, Montiel-Company JM, Candel-Martí E, Almerich-Silla JM, Peñarrocha-Diago M, Bellot-Arcís C. Med Oral Patol Oral Cir Bucal. 2016 Nov 1;21(6):e703-e712.

Corticotomies and orthodontic tooth movement: a systematic review. Patterson BM, Dalci O, Darendeliler MA, Papadopoulou AK. J Oral Maxillofac Surg. 2016 Mar;74(3):453–73.

Efficacy of surgical and non-surgical interventions on accelerating orthodontic tooth movement: a systematic review. Kalemaj Z, DebernardI CL, Buti J. Eur J Oral Implantol. 2015 Spring;8(1):9–4.

Surgically facilitated orthodontic treatment: a systematic review. Hoogeveen EJ, Jansma J, Ren Y. Am J Orthod Dentofacial Orthop. 2014 Apr;145(4 Suppl):S51–64.

Low level laser therapy

Efficacy of low-level laser therapy in accelerating tooth movement, preventing relapse and managing acute pain during orthodontic treatment in humans: a systematic review. Sonesson M, De Geer E, Subraian J, Petrén S. BMC Oral Health. 2016 Jul 7;17(1):11.

Efficiency of low-level laser therapy within induced dental movement: A systematic review and meta-analysis. de Almeida VL, de Andrade Gois VL, Andrade RN, Cesar CP, de Albuquerque-Junior RL, de Mello Rode S, Paranhos LR. J Photochem Photobiol B. 2016 May;158:258–66.

Efficacy of low-level laser therapy for accelerating tooth movement during orthodontic treatment: a systematic review and meta-analysis. Ge MK, He WL, Chen J, Wen C, Yin X, Hu ZA, Liu ZP, Zou SJ. Lasers Med Sci. 2015 Jul;30(5):1609–18.

The effectiveness of low-level laser therapy in accelerating orthodontic tooth movement: a meta-analysis. Long H, Zhou Y, Xue J, Liao L, Ye N, Jian F, Wang Y, Lai W. Lasers Med Sci. 2015 Apr;30 (3):1161–70.

The co-editors would like to thank Dr. Surbhi Singh for her excellent assistance with the organization of this section.

Systematic literature review: influence of low-level laser on orthodontic movement and pain control in humans. Sousa MV, Pinzan A, Consolaro A, Henriques JF, de Freitas MR. Photomed Laser Surg. 2014 Nov;32(11):592–9.

Tooth movement in orthodontic treatment with low-level laser therapy: a systematic review of human and animal studies. Carvalho-Lobato P, Garcia VJ, Kasem K, Ustrell-Torrent JM, Tallon-Walton V, Manzanares-Cespedes MC. Photomed Laser Surg. 2014 May;32(5):302–9.

Influence of low-level laser therapy on the rate of orthodontic movement: a literature review. Torri S, Weber JB. Photomed Laser Surg. 2013 Sep;31(9):411–21.

Pharmacological agents

The influence of teriparatide in induced tooth movement: A systematic review. Souza-Silva BN, Rodrigues JA, Moreira JC, Matos FS, Cesar CP, Repeke CE, Paranhos LR. J Clin Exp Dent. 2016 Dec 1;8(5):e615–e621.

Piezocision

Efficacy of piezocision on accelerating orthodontic tooth movement: A systematic review. Yi J, Xiao J, Li Y, Li X, Zhao Z. Angle Orthod. 2017 Jul;87(4):491–498.

Influence of piezotomy and osteoperforation of the alveolar process on the rate of orthodontic tooth movement: a systematic review. Hoffmann S, Papadopoulos N, Visel D, Visel T, Jost-Brinkmann PG, Prager TM. J Orofac Orthop. 2017 Jul;78(4):301–311.

Unspecified or multiple interventions

Effectiveness of adjunctive interventions for accelerating orthodontic tooth movement: a systematic review of systematic reviews. Yi J, Xiao J, Li H, Li Y, Li X, Zhao Z. J Oral Rehabil. 2017 Aug;44(8):636–654.

Non-surgical adjunctive interventions for accelerating tooth movement in patients undergoing fixed orthodontic treatment. El-Angbawi A, McIntyre GT, Fleming PS, Bearn DR. Cochrane Database Syst Rev. 2015 Nov 18;(11):CD010887.

Effectiveness of non-conventional methods for accelerated orthodontic tooth movement: a systematic review and meta-analysis. Gkantidis N, Mistakidis I, Kouskoura T, Pandis N. J Dent. 2014 Oct;42(10):1300–19.

Interventions for accelerating orthodontic tooth movement: a systematic review. Long H, Pyakurel U, Wang Y, Liao L, Zhou Y, Lai W. Angle Orthod. 2013 Jan;83(1):164–71.

Activator

Please see Functional and orthopedic appliances.

Adherence

Please see Compliance.

Adhesives and bonding agents

Bands

Adhesives for fixed orthodontic bands. Millett DT, Glenny AM, Mattick RC, Hickman J, Mandall NA. Cochrane Database Syst Rev. 2016 Oct 25;(10):CD004485.

Adhesives for fixed orthodontic bands - Millett DT, Glenny AM, Mattick CR, Hickman J, Mandall NA. Cochrane Database Syst Rev. 2007 Apr 18;(2):CD004485.

Brackets

The effect of antimicrobial agents on bond strength of orthodontic adhesives: a meta-analysis of in vitro studies. Altmann AS, Collares FM, Leitune VC, Samuel SM. Orthod Craniofac Res. 2016 Feb;19(1):1–9.

Orthodontic bonding to porcelain: a systematic review. Grewal Bach GK, Torrealba Y, Lagravere MO. Angle Orthod. 2014 May;84(3):555–60.

Effect of orthodontic debonding and adhesive removal on the enamel - current knowledge and future perspectives - a systematic review. Janiszewska-Olszowska J, Szatkiewicz T, Tomkowski R, Tandecka K, Grocholewicz K. Med Sci Monit. 2014 Oct 20;20:1991–2001.

Self-etch primers and conventional acid-etch technique for orthodontic bonding: a systematic review and meta-analysis. Fleming PS, Johal A, Pandis N. Am J Orthod Dentofacial Orthop. 2012 Jul;142(1):83–94.

Retention of orthodontic brackets bonded with resin-modified GIC versus composite resin adhesives—a quantitative systematic review of clinical trials. Mickenautsch S, Yengopa V, Banerjee A. Clin Oral Investig. 2012 Feb;16(1):1–14.

Adhesives for bonded molar tubes during fixed brace treatment. Millett DT, Mandall NA, Mattick RC, Hickman J, Glenny AM Cochrane Database Syst Rev. 2011 Jun 15;(6):CD00823.

The effect of antisialogogues in dentistry: a systematic review with a focus on bond failure in orthodontics. Kuijpers MA, Vissink A, Ren Y, Kuijpers-Jagtman AM. J Am Dent Assoc. 2010 Aug;141(8):954–65.

In-vitro orthodontic bond strength testing: a systematic review and meta-analysis. Finnema KJ, Ozcan M, Post WJ, Ren Y, Dijkstra PU. Am J Orthod Dentofacial Orthop. 2010 May;137(5):615–622.e3.

Adhesives for fixed orthodontic brackets. Mandall NA, Millett DT, Mattick CR, Hickman J, Macfarlane TV, Worthington HV. Cochrane Database Syst Rev 2003;(2):CD002282.

Orthodontic adhesives: a systematic review. Mandall NA, Millett DT, Mattick CR, Hickman J, Worthington HV, Macfarlane TV. J Orthod 2002;29(3):205–10.

Curing lights

Curing lights for orthodontic bonding: a systematic review and meta-analysis. Fleming PS, Eliades T, Katsaros C, Pandis N. Am J Orthod Dentofacial Orthop. 2013 Apr;143(4 Suppl):S92–103.

Agenesis and anomalies

Cleft lip and palate

Please see Cleft lip and palate.

Lateral incisors

Prosthetic replacement vs space closure for maxillary lateral incisor agenesis: A systematic review. Silveira GS, de Almeida NV, Pereira DM, Mattos CT, Mucha JN. Am J Orthod Dentofacial Orthop. 2016 Aug;150(2):228–37.

Treatment options for congenitally missing lateral incisors. Kiliaridis S, Sidira M, Kirmanidou Y, Michalakis K. Eur J Oral Implantol. 2016;9 Suppl 1:S5–24.

Third molars

Morphologic and Demographic Predictors of Third Molar Agenesis: A Systematic Review and Meta-analysis. Carter K, Worthington S.J Dent Res. 2015 Jul;94(7):886–94.

Airway

Please also see Obstructive sleep apnea.

Craniofacial and upper airway morphology in adult obstructive sleep apnea patients: A systematic review and meta-analysis of cephalometric studies. Neelapu BC, Kharbanda OP, Sardana HK, Balachandran R, Sardana V, Kapoor P, Gupta A, Vasamsetti S. Sleep Med Rev. 2017 Feb;31:79–90.

Efficiency of bimaxillary advancement surgery in increasing the volume of the upper airways: a systematic review of observational studies and meta-analysis. Rosário HD, Oliveira GM, Freires IA, de Souza Matos F, Paranhos LR. Eur Arch Otorhinolaryngol. 2017 Jan;274(1):35–44.

Reliability of upper pharyngeal airway assessment using dental CBCT: a systematic review. Zimmerman JN, Lee J, Pliska BT. Eur J Orthod. 2017 Oct 1;39(5):489–496.

Volumetric upper airway changes after rapid maxillary expansion: a systematic review and meta-analysis. Buck LM, Dalci O, Darendeliler MA, Papageorgiou SN, Papadopoulou AK. Eur J Orthod. 2017 Oct 1;39(5):463–473.

Efficiency of bimaxillary advancement surgery in increasing the volume of the upper airways: a systematic review of observational studies and meta-analysis. Rosário HD, Oliveira GM, Freires IA, de Souza Matos F, Paranhos LR. Eur Arch Otorhinolaryngol. 2017 Jan;274(1):35–44.

Effect of Head and Tongue Posture on the Pharyngeal Airway Dimensions and Morphology in Three-Dimensional Imaging: A Systematic Review.Gurani SF, Di Carlo G, Cattaneo PM, Thorn JJ, Pinholt EM. J Oral Maxillofac Res. 2016 Mar 31;7(1):e1.

Effect of surgically assisted rapid maxillary expansion on upper airway volume: a systematic review. Buck LM, Dalci O, Darendeliler MA, Papadopoulou AK. J Oral Maxillofac Surg. 2016 May;74(5):1025–43.

The upper airway dimensions in different sagittal craniofacial patterns: a systematic review. Indriksone I, Jakobsone G. Stomatologija. 2014;16(3):109–17.

Effects of orthognathic surgery on oropharyngeal airway: a meta-analysis. Mattos CT, Vilani GN, Sant'Anna EF, Ruellas AC, Maia LC. Int J Oral Maxillofac Surg. 2011 Dec;40(12):1347–56.

Does rapid maxillary expansion have long-term effects on airway dimensions and breathing? Baratieri C, Alves M Jr, de Souza MM, de Souza Araujo MT, Maia LC. Am J Orthod Dentofacial Orthop. 2011 Aug;140(2):146–56.

Aligners

Please see Clear aligners.

Alternating rapid maxillary expansion and constriction (ALT RAMEC)

Please see Crossbite (posterior).

Anchorage/temporary anchorage devices (TADs)

Class II

Comparison of the effects of mini-implant and traditional anchorage on patients with maxillary dentoalveolar protrusion. Xu Y, Xie J. Angle Orthod. 2017 Mar;87(2):320–327.

Can the use of skeletal anchors in conjunction with fixed functional appliances promote skeletal changes? A systematic review and meta-analysis. Elkordy SA, Aboelnaga AA, Fayed MM, AboulFotouh MH, Abouelezz AM. Eur J Orthod. 2016 Oct;38(5):532–45.

Are orthodontic distalizers reinforced with the temporary skeletal anchorage devices effective? Fudalej P, Antoszewska J. Am J Orthod Dentofacial Orthop. 2011 Jun;139(6):722–9. June, 2011.

Intraoral distalizer effects with conventional and skeletal anchorage: a meta-analysis. Grec RH, Janson G, Branco NC, Moura-Grec PG, Patel MP, Castanha Henriques JF. Am J Orthod Dentofacial Orthop. 2013 May;143(5):602–15.

Comparison of anchorage capacity between implant and headgear during anterior segment retraction. Li F, Hu HK, Chen JW, Liu ZP, Li GF, He SS, Zou SJ, Ye QS. Angle Orthod. 2011 Sep;81(5):915–22.

Class III

Bone- and dentoalveolar-anchored dentofacial orthopedics for Class III malocclusion: new approaches, similar objectives? a systematic review. Morales-Fernandez M, Iglesias-Linares A, Yanez-Vico RM, Mendoza-Mendoza A, Solano-Reina E. Angle Orthod. 2013 May;83(3):540–52.

Effectiveness of interceptive treatment of class III malocclusions with skeletal anchorage: A systematic review and meta-analysis. Rodriguez de Guzman-Barrera J, Saez Martínez C, Boronat-Catala M, Montiel-Company. JM, Paredes-Gallardo V, Gandía-Franco JL, Almerich-Silla JM, Bellot-Arcís C. PLoS One. 2017 Mar 22;12(3):e0173875.

Effectiveness of TAD-anchored maxillary protraction in late mixed dentition. Feng X, Li J, Li Y, Zhao Z, Zhao S, Wang J. Angle Orthod. 2012 Nov;82(6):1107–14.

Effectiveness/ success rates

Comparison of the success rate between self-drilling and self-tapping miniscrews: a systematic review and meta-analysis. Yi J, Ge M, Li M, Li C, Li Y, Li X, Zhao Z. Eur J Orthod. 2017 Jun 1;39(3):287–293.

Effectiveness of orthodontic miniscrew implants in anchorage reinforcement during en-masse retraction: A systematic review and meta-analysis. Antoszewska-Smith J, Sarul M, Lyczek J, Konopka T, Kawala B. Am J Orthod Dentofacial Orthop. 2017 Mar;151(3):440–455.

Temporary anchorage devices (TADs) in orthodontics: review of the factors that influence the clinical success rate of the mini-implants. Leo M, Cerroni L, Pasquantonio G, Condo SG, Condo R. Clin Ter. 2016 May-Jun;167(3):e70–7.

Prognostic factors associated with the success rates of posterior orthodontic miniscrew implants: A subgroup meta-analysis. Hong SB, Kusnoto B, Kim EJ, BeGole EA, Hwang HS, Lim HJ. Korean J Orthod. 2016 Mar;46(2):111–26.

Reinforcement of anchorage during orthodontic brace treatment with implants or other surgical methods. Jambi S, Walsh T, Sandler J, Benson PE, Skeggs RM, O'Brien KD. Cochrane Database Syst Rev. 2014 Aug 19;(8):CD005098.

Determinants for success rates of temporary anchorage devices in orthodontics: a meta-analysis (n > 50). Dalessandri D, Salgarello S, Dalessandri M, Lazzaroni E, Piancino M, Paganelli C, Maiorana C, Santoro F. Eur J Orthod. 2014 Jun;36(3):303–13.

Bone anchor systems for orthodontic application: a systematic review. Tsui WK, Chua HD, Cheung LK. Int J Oral Maxillofac Surg. 2012 Nov;41(11):1427–38.

Insertion torque and success of orthodontic mini-implants: a systematic review. Meursinge Reynders RA, Ronchi L, Ladu L, van Etten-Jamaludin F, Bipat S. Am J Orthod Dentofacial Orthop. 2012 Nov;142(5):596–614.

Failure rates and associated risk factors of orthodontic miniscrew implants: a meta-analysis. Papageorgiou SN, Zogakis IP, Papadopoulos MA. Am J Orthod Dentofacial Orthop. 2012 Nov;142(5):577–595.

Clinical effectiveness of orthodontic miniscrew implants: a meta-analysis. Papadopoulos MA, Papageorgiou SN, Zogakis IP. J Dent Res. 2011 Aug;90(8):969–76.

Survival and failure rates of orthodontic temporary anchorage devices: a systematic review. Schatzle M, Mannchen R, Zwahlen M, Lang NP. Clin Oral Implants Res. 2009 Dec;20(12):1351–9.

Mini-implants in orthodontics: a systematic review of the literature. Reynders R, Ronchi L, Bipat S. Am J Orthod Dentofacial Orthop. 2009 May;135(5): 564.e1–19; discussion 564–5.

Critical factors for the success of orthodontic mini-implants: a systematic review. Chen Y, Kyung HM, Zhao WT, Yu WJ. Am J Orthod Dentofacial Orthop. 2009 Mar;135(3):284–91.

Skeletal anchorage in orthodontics--a review of various systems in animal and human studies. Janssen KI, Raghoebar GM, Vissink A, Sandham A. Int J Oral Maxillofac Implants. 2008 Jan-Feb;23(1):75–88.

Orthodontic anchorage: a systematic review. Feldmann I, Bondemark L. Angle Orthod. 2006 May;76(3):493–501.

Implants for orthodontic anchorage. Meta-analysis. Labanauskaite B, Jankauskas G, Vasiliauskas A, Haffar N. Stomatologija. 2005;7(4):128–32.

Insertion/ location factors

How do geometry-related parameters influence the clinical performance of orthodontic mini-implants? A systematic review and meta-analysis. Cunha AC, da Veiga AMA, Masterson D, Mattos CT, Nojima LI, Nojima MCG, Maia LC. Int J Oral Maxillofac Surg. 2017 Dec;46(12):1539–1551.

Barriers and facilitators to the implementation of orthodontic mini implants in clinical practice: a systematic review. Meursinge Reynders R, Ronchi L, Ladu L, Di Girolamo N, de Lange J, Roberts N, Mickan S. Syst Rev. 2016 Sep 23;5(1):163.

Insertion torque recordings for the diagnosis of contact between orthodontic mini-implants and dental roots: a systematic review. Meursinge Reynders R, Ladu L, Ronchi L, Di Girolamo N, de Lange J, Roberts N, Pluddemann A. Syst Rev. 2016 Mar 31;5:50.

Does cortical thickness influence the primary stability of miniscrews? A systematic review and meta-analysis. Marquezan M, Mattos CT, Sant'Anna EF, de Souza MM, Maia LC. Angle Orthod. 2014 Nov;84(6):1093–103.

Paramedian vertical palatal bone height for mini-implant insertion: a systematic review. Winsauer H, Vlachojannis C, Bumann A, Vlachojannis J, Chrubasik S. Eur J Orthod. 2014 Oct;36(5):541–9.

Insertion torque and orthodontic mini-implants: a systematic review of the artificial bone literature. Meursinge Reynders R, Ronchi L, Ladu L, Van Etten-Jamaludin F, Bipat S. Proc Inst Mech Eng H. 2013 Nov;227(11):1181–202.

Positional guidelines for orthodontic mini-implant placement in the anterior alveolar region: a systematic review. Alsamak S, Psomiadis S, Gkantidis N. Int J Oral Maxillofac Implants. 2013 Mar-Apr;28(2):470–9.

Assessment of potential orthodontic mini-implant insertion sites based on anatomical hard tissue parameters: a systematic review. AlSamak S, Gkantidis N, Bitsanis E, Christou P. Int J Oral Maxillofac Implants. 2012 Jul-Aug;27(4): 875–87.

Does bone mineral density influence the primary stability of dental implants? A systematic review. Marquezan M, Osorio A, Sant'Anna E, Souza MM, Maia L. Clin Oral Implants Res. 2012 Jul;23(7):767–74.

Loading of implants

Systematic review of the experimental use of temporary skeletal anchorage devices in orthodontics. Cornelis MA, Scheffler NR, De Clerck HJ, Tulloch JF, Behets CN. Am J Orthod Dentofacial Orthop. 2007 Apr;131(4 Suppl): S52–8. April, 2007.

Implant vs screw loading protocols in orthodontics. Ohashi E, Pecho OE, Moron M, Lagravere MO. Angle Orthod. 2006 Jul;76(4):721–7.

Openbite

Effect of molar intrusion with temporary anchorage devices in patients with anterior open bite: a systematic review. Alsafadi AS, Alabdullah MM, Saltaji H, Abdo A, Youssef M. Prog Orthod. 2016;17:9.

TADs as dental implants

Mini implants for definitive prosthodontic treatment: a systematic review. Bidra AS, Almas K. J Prosthet Dent. 2013 Mar;109(3):156–64.

Anterior crossbite

Please see Class III.

Anterior openbite

Please see Openbite.

Antimicrobial agents

Effects of chlorhexidine varnish on caries during orthodontic treatment: a systematic review and meta-analysis. Okada EM, Ribeiro LN, Stuani MB, Borsatto MC, Fidalgo TK, Paula-Silva FW, Küchler. EC. Braz Oral Res. 2016 Nov 28;30(1):e115.

The antimicrobial effect of chlorhexidine varnish on mutans streptococci in patients with fixed orthodontic appliances: a systematic review of clinical efficacy. Tang X, Sensat ML, Stoltenberg JL. Int J Dent Hyg. 2016 Feb;14(1):53–61.

Assessment of the effectiveness of mouthwashes in reducing cariogenic biofilm in orthodontic patients: a systematic review. Pithon MM, Sant'Anna LI, Baiao FC, dos Santos RL, Coqueiro Rda S, Maia LC. J Dent. 2015 Mar;43(3):297–308.

Caries-Inhibiting Effect of Preventive Measures during Orthodontic Treatment with Fixed Appliances. A Systematic Review Derks A, Katsaros C, Frencken JE, Van't Hof MA, Kuijpers-Jagtman AM. Caries Res 2004;38(5):413–20.

Appliances

Please see Brackets or Functional and orthopedic appliances.

Arch width

Please see Intra-arch width.

Arch-wires

A systematic review and meta-analysis of experimental clinical evidence on initial aligning archwires and archwire sequences. Papageorgiou SN, Konstantinidis I, Papadopoulou K, Jager A, Bourauel C. Orthod Craniofac Res. 2014 Nov;17(4):197–215.

Initial arch wires for tooth alignment during orthodontic treatment with fixed appliances. Jian F, Lai W, Furness S, McIntyre GT, Millett DT, Hickman J, Wang Y. Cochrane Database Syst Rev. 2013 Apr 30;(4):CD007859.

A systematic review of clinical trials of aligning archwires. Riley M, Bearn DR. J Orthod. 2009 Mar;36(1):42–51.

Auto transplantation

Success rate of autotransplantation of teeth with an open apex: systematic review and meta-analysis. Atala-Acevedo C, Abarca J, Martinez-Zapata MJ, Diaz J, Olate S, Zaror C. J Oral Maxillofac Surg. 2017 Jan;75(1):35–50.

Autotransplantation of teeth using computer-aided rapid prototyping of a three-dimensional replica of the donor tooth: a systematic literature review. Verweij JP, Jongkees FA, Anssari Moin D, Wismeijer D, Van Merkesteyn JPR. Int J Oral Maxillofac Surg. 2017 Nov;46(11):1466–1474.

Long-term prognosis of tooth autotransplantation a systematic review and meta-analysis. Machado LA, do Nascimento RR, Ferreira DM, Mattos CT, Vilella OV. Int J Oral Maxillofac Surg. 2016 May;45(5):610–7.

Occlusal rehabilitation in patients with congenitally missing teeth-dental implants, conventional prosthetics, tooth auto transplant, and preservation of deciduous teeth-a systematic review. Terheyden H, Wusthoff F. Int J Implant Dent. 2015 Dec;1(1):30.

Biology of tooth movement

Biomarkers of Orthodontic Tooth Movement in Gingival Crevicular Fluid: A Systematic Review. Alhadlaq AM. J Contemp Dent Pract. 2015 Jul 1;16(7):578–87.

Effect of orthodontic forces on cytokine and receptor levels in gingival crevicular fluid: a systematic review. Kapoor P, Kharbanda OP, Monga N, Miglani R, Kapila S. Prog Orthod. 2014 Dec 9;15:65.

Is gingival crevicular fluid volume sensitive to orthodontic tooth movement? A systematic review of split-mouth longitudinal studies. Perinetti G, Primozic J, Castaldo A, Di Lenarda R, Contardo L. Orthod Craniofac Res. 2013 Feb;16(1):1–19.

Bionator

Please see Functional and orthopedic appliances.

Bisphosphonates

Effects of bisphosphonates in orthodontic therapy: systematic review. Rodolfino D, Saccucci M, Filippakos A, Gerxhani R, Lopez G, Felice F, D'Arcangelo C. J Biol Regul Homeost Agents. 2012 Apr-Jun;26(2 Suppl):29–33.

Influence of bisphosphonates in orthodontic therapy: systematic review. Iglesias-Linares A, Yanez-Vico RM, Solano-Reina E, Torres-Lagares D, Gonzalez Moles MA. J Dent. 2010 Aug;38(8):603–11.

Bond strength

Please see Adhesives and bonding agents.

Botulinum toxin

Botulinum toxin for the treatment of excessive gingival display: a systematic review. Marwan W, Nasr MD, Samer F, Jabbour MD, Joseph A, Sidaoui MD, Roger N, Haber MD, Elio G, Kechichian MD. Aesthetic Surg J 2016;36(1):82–88.

Efficacy of botulinum toxins on bruxism: an evidence-based review. Long H, Liao Z, Wang Y, Liao L, Lai W. Int Dent J. 2012 Feb;62(1):1–5.

Brackets

Lingual

Clinical outcomes of lingual orthodontic treatment: A systematic review. Mistakidis I, Katib H, Vasilakos G, Kloukos D, Gkantidis N. Eur J Orthod. 2016 Oct;38(5):447–58.

Adverse effects of lingual and buccal orthodontic techniques: A systematic review and meta-analysis. Ata-Ali F, Ata-Ali J, Ferrer-Molina M, Cobo T, De Carlos F, Cobo J. Am J Orthod Dentofacial Orthop. 2016 Jun;149(6):820–9.

Comparison of adverse effects between lingual and labial orthodontic treatment. Long H, Zhou Y, Pyakurel U, Liao L, Jian F, Xue J, Ye N, Yang X, Wang Y, Lai W. Angle Orthod. 2013 Nov;83(6):1066–73

Microbiota

The influence of orthodontic fixed appliances on the oral microbiota: a systematic review. Freitas AO, Marquezan M, Nojima Mda C, Alviano DS, Maia LC. Dental Press J Orthod. 2014 Mar–Apr;19(2):46–55.

Polycarbonate brackets

Bisphenol-A and residual monomer leaching from orthodontic adhesive resins and polycarbonate brackets: a systematic review Kloukos D, Pandis N, Eliades T. Am J Orthod Dentofacial Orthop. 2013 Apr;143(4 Suppl):S104–12. e1–2.

Prescriptions, torque, and tip

Treatment effects of various prescriptions and techniques for fixed orthodontic appliances: A systematic review. Mousoulea S, Papageorgiou SN, Eliades T. J Orofac Orthop. 2017 Sep;78(5):403–414.

Clinical effects of pre-adjusted edgewise orthodontic brackets: A systematic review and meta-analysis. Papageorgiou SN, Konstantinidis I, Papadopoulou K, Jager A, Bourauel C. Eur J Orthod. 2014 Jun;36(3):350–63.

Torque expression in stainless steel orthodontic brackets. A systematic review. Archambault A, Lacoursiere R, Badawi H, Major PW, Carey J, Flores-Mir C. Angle Orthod. 2010 Jan;80(1):201–10.

Release of metal ions

Release of metal ions from orthodontic appliances by in vitro studies: a systematic literature review. Mikulewicz M, Chojnacka K. Biol Trace Elem Res. 2011 Mar;139(3):241–56.

Self-ligating brackets

Differences between active and passive self-ligating brackets for orthodontic treatment: Systematic review and meta-analysis based on randomized clinical trials. Yang X, He Y, Chen T, Zhao M, Yan Y, Wang H, Bai D. J Orofac Orthop. 2017 Mar;78(2):121–128.

Effects of self-ligating brackets on oral hygiene and discomfort: a systematic review and meta-analysis of randomized controlled clinical trials. Yang X, Su N, Shi Z, Xiang Z, He Y, Han X, Bai D. Int J Dent Hyg.2017 Feb;15(1):16–22.

Torque expression in self-ligating orthodontic brackets and conventionally ligated brackets: A systematic review. Al-Thomali Y, Mohamed RN, Basha S. J Clin Exp Dent. 2017 Jan 1;9(1):e123–e128.

Root resorption during orthodontic treatment with self-ligating or conventional brackets: a systematic review and meta-analysis. Yi J, Li M, Li Y, Li X, Zhao Z. BMC Oral Health. 2016 Nov 21;16(1):125.

Initial orthodontic alignment effectiveness with self-ligating and conventional appliances: a network meta-analysis in practice. Pandis N, Fleming PS, Spineli LM, Salanti. Am J Orthod Dentofacial Orthop. 2014 Apr;145(4 Suppl):S152–63.

Are self-ligating brackets related to less formation of Streptococcus mutans colonies? A systematic review. do Nascimento LE, de Souza MM, Azevedo AR, Maia LC. Dental Press J Orthod. 2014 Jan–Feb;19(1):60–8.

Systematic review on self-ligating vs. conventional brackets: initial pain, number of visits, treatment time. Celar A, Schedlberger M, Dorfler P, Bertl M. J Orofac Orthop. 2013 Jan;74(1):40–51.

Systematic review of self-ligating brackets. Chen SS, Greenlee GM, Kim JE, Smith CL, Huang GJ. Am J Orthod Dentofacial Orthop. 2010 Jun;137(6):726.e1–726.e18.

Self-ligating brackets in orthodontics. A systematic review. Fleming PS, Johal A. Angle Orthod. 2010 May;80(3):575–84.

Frictional resistance in self-ligating orthodontic brackets and conventionally ligated brackets. A systematic review. Ehsani S, Mandich MA, El-Bialy TH, Flores-Mir C. Angle Orthod. 2009 May;79(3):592–601.

Bruxism

A systematic review of etiological and risk factors associated with bruxism. Feu D, Catharino F, Quintao CC, Almeida MA. J Orthod. 2013 Jun;40(2):163–71.

Efficacy of botulinum toxins on bruxism: an evidence-based review. Long H, Liao Z, Wang Y, Liao L, Lai W. Int Dent J. 2012 Feb;62(1):1–5.

Occlusal splints for treating sleep bruxism (tooth grinding). Macedo CR, Silva AB, Machado MA, Saconato H, Prado GF. Cochrane Database Syst Rev. 2007 Oct 17;(4):CD005514.

Stabilization splint therapy for the treatment of temporomandibular myofascial pain: A systematic review. Al-Ani Z, Gray RJ, Davies SJ, Sloan P, Glenny AM. J Dent Educ. 2005 Nov;69(11):1242–50.

Canine impaction and transmigration

Canine impaction

Open versus closed surgical exposure of palatally impacted maxillary canines: comparison of the different treatment outcomes-A systematic review. Sampaziotis D, Tsolakis IA, Bitsanis E, Tsolakis AI. Eur J Orthod. 2017 May 9. doi: 10.1093/ejo/cjw077. [Epub ahead of print].

Impacted and transmigrant mandibular canines incidence, aetiology, and treatment: A systematic review. Dalessandri D, Parrini S, Rubiano R, Gallone D, Migliorati M. Eur J Orthod. 2017 Apr 1;39(2):161–169.

Periodontal status after surgical-orthodontic treatment of labially impacted canines with different surgical techniques: A systematic review. Incerti-Parenti S, Checchi V, Ippolito DR, Gracco A, Alessandri-Bonetti G. Am J Orthod Dentofacial Orthop. 2016 Apr;149(4):463–72.

A systematic review of the interceptive treatment of palatally displaced maxillary canines. Naoumova J, Kurol J, Kjellberg H. Eur J Orthod. 2011 Apr;33(2):143–9.

Canine transmigration

Impacted and transmigrant mandibular canines incidence, aetiology, and treatment: A systematic review. Dalessandri D, Parrini S, Rubiano R, Gallone D, Migliorati M. Eur J Orthod. 2017 Apr 1;39(2):161–169.

Mandibular Canine Transmigration: Report of Three Cases and Literature Review. Bhullar MK, Aggarwal I, Verma R, Uppal AS. J Int Soc Prev Community Dent. 2017 Jan-Feb;7(1):8–4.

Caries

Please also see White spot lesions.

Effects of chlorhexidine varnish on caries during orthodontic treatment: a systematic review and meta-analysis. Okada EM, Ribeiro LN, Stuani MB, Borsatto MC, Fidalgo TK, Paula-Silva FW, KuchlerEC. Braz Oral Res. 2016 Nov 28;30(1):e115.

The antimicrobial effect of chlorhexidine varnish on mutans streptococci in patients with fixed orthodontic appliances: a systematic review of clinical efficacy. Tang X, Sensat ML, Stoltenberg JL. Int J Dent Hyg. 2016 Feb;14(1):53–61.

Enamel roughness and incidence of caries after interproximal enamel reduction: a systematic review. Koretsi V, Chatzigianni A, Sidiropoulou S. Orthod Craniofac Res. 2014 Feb;17(1):1–13.

Long-term remineralizing effect of casein phosphopeptide-amorphous calcium phosphate (CPP-ACP) on early caries lesions in vivo: a systematic review. Li J, Xie X, Wang Y, Yin W, Antoun JS, Farella M, Mei L. J Dent. 2014 Jul;42(7):769–77.

Fluorides for the prevention of early tooth decay (demineralised white lesions) during fixed brace treatment. Benson PE, Parkin N, Dyer F, Millett DT, Furness S, Germain P. Cochrane Database Syst Rev. 2013 Dec 12;(12):CD003809.

Dental crowding as a caries risk factor: a systematic review. Hafez HS, Shaarawy SM, Al-Sakiti AA, Mostafa YA. Am J Orthod Dentofacial Orthop. 2012 Oct;142(4):443–50.

Caries-inhibiting effect of preventive measures during orthodontic treatment with fixed appliances. a systematic review. Derks A, Katsaros C, Frencken JE, Van't Hof MA, Kuijpers-Jagtman AM. Caries Res 2004;38(5):413–20.

CBCT

Please see Diagnostic records.

Cephalometry

Please see Diagnostic records.

Chin cup

Please see Class III and Functional and orthopedic appliances.

Class II

Early treatment

Early orthodontic treatment for Class II malocclusion reduces the chance of incisal trauma: Results of a Cochrane systematic review. Thiruvenkatachari B, Harrison J, Worthington H, O'Brien K. Am J Orthod Dentofacial Orthop. 2015 Jul;148(1):47–59.

Orthodontic treatment for prominent upper front teeth (Class II malocclusion) in children. Thiruvenkatachari B, Harrison JE, Worthington HV, O'Brien KD. Cochrane Database Syst Rev. 2013 Nov 13;(11):CD003452.

Orthodontic treatment for prominent upper front teeth in children. More recent review. Harrison JE, O'Brien KD, Worthington HV. Cochrane Database Syst Rev. 2007 Jul 18;(3):CD003452.

Elastics

Correction of Class II malocclusion with Class II elastics: A systematic review. Janson G, Sathler R, Fernandes TM, Branco NC, Freitas MR. Am J Orthod Dentofacial Orthop. 2013 Mar;143(3):383–92.

Extraction

Changes in apical base sagittal relationship in Class II malocclusion treatment with and without premolar extractions: A systematic review and meta-analysis. Janson G, Aliaga-Del Castillo A, Niederberger A. Angle Orthod. 2017 Mar;87(2):338–355.

Soft-tissue changes in Class II malocclusion patients treated with extractions: A systematic review. Janson G, Mendes LM, Junqueira CH, Garib DG. Eur J Orthod. 2016 Dec;38(6):631–637.

Functional appliances

Changes in airway dimensions following functional appliances in growing patients with skeletal class II malocclusion: A systematic review and meta-analysis. Xiang M, Hu B, Liu Y, Sun J, Song J. Int J Pediatr Otorhinolaryngol. 2017 Jun;97:170–180.

Effect of functional appliances on the airway dimensions in patients with skeletal class II malocclusion: A systematic review. Kannan A, Sathyanarayana HP, Padmanabhan S. J Orthod Sci. 2017 Apr–Jun;6(2):54–64.

A comparison of the efficacy of fixed versus removable functional appliances in children with Class II malocclusion: A systematic review. Pacha MM, Fleming PS, Johal A. Eur J Orthod. 2016 Dec;38(6):621–630.

Can the use of skeletal anchors in conjunction with fixed functional appliances promote skeletal changes? A systematic review and meta-analysis. Elkordy SA, Aboelnaga AA, Fayed MM, AboulFotouh MH, Abouelezz AM. Eur J Orthod. 2016 Oct;38(5):532–45.

The effectiveness of the Herbst appliance for patients with Class II malocclusion: A meta-analysis. Yang X, Zhu Y, Long H, Zhou Y, Jian F, Ye N, Gao M, Lai W. Eur J Orthod. 2016 Jun;38(3):324–33.

Effectiveness of orthodontic treatment with functional appliances on maxillary growth in the short term: A systematic review and meta-analysis. Nucera R, Lo Giudice A, Rustico L, Matarese G, Papadopoulos MA, Cordasco G. Am J Orthod Dentofacial Orthop. 2016 May;149(5):600–611.e3.

Treatment effects of fixed functional appliances in patients with Class II malocclusion: A systematic review and meta-analysis. Zymperdikas VF, Koretsi V, Papageorgiou SN, Papadopoulos MA. Eur J Orthod. 2016 Apr;38(2):113–26.

Fixed functional appliances show definite skeletal and dental changes in the short term. McGuinness N. Eur J Orthod. 2016 Apr;38(2):127–8.

Stability of Class II fixed functional appliance therapy-A systematic review and meta-analysis. Bock NC, von Bremen J, Ruf S. Eur J Orthod. 2016 Apr;38(2):129–39.

Class II functional orthopaedic treatment: A systematic review of systematic reviews. D'Anto V, Bucci R, Franchi L, Rongo R, Michelotti A, Martina R.J Oral Rehabil. 2015 Aug;42(8):624–42.

Treatment effects of removable functional appliances in patients with Class II malocclusion: A systematic review and meta-analysis. Koretsi V, Zymperdikas VF, Papageorgiou SN, Papadopoulos MA. Eur J Orthod. 2015 Aug;37(4):418–34.

Meta-analysis on the mandibular dimensions effects of the MARA appliance in patients with Class II malocclusions. Al-Jewair TS. Angle Orthod. 2015 Jul;85(4):706–14.

Meta-analysis of skeletal mandibular changes during Frankel appliance treatment. Perillo L, Cannavale R, Ferro F, Franchi L, Masucci C, Chiodini P, Baccetti T. Eur J Orthod. 2011 Feb;33(1):84–92.

Effectiveness of orthodontic treatment with functional appliances on mandibular growth in the short term. Marsico E, Gatto E, Burrascano M, Matarese G, Cordasco G. Am J Orthod Dentofacial Orthop. 2011 Jan;139(1):24–36.

Skeletal and dental changes in Class II division 1 malocclusions treated with splint-type Herbst appliances. A systematic review. Flores-Mir C, Ayeh A, Goswani A, Charkhandeh S. Angle Orthod. 2007 Mar;77(2):376–81.

A systematic review of cephalometric facial soft tissue changes with the Activator and Bionator appliances in Class II division 1 subjects. Flores-Mir C, Major PW. Eur J Orthod. 2006 Dec;28(6):586–93.

Mandibular changes produced by functional appliances in Class II malocclusion: A systematic review. Cozza P, Baccetti T, Franchi L, De Toffol L, McNamara JA Jr. Am J Orthod Dentofacial Orthop. 2006 May;129(5):599. e1–12.

Analysis of efficacy of functional appliances on mandibular growth. Chen JY, Will LA, Niederman R. Am J Orthod Dentofacial Orthop 2002;122(5):470–6.

Headgear

Effectiveness of early orthopaedic treatment with headgear: A systematic review and meta-analysis. Papageorgiou SN, Kutschera E, Memmert S, Golz L, Jager A, Bourauel C, Eliades T. Eur J Orthod. 2017 Apr 1;39(2):176–187.

Effects of cervical headgear appliance: A systematic review. Henriques FP, Janson G, Henriques JF, Pupulim DC. Dental Press J Orthod. 2015 Jul-Aug;20(4):76–81.

Class II malocclusion treatment using high-pull headgear with a splint: A systematic review. Jacob HB, Buschang PH, dos Santos-Pinto A. Dental Press J Orthod. 2013 Mar 15;18(2):21. e1–7.

Comparison of anchorage capacity between implant and headgear during anterior segment retraction. Li F, Hu HK, Chen JW, Liu ZP, Li GF, He SS, Zou SJ, Ye QS. Angle Orthod. 2011 Sep;81(5):915–22.

Orthognathic surgery

Effects of mandibular advancement surgery on the temporomandibular joint and muscular and articular adaptive changes--a systematic review. Bermell-Baviera A, Bellot-Arcis C, Montiel-Company JM, Almerich-Silla JM. Int J Oral Maxillofac Surg. 2016 May;45(5):545–52.

Stability

Predictive factors of sagittal stability after treatment of Class II malocclusions. Maniewicz Wins S, Antonarakis GS, Kiliaridis S. Angle Orthod. 2016 Nov;86(6):1033–1041.

Stability of Class II fixed functional appliance therapy-A systematic review and meta-analysis. Bock NC, von Bremen J, Ruf S. Eur J Orthod. 2016 Apr;38(2):129–39.

Temporary anchorage devices (TADs)

Comparison of the effects of mini-implant and traditional anchorage on patients with maxillary dentoalveolar protrusion. Xu Y, Xie J. Angle Orthod. 2017 Mar;87(2):320–327.

Can the use of skeletal anchors in conjunction with fixed functional appliances promote skeletal changes? A systematic review and meta-analysis. Elkordy SA, Aboelnaga AA, Fayed MM, AboulFotouh MH, Abouelezz AM. Eur J Orthod. 2016 Oct;38(5):532–45.

Are orthodontic distalizers reinforced with the temporary skeletal anchorage devices effective? Fudalej P, Antoszewska J. Am J Orthod Dentofacial Orthop. 2011 Jun;139(6):722–9.

Intraoral distalizer effects with conventional and skeletal anchorage: a meta-analysis. Grec RH, Janson G, Branco NC, Moura-Grec PG, Patel MP, Castanha Henriques JF. Am J Orthod Dentofacial Orthop. 2013 May;143(5):602–15.

Comparison of anchorage capacity between implant and headgear during anterior segment retraction. Li F, Hu HK, Chen JW, Liu ZP, Li GF, He SS, Zou SJ, Ye QS. Angle Orthod. 2011 Sep;81(5):915–22.

Class III

Alternating rapid maxillary expansion and constriction (ALT RAMEC)

Is alternate rapid maxillary expansion and constriction an effective protocol in the treatment of Class III malocclusion? A systematic review. Pithon MM, Santos NL, Santos CR, Baiao FC, Pinheiro MC, Matos M Neto, Souza IA, Paula RP. Dental Press J Orthod. 2016 Nov-Dec;21(6):34–42.

Early treatment

Early orthodontic treatment for Class III malocclusion: A systematic review and meta-analysis. Woon SC, Thiruvenkatachari B. Am J Orthod Dentofacial Orthop. 2017 Jan;151(1):28–52.

Functional and orthopedic appliances

Skeletal and dental effects of Class III orthopaedic treatment: A systematic review and meta-analysis. Rongo R, D'Antò V, Bucci R, Polito I, Martina R, Michelotti A. J Oral Rehabil. 2017 Jul;44(7):545–562.

The effect of chin-cup therapy in Class III malocclusion: a systematic review. Mousoulea S, Tsolakis I, Ferdianakis E, Tsolakis AI. Open Dent J. 2016 Dec 9;10:664–679.

Is alternate rapid maxillary expansion and constriction an effective protocol in the treatment of Class III malocclusion? A systematic review. Pithon MM, Santos NL, Santos CR, Baiao FC, Pinheiro MC, Matos M Neto, Souza IA, Paula RP. Dental Press J Orthod. 2016 Nov–Dec;21(6):34–42.

Methodological quality and outcome of systematic reviews reporting on orthopaedic treatment for class III malocclusion: Overview of systematic reviews. Jamilian A, Cannavale R, Piancino MG, Eslami S, Perillo L. J Orthod. 2016 Jun;43(2):102–20.

Effectiveness of maxillary protraction using facemask with or without maxillary expansion: asystematic review and meta-analysis. Foersch M, Jacobs C, Wriedt S, Hechtner M, Wehrbein H. Clin Oral Investig. 2015 Jul;19(6):1181–92.

Clinical effectiveness of chin cup treatment for the management of Class III malocclusion in pre-pubertal patients: a systematic review and meta-analysis. Chatzoudi MI, Ioannidou-Marathiotou I, Papadopoulos MA. Prog Orthod. 2014 Dec 2;15:62.

Treatment effectiveness of Frankel function regulator on the Class III malocclusion: a systematic review and meta-analysis. Yang X, Li C, Bai D, Su N, Chen T, Xu Y, Han X. Am J Orthod Dentofacial Orthop. 2014 Aug;146(2):143–54.

Efficacy of orthopedic treatment with protraction facemask on skeletal Class III malocclusion: a systematic review and meta-analysis. Cordasco G, Matarese G, Rustico L, Fastuca S, Caprioglio A, Lindauer SJ, Nucera R. Orthod Craniofac Res. 2014 Aug;17(3):133–43.

Orthodontic treatment for prominent lower front teeth (Class III malocclusion) in children. Watkinson S, Harrison JE, Furness S, Worthington HV. Cochrane Database Syst Rev. 2013 Sep 30;(9):CD003451.

Orthopedic treatment outcomes in Class III malocclusion. A systematic review. Toffol LD, Pavoni C, Baccetti T, Franchi L, Cozza P. Angle Orthod. 2008 May;78(3):561–73.

Skeletal and dental effects of maxillary protraction in patients with angle class III malocclusion: A meta-analysis. Jager A, Braumann B, Kim C, Wahner S. J Orofac Orthop 2001;62(4):275–84.

The effectiveness of protraction face mask therapy: A meta-analysis. Kim JH, Viana MA, Graber TM, Omerza FF, BeGole EA. Am J Orthod Dentofacial Orthop 1999;115(6):675–85.

Orthognathic surgery

Relation between soft tissue and skeletal changes after mandibular setback surgery: A systematic review and meta-analysis. Kaklamanos EG, Kolokitha OE. J Craniomaxillofac Surg. 2016 Apr;44(4):427–35.

Soft tissue profile changes after bilateral sagittal split osteotomy for mandibular setback: A systematic review. Joss CU, Joss-Vassalli IM, Berge SJ, Kuijpers-Jagtman AM. J Oral Maxillofac Surg. 2010 Nov;68(11):2792–801.

Stability

Stability factors after double-jaw surgery in Class III malocclusion. A systematic review. Mucedero M, Coviello A, Baccetti T, Franchi L, Cozza P. Angle Orthod. 2008 Nov;78(6):1141–52.

Temporary anchorage devices (TADs)

Bone- and dentoalveolar-anchored dentofacial orthopedics for Class III malocclusion: new approaches, similar objectives? a systematic review. Morales-Fernandez M, Iglesias-Linares A, Yanez-Vico RM, Mendoza-Mendoza A, Solano-Reina E. Angle Orthod. 2013 May;83(3):540–52.

Effectiveness of interceptive treatment of class III malocclusions with skeletal anchorage: A systematic review and meta-analysis. Rodríguez de Guzmán-Barrera J, Sáez Martínez C, Boronat-Catalá M, Montiel-Company. JM, Paredes-Gallardo V, Gandía-Franco JL, Almerich-Silla JM, Bellot-Arcís C. PLoS One. 2017 Mar 22;12(3):e0173875.

Effectiveness of TAD-anchored maxillary protraction in late mixed dentition. Feng X, Li J, Li Y, Zhao Z, Zhao S, Wang J. Angle Orthod. 2012 Nov;82(6):1107–14.

Treatment timing

Orthodontic treatment for prominent lower front teeth (Class III malocclusion) in children. Watkinson S, Harrison JE, Furness S, Worthington HV. Cochrane Database Syst Rev. 2013 Sep 30;(9):CD003451.

Treatments for adults with prominent lower front teeth. Minami-Sugaya H, Lentini-Oliveira DA, Carvalho FR, Machado MA, Marzola C, Saconato H, Prado GF. Cochrane Database Syst Rev. 2012 May 16;(5):CD006963.

Prediction of the outcome of orthodontic treatment of Class III malocclusions--A systematic review. Fudalej P, Dragan M, Wedrychowska-Szulc B. Eur J Orthod. 2011 Apr;33(2):190–7.

Clear aligners

Efficiency, effectiveness and treatment stability of clear aligners: A systematic review and meta-analysis. Zheng M, Liu R, Ni Z, Yu Z. Orthod Craniofac Res. 2017 Aug;20(3):127–133.

Periodontal health during clear aligners treatment: A systematic review. Rossini G, Parrini S, Castroflorio T, Deregibus A, Debernardi CL. Eur J Orthod. 2015 Oct;37(5):539–43.

Efficacy of clear aligners in controlling orthodontic tooth movement: A systematic review. Rossini G, Parrini S, Castroflorio T, Deregibus A, Debernardi CL. Angle Orthod. 2015 Sep;85(5):881–9.

The treatment effects of Invisalign orthodontic aligners: A systematic review. Lagravere MO, Flores-Mir C. J Am Dent Assoc. 2005 Dec;136(12):1724–9.

Cleft lip and palate

Arch dimension

Effects of labial adhesion on maxillary arch dimensions and nasolabial esthetics in cleft lip and palate: A systematic review. Thierens L, Brusselaers N, De Roo N, De Pauw G. Oral Dis. 2017 Oct;23(7):889–896.

Is cleft severity related to maxillary growth in patients with unilateral cleft lip and palate? Chiu YT, Liao YF. Cleft Palate Craniofac J. 2012 Sep;49(5):535–40.

Distraction osteogenesis

Maxillary distraction osteogenesis versus orthognathic surgery for cleft lip and palate patients. Kloukos D, Fudalej P, Sequeira- Byron P, Katsaros C. Cochrane Database Syst Rev. 2016 Sep 30;(9):CD010403.

Distraction osteogenesis in the management of severe maxillary hypoplasia in cleft lip and palate patients. Scolozzi, P. J Craniofac Surg. 2008 Sep;19(5):1199–214.

Genetics

Genome-wide meta-analyses of nonsyndromic orofacial clefts identify novel associations between FOXE1 and all orofacial clefts, and TP63 and cleft lip with or without cleft palate. Leslie EJ, Carlson JC, Shaffer JR, Butali A, Buxó CJ, Castilla EE, Christensen K, Deleyiannis FW, Leigh Field L, Hecht JT, Moreno L, Orioli IM, Padilla C, Vieira AR, Wehby GL, Feingold E, Weinberg SM, Murray JC, Beaty TH, Marazita ML. Hum Genet. 2017 Mar;136(3):275–286.

Association between polymorphism of TGFA Taq I and cleft lip and/or palate: A meta-analysis. Feng C, Zhang E, Duan W, Xu Z, Zhang Y, Lu L. BMC Oral Health. 2014 Jul 11;14:88.

Imaging

Three-dimensional imaging methods for quantitative analysis of facial soft tissues and skeletal morphology in patients with orofacial clefts: A systematic review. Kuijpers MA, Chiu YT, Nada RM, Carels CE, Fudalej PS. PLoS One. 2014 Apr 7;9(4):e93442.

Quality of life

Oral health-related quality of life in non-syndromic cleft lip and/or palate patients: A systematic review. Antonarakis GS, Patel RN, Tompson B. Community Dent Health. 2013 Sep;30(3):189–95.

Tooth agenesis and anomalies

Mesiodistal tooth size in non-syndromic unilateral cleft lip and palate patients: A meta-analysis. Antonarakis GS, Tsiouli K, Christou P. Clin Oral Investig. 2013 Mar;17(2):365–77.

Prevalence of dental anomalies in nonsyndromic individuals with cleft lip and palate: A systematic review and meta-analysis. Tannure PN, Oliveira CA, Maia LC, Vieira AR, Granjeiro JM, Costa Mde C. Cleft Palate Craniofac J. 2012 Mar;49(2):194–20.

Treatment outcome

Predictive validity of the GOSLON Yardstick index in patients with unilateral cleft lip and palate: A systematic review. Buj-Acosta C, Paredes-Gallardo V, Montiel-Company JM, Albaladejo A, Bellot-Arcís C. PLoS One. 2017 Jun 1;12(6):e0178497.

A scoping review of outcomes related to orthodontic treatment measured in cleft lip and palate. Tsichlaki A, O'Brien K, Johal A, Fleming PS. Orthod Craniofac Res. 2017 May;20(2):55–64.

Effectiveness of pre-surgical infant orthopedic treatment for cleft lip and palate patients: A systematic review and meta-analysis. Papadopoulos MA, Koumpridou EN, Vakalis ML, Papageorgiou SN. Orthod Craniofac Res. 2012 Nov;15(4):207–36.

Long-term effects of presurgical infant orthopedics in patients with cleft lip and palate: A systematic review. Uzel A, Alparslan ZN. Cleft Palate Craniofac J. 2011 Sep;48(5):587–95.

Impact of primary palatoplasty on the maxillomandibular sagittal relationship in patients with unilateral cleft lip and palate: A systematic review and meta-analysis. Bichara LM, Araujo RC, Flores-Mir C, Normando D. Int J Oral Maxillofac Surg. 2015 Jan;44(1):50–6.

Treatment outcome in unilateral cleft lip and palate evaluated with the GOSLON yardstick: A meta-analysis of 1236 patients. Nollet PJ, Katsaros C, Van't Hof MA, Kuijpers-Jagtman AM. Plast Reconstr Surg. 2005 Oct;116(5):1255–62.

Compliance

Compliance with removable orthodontic appliances and adjuncts: A systematic review and meta-analysis. Al-Moghrabi D, Salazar FC, Pandis N, Fleming PS. Am J Orthod Dentofacial Orthop. 2017 Jul;152(1):17–32.

A systematic review of randomized controlled trials of interventions to improve adherence among orthodontic patients aged 12 to 18. Aljabaa A, McDonald F, Newton JT. Angle Orthod. 2015 Mar;85(2):305–13.

Factors affecting children's adherence to regular dental attendance: A systematic review. Badri P, Saltaji H, Flores-Mir C, Amin M. J Am Dent Assoc. 2014 Aug;145(8):817–28.

Non-compliance maxillary molar distalizing appliances: an overview of the last decade. Fontana M, Cozzani M, Caprioglio A. Prog Orthod. 2012 Sep;13(2):173–84.

Cone beam computed tomography (CBCT)

Please see Diagnostic records.

Continuous positive airway pressure (CPAP)

Please see Obstructive sleep apnea.

Corticotomy

Please see Accelerated tooth movement.

Coronectomy

Coronectomy vs. total removal for third molar extraction: A systematic review. Long H, Zhou Y, Liao L, Pyakurel U, Wang Y, Lai W. J Dent Res. 2012 Jul;91(7):659–65.

Crossbites (anterior)

Please see Class III.

Crossbites (posterior)

Alternating rapid maxillary expansion and constriction (ALT RAMEC)

Is alternate rapid maxillary expansion and constriction an effective protocol in the treatment of Class III malocclusion? A systematic review. Pithon MM, Santos NL, Santos CR, Baiao FC, Pinheiro MC, Matos M Neto, Souza IA, Paula RP. Dental Press J Orthod. 2016 Nov-Dec;21(6):34–42.

Diagnostic methods

Diagnostic methods for assessing maxillary skeletal and dental transverse deficiencies: A systematic review. Sawchuk D, Currie K, Vich ML, Palomo JM, Flores-Mir C. Korean J Orthod. 2016 Sep;46(5):331–42.

Early treatment

Functional changes after early treatment of unilateral posterior cross-bite associated with mandibular shift: A systematic review. Tsanidis N, Antonarakis GS, Kiliaridis S. J Oral Rehabil. 2016 Jan;43(1):59–68.
Early correction of anterior crossbites: A systematic review. Borrie F, Bearn D. J Orthod. 2011 Sep;38(3):175–84.

Effect of expansion on other structures

Volumetric upper airway changes after rapid maxillary expansion: A systematic review and meta-analysis. Buck LM, Dalci O, Darendeliler MA, Papageorgiou SN, Papadopoulou AK. Eur J Orthod. 2017 Oct 1;39(5):463–473.
Association between posterior crossbite, skeletal, and muscle asymmetry: a systematic review. Iodice G, Danzi G, Cimino R, Paduano S, Michelotti A. Eur J Orthod. 2016 Dec;38(6):638–651.
Effect of surgically assisted rapid maxillary expansion on upper airway volume: a systematic review. Buck LM, Dalci O, Darendeliler MA, Papadopoulou AK. J Oral Maxillofac Surg. 2016 May;74(5):1025–43.
Effects of rapid maxillary expansion on the midpalatal suture: A systematic review. Liu S, Xu T, Zou W. Eur J Orthod. 2015 Dec;37(6):651–5.
Effect of non-surgical maxillary expansion on the nasal septum deviation: A systematic review. Aziz T, Ansari K, Lagravere MO, Major MP, Flores-Mir C. Prog Orthod. 2015;16:15.
Association between posterior crossbite, masticatory muscle pain, and disc displacement: a systematic review. Iodice G, Danzi G, Cimino R, Paduano S, Michelotti A. Eur J Orthod. 2013 Dec;35(6):737–44.
Does rapid maxillary expansion have long-term effects on airway dimensions and breathing? Baratieri C, Alves M Jr, de Souza MM, de Souza Araujo MT, Maia LC. Am J Orthod Dentofacial Orthop. 2011 Aug;140(2):146–56.

Effectiveness and treatment outcomes

Do different maxillary expansion appliances influence the outcomes of the treatment? Algharbi M, Bazargani F, Dimberg L. Eur J Orthod. 2017 doi: 10.1093/ejo/cjx035. [Epub ahead of print].
Dental and skeletal effects of palatal expansion techniques: a systematic review of the current evidence from systematic reviews and meta-analyses. Bucci R, D'Anto V, Rongo R, Valletta R, Martina R, Michelotti A. J Oral Rehabil. 2016 Jul;43(7):543–64.

Rapid maxillary expansion effects in Class II malocclusion: a systematic review. Feres MF, Raza H, Alhadlaq A, El-Bialy T. Angle Orthod. 2015 Nov;85(6):1070–9.

Orthodontic treatment for posterior Crossbites. Agostino P, Ugolini A, Signori A, Silvestrini-Biavati A, Harrison JE, Riley P. Cochrane Database Syst Rev. 2014 Aug 8;(8):CD000979.

The effectiveness of non-surgical maxillary expansion: a meta-analysis. Zhou Y, Long H, Ye N, Xue J, Yang X, Liao L, Lai W. Eur J Orthod. 2014 Apr;36(2):233–42.

Meta-analysis of immediate changes with rapid maxillary expansion treatment. Lagravere MO, Heo G, Major PW, Flores-Mir C. J Am Dent Assoc. 2006 Jan;137(1):44–53.

Long-term skeletal changes with rapid maxillary expansion: a systematic review. Lagravere MO, Major PW, Flores-Mir C. Angle Orthod. 2005 Nov;75(6):1046–52.

Long-term dental arch changes after rapid maxillary expansion treatment: a systematic review. Lagravere MO, Major PW, Flores-Mir C. Angle Orthod. 2005 Mar;75(2):155–61.

Skeletal and dental changes with fixed slow maxillary expansion treatment: a systematic review. Lagravere MO, Major PW, Flores-Mir C. J Am Dent Assoc. 2005 Feb;136(2):194–9.

Maxillary expansion: a meta analysis. Schiffman PH, Tuncay OC. Clin Orthod Res 2001;4(2):86–96.

Retention

Retention period after treatment of posterior crossbite with maxillary expansion: a systematic review. Costa JG, Galindo TM, Mattos CT, Cury-Saramago AA. Dental Press J Orthod. 2017 Mar-Apr;22(2):35–44.

Stability

Transverse Expansion and Stability after Segmental Le Fort I Osteotomy versus Surgically Assisted Rapid Maxillary Expansion: a systematic Review. Starch-Jensen T, Blaehr TL. J Oral Maxillofac Res. 2016 Dec 28;7(4):e1.

Surgically assisted maxillary expansion

Following Surgically Assisted Rapid Palatal Expansion, Do Tooth-Borne or Bone-Borne Appliances Provide More Skeletal Expansion and Dental Expansion? Hamedi-Sangsari A, Chinipardaz Z, Carrasco L. J Oral Maxillofac Surg. 2017 Oct;75(10):2211–2222.

Surgically Assisted Rapid Palatomaxillary Expansion with or Without Pterygomaxillary Disjunction: a systematic Review and Meta-Analysis.Hamedi Sangsari A, Sadr-Eshkevari P, Al-Dam A, Friedrich RE, Freymiller E, Rashad A. J Oral Maxillofac Surg. 2016 Feb;74(2):338–48.

Long-term dental and skeletal changes in patients submitted to surgically assisted rapid maxillary expansion: a meta-analysis. Vilani GN, Mattos CT, de Oliveira Ruellas AC, Maia LC. Oral Surg Oral Med Oral Pathol Oral Radiol. 2012 Dec;114(6):689–97.

A systematic review of the effects of bone-borne surgical assisted rapid maxillary expansion. Verstraaten J, Kuijpers-Jagtman AM, Mommaerts MY, Berg SJ, Nada RM, Schols JG. J Craniomaxillofac Surg. 2010 Apr;38(3):166–74.

Crowding

Early vs late orthodontic treatment of tooth crowding by first premolar extraction: a systematic review. Lopes Filho H, Maia LH, Lau TC, de Souza MM, Maia LC. Angle Orthod. 2015 May;85(3):510–7.

The role of mandibular third molars on lower anterior teeth crowding and relapse after orthodontic treatment: a systematic review. Zawawi KH, Melis M ScientificWorldJournal. 2014;2014:615429.

Is there justification for prophylactic extraction of third molars? a systematic review. Costa MG, Pazzini CA, Pantuzo MC, Jorge ML, Marques LS. Braz Oral Res. 2013 Mar-Apr;27(2):183–8.

Dental crowding as a caries risk factor: a systematic review. Hafez HS, Shaarawy SM, Al-Sakiti AA, Mostafa YA. Am J Orthod Dentofacial Orthop. 2012 Oct;142(4):443–50.

Dental arch space changes following premature loss of primary first molars: a systematic review. Tunison W, Flores-Mir C, ElBadrawy H, Nassar U, El-Bialy T. Pediatr Dent. 2008 Jul-Aug;30(4):297–302.

Curing lights

Please see Adhesives and bonding agents.

Deep bite

Stability of deep-bite correction: A systematic review. Huang GJ, Bates SB, Ehlert AA, Whiting DP, Chen SS, Bollen AM. J World Fed Orthod. 2012 Sep 1;1(3):e89–e86.

Orthodontic treatment for deep bite and retroclined upper front teeth in children. Millett DT, Cunningham SJ, O'Brien KD, Benson P, Williams A, de Oliveira CM. Cochrane Database Syst Rev. 2006 Oct 18;(4):CD005972.

Demineralization

Please see Caries and White spot lesions.

Dental trauma

Clinical factors and socio-demographic characteristics associated with dental trauma in children: a systematic review and meta-analysis. Correa-Faria P, Martins CC, Bonecker M, Paiva SM, Ramos-Jorge ML, Pordeus IA. Dent Traumatol. 2016 Oct;32(5):367–78.

Early orthodontic treatment for Class II malocclusion reduces the chance of incisal trauma: Results of a Cochrane systematic review. Thiruvenkatachari B, Harrison J, Worthington H, O'Brien K. Am J Orthod Dentofacial Orthop. 2015 Jul;148(1):47–59.

Over two hundred million injuries to anterior teeth attributable to large overjet: a meta-analysis. Petti S. Dent Traumatol. 2015 Feb;31(1):1–8.

Emergency orthodontic treatment after the traumatic intrusive luxation of maxillary incisors. Chaushu S, Shapira J, Heling I, Becker A. Am J Orthod Dentofacial Orthop 2004;126(2):162–72.

A systematic review of the relationship between overjet size and traumatic dental injuries. Nguyen QV, Bezemer PD, Habets L, Prahl-Andersen B. Eur J Orthod 1999;21(5):503–15.

Diagnostic records

CBCT

Reliability of upper pharyngeal airway assessment using dental CBCT: a systematic review. Zimmerman JN, Lee J, Pliska BT. Eur J Orthod. 2017 Oct 1;39(5):489–496.

Effect of Head and Tongue Posture on the Pharyngeal Airway Dimensions and Morphology in Three-Dimensional Imaging: A Systematic Review. Gurani SF, Di Carlo G, Cattaneo PM, Thorn JJ, Pinholt EM. J Oral Maxillofac Res. 2016 Mar 31;7(1):e1.

Reliability and reproducibility of three-dimensional cephalometric landmarks using CBCT: a systematic review. Lisboa Cde O, Masterson D, da Motta AF, Motta AT. J Appl Oral Sci. 2015 Mar–Apr;23(2):112–9.

Three-dimensional cephalometric analysis in orthodontics: a systematic review. Pittayapat P, Limchaichana-Bolstad N, Willems G, Jacobs R. Orthod Craniofac Res. 2014 May;17(2):69–91.

Three-dimensional imaging methods for quantitative analysis of facial soft tissues and skeletal morphology in patients with orofacial clefts: a systematic review. Kuijpers MA, Chiu YT, Nada RM, Carels CE, Fudalej PS. PLoS One. 2014 Apr 7;9(4):e93442.

CBCT assessment of upper airway changes and treatment outcomes of obstructive sleep apnoea: a systematic review. Alsufyani NA, Al-Saleh MA, Major PW. Sleep Breath. 2013 Sep;17(3):911–23.

Evidence supporting the use of cone-beam computed tomography in orthodontics. van Vlijmen OJ, Kuijpers MA, Berge SJ, Schols JG, Maal TJ, Breuning H, Kuijpers-Jagtman AM. J Am Dent Assoc. 2012 Mar;143(3):241–52.

Digital three-dimensional image fusion processes for planning and evaluating orthodontics and orthognathic surgery. A systematic review. Plooij JM, Maal TJ, Haers P, Borstlap WA, Kuijpers-Jagtman AM, Berge SJ. Int J Oral Maxillofac Surg. 2011 Apr;40(4):341–52.

Cephalometry (2D)

Validity of 2D lateral cephalometry in orthodontics: a systematic review. Durao AR, Pittayapat P, Rockenbach MI, Olszewski R, Ng S, Ferreira AP, Jacobs R. Prog Orthod. 2013 Sep 20;14:31.

Landmark identification error in posteroanterior cephalometric radiography. A systematic review. Leonardi R, Annunziata A, Caltabiano M. Angle Orthod. 2008 Jul;78(4):761–5.

Digital models

Accuracy and reproducibility of dental measurements on tomographic digital models: a systematic review and meta-analysis. Ferreira JB, Christovam IO, Alencar DS, da Motta AFJ, Mattos CT, Cury-Saramago A. Dentomaxillofac Radiol. 2017 Apr 26:20160455.

Diagnostic accuracy and measurement sensitivity of digital models for orthodontic purposes: A systematic review. Rossini G, Parrini S, Castroflorio T, Deregibus A, Debernardi CL. Am J Orthod Dentofacial Orthop. 2016 Feb;149(2):161–70.

Variation of orthodontic treatment decision-making based on dental model type: A systematic review. Pacheco-Pereira C, De Luca Canto G, Major PW, Flores-Mir C. Angle Orthod. 2015 May;85(3):501–9.

Growth prediction

Methods to quantify soft tissue-based cranial growth and treatment outcomes in children: a systematic review. Brons S, van Beusichem ME, Bronkhorst EM, Draaisma JM, Berge SJ, Schols JG, Kuijpers-Jagtman AM. PLoS One. 2014 Feb 27;9(2):e89602.

The diagnostic performance of dental maturity for identification of the circumpubertal growth phases: a meta-analysis. Perinetti G, Westphalen GH, Biasotto M, Salgarello S, Contardo L. Prog Orthod. 2013 May 23;14:8.

Use of skeletal maturation based on hand-wrist radiographic analysis as a predictor of facial growth: a systematic review. Flores-Mir C, Nebbe B, Major PW. Angle Orthod 2004;74(1):118–24.

Intraoral scanners

Validity and reliability of intraoral scanners compared to conventional gypsum models measurements: a systematic review. Aragón ML, Pontes LF, Bichara LM, Flores-Mir C, Normando D. Eur J Orthod. 2016 Aug;38(4):429–34.

Miscellaneous

Records needed for orthodontic diagnosis and treatment planning: a systematic review. Rischen RJ, Breuning KH, Bronkhorst EM, Kuijpers-Jagtman AM. PLoS One. 2013 Nov 12;8(11):e74186.

Subjective and objective perception of orthodontic treatment need: a systematic review. Livas C, Delli K. Eur J Orthod. 2013 Jun;35(3):347–53.

Digital models

Please see Diagnostic records.

Distraction osteogenesis

Cleft lip and palate and other midfacial hypoplasia

Maxillary distraction osteogenesis versus orthognathic surgery for cleft lip and palate patients. Kloukos D, Fudalej P, Sequeira-Byron P, Katsaros C. Cochrane Database Syst Rev. 2016 Sep 30;(9):CD010403.

Le Fort III distraction osteogenesis versus conventional Le Fort III osteotomy in correction of syndromic midfacialhypoplasia: a systematic review. Saltaji H, Altalibi M, Major MP, Al-Nuaimi MH, Tabbaa S, Major PW, Flores-Mir C. J Oral Maxillofac Surg. 2014 May;72(5):959–72.

Distraction osteogenesis in the management of severe maxillary hypoplasia in cleft lip and palate patients. Scolozzi, P. J Craniofac Surg. 2008 Sep;19(5):1199–214.

Low intensity pulsed ultrasound

Effect of low-intensity pulsed ultrasound on distraction osteogenesis treatment time: a meta-analysis of randomized clinical trials. Raza H, Saltaji H, Kaur H, Flores-Mir C, El-Bialy T. J Ultrasound Med. 2016 Feb;35(2):349–58.

Obstructive sleep apnea

Distraction osteogenesis as a treatment of obstructive sleep apnea syndrome: A systematic review. Tsui WK, Yang Y, Cheung LK, Leung YY. Medicine (Baltimore). 2016 Sep;95(36):e4674.

Stability

Mandibular distraction osteogenesis: a systematic review of stability and the effects on hard and soft tissues. Rossini G, Vinci B, Rizzo R, Pinho TM, Deregibus A. Int J Oral Maxillofac Surg. 2016 Nov;45(11):1438–1444.

Skeletal stability and complications of bilateral sagittal split osteotomies and mandibular distraction osteogenesis: an evidence-based review. Ow A, Cheung LK. J Oral Maxillofac Surg. 2009 Nov;67(11):2344–53.

Early treatment

Please see Class II and Class III and Crossbites (posterior).

Education

Computer-assisted learning in orthodontic education: a systematic review and meta-analysis. Al-Jewair TS, Azarpazhooh A, Suri S, Shah PS. J Dent Educ. 2009 Jun;73(6):730–9.

Elastics

Correction of Class II malocclusion with Class II elastics: A systematic review. Janson G, Sathler R, Fernandes TM, Branco NC, Freitas MR. Am J Orthod Dentofacial Orthop. 2013 Mar;143(3):383–92.

Electric toothbrush

Please see Powered toothbrush.

Enamel

Please see Caries and White spot lesions.

Endodontically treated teeth

Radiographic comparison of the extent of orthodontically induced external apical root resorption in vital and root-filled teeth: a systematic review. Walker SL, Tieu LD, Flores-Mir C. Eur J Orthod. 2013 Dec;35(6):796–802.
Root resorption of endodontically treated teeth following orthodontic treatment: a meta-analysis. Ioannidou-Marathiotou I, Zafeiriadis AA, Papadopoulos MA. Clin Oral Investig. 2013 Sep;17(7):1733–44.

Epidemiology

Impacted and transmigrant mandibular canines incidence, aetiology, and treatment: a systematic review. Dalessandri D, Parrini S, Rubiano R, Gallone D, Migliorati M. Eur J Orthod. 2017 Apr 1;39(2):161–169.
Prevalence of peg-shaped maxillary permanent lateral incisors: A meta-analysis. Hua F, He H, Ngan P, Bouzid W. Am J Orthod Dentofacial Orthop. 2013 Jul;144(1):97–109.
Prevalence of dental anomalies in nonsyndromic individuals with cleft lip and palate: a systematic review and meta-analysis. Tannure PN, Oliveira CA, Maia LC, Vieira AR, Granjeiro JM, Costa Mde C. Cleft Palate Craniofac J. 2012 Mar;49(2):194–200.
Prevalence of tooth transposition. A meta-analysis. Papadopoulos MA, Chatzoudi M, Kaklamanos EG. Angle Orthod. 2010 Mar;80(2):275–85.
Prevalence of nickel hypersensitivity in orthodontic patients: a meta-analysis. Kolokitha OE, Kaklamanos EG, Papadopoulos MA. Am J Orthod Dentofacial Orthop. 2008 Dec;134(6):722.e1–722.
A meta-analysis of the prevalence of dental agenesis of permanent teeth. Polder BJ, Van't Hof MA, Van der Linden FP, Kuijpers-Jagtman AM. Community Dent Oral Epidemiol 2004;32(3):217–26.

Essix retainer

Please see Retention and relapse.

Extraction

Airway

The effect of teeth extraction for orthodontic treatment on the upper airway: a systematic review. Hu Z, Yin X, Liao J, Zhou C, Yang Z, Zou S. Sleep Breath. 2015 May;19(2):441–51.

Bimaxillary protrusion

Early vs late orthodontic treatment of tooth crowding by first premolar extraction: A systematic review. Lopes Filho H, Maia LH, Lau TC, de Souza MM, Maia LC. Angle Orthod. 2015 May;85(3):510–7.

Soft tissue changes following the extraction of premolars in nongrowing patients with bimaxillary protrusion. A systematic review. Leonardi R, Annunziata A, Licciardello V, Barbato E. Angle Orthod. 2010 Jan;80(1):211–6.

Class II

Changes in apical base sagittal relationship in Class II malocclusion treatment with and without premolar extractions: A systematic review and meta-analysis. Janson G, Aliaga-Del Castillo A, Niederberger A. Angle Orthod. 2017 Mar;87(2):338–355.

Soft-tissue changes in Class II malocclusion patients treated with extractions: a systematic review. Janson G, Mendes LM, Junqueira CH, Garib DG. Eur J Orthod. 2016 Dec;38(6):631–637.

First molars

The timing of extraction of non-restorable first permanent molars: a systematic review. Eichenberger M, Erb J, Zwahlen M, Schätzle M. Eur J Paediatr Dent. 2015 Dec;16(4):272–8.

Incisors

Interproximal wear versus incisors extraction to solve anterior lower crowding: a systematic review. Almeida NV, Silveira GS, Pereira DM, Mattos CT, Mucha JN. Dental Press J Orthod. 2015 Jan-Feb;20(1):66–73.

Mandibular incisor extraction: a systematic review of an uncommon extraction choice in orthodontic treatment. Zhylich D, Suri S. J Orthod. 2011 Sep;38(3):185–95.

Third molars

Does Orthodontic Extraction Treatment Improve the Angular Position of Third Molars? A Systematic Review. Livas C, Delli K. J Oral Maxillofac Surg. 2017 Mar;75(3):475–483.

Extrusion

Intrusive luxation of permanent teeth: a systematic review of factors important for treatment decision-making. AlKhalifa JD, AlAzemi AA. Dent Traumatol. 2014 Jun;30(3):169–75.

Implant site development by orthodontic extrusion. A systematic review. Korayem M, Flores-Mir C, Nassar U, Olfert K. Angle Orthod. 2008 Jul;78(4):752–60.

Face mask

Please see Functional and orthopedic appliances and Class III.

Fluoride

Please see Caries and White spot lesions.

Force levels

Optimal force for maxillary protraction facemask therapy in the early treatment of class III malocclusion. Yepes E, Quintero P, Rueda ZV, Pedroza A. Eur J Orthod. 2014 Oct;36(5):586–94.

Optimum force magnitude for orthodontic tooth movement: a systematic literature review. Ren Y, Maltha JC, Kuijpers-Jagtman AM. Angle Orthod 2003;73(1):86–92.

Frankel function regulator

Please see Functional and orthopedic appliances.

Frenum

Facts and myths regarding the maxillary midline frenum and its treatment: a systematic review of the literature. Delli K, Livas C, Sculean A, Katsaros C, Bornstein MM. Quintessence Int. 2013 Feb;44(2):177–87.

Functional and orthopedic appliances

Class II

Changes in airway dimensions following functional appliances in growing patients with skeletal class II malocclusion: A systematic review and meta-analysis. Xiang M, Hu B, Liu Y, Sun J, Song J. Int J Pediatr Otorhinolaryngol. 2017 Jun;97:170–180.

Effectiveness of early orthopaedic treatment with headgear: a systematic review and meta-analysis. Papageorgiou SN, Kutschera E, Memmert S, Golz L, Jäger A, Bourauel C, Eliades T. Eur J Orthod. 2017 Apr 1;39(2):176–187.

Effect of functional appliances on the airway dimensions in patients with skeletal class II malocclusion: A systematic review. Kannan A, Sathyanarayana HP, Padmanabhan S. J Orthod Sci. 2017 Apr–Jun;6(2):54–64.

A comparison of the efficacy of fixed versus removable functional appliances in children with Class II malocclusion: A systematic review. Pacha MM, Fleming PS, Johal A. Eur J Orthod. 2016 Dec;38(6):621–630.

Can the use of skeletal anchors in conjunction with fixed functional appliances promote skeletal changes? A systematic review and meta-analysis. Elkordy SA, Aboelnaga AA, Fayed MM, AboulFotouh MH, Abouelezz AM. Eur J Orthod. 2016 Oct;38(5):532–45.

The effectiveness of the Herbst appliance for patients with Class II malocclusion: a meta-analysis. Yang X, Zhu Y, Long H, Zhou Y, Jian F, Ye N, Gao M, Lai W. Eur J Orthod. 2016 Jun;38(3):324–33.

Effectiveness of orthodontic treatment with functional appliances on maxillary growth in the short term: A systematic review and meta-analysis. Nucera R, Lo Giudice A, Rustico L, Matarese G, Papadopoulos MA, Cordasco G. Am J Orthod Dentofacial Orthop. 2016 May;149(5):600–611.e3.

Treatment effects of fixed functional appliances in patients with Class II malocclusion: a systematic review and meta-analysisZymperdikas VF, Koretsi V, Papageorgiou SN, Papadopoulos MA. Eur J Orthod. 2016 Apr;38(2):113–26.

Fixed functional appliances show definite skeletal and dental changes in the short term. McGuinness N. Eur J Orthod. 2016 Apr;38(2):127–8.

Stability of Class II fixed functional appliance therapy-a systematic review and meta-analysis. Bock NC, von Bremen J, Ruf S. Eur J Orthod. 2016 Apr;38(2):129–39.

Class II functional orthopaedic treatment: a systematic review of systematic reviews. D'Anto V, Bucci R, Franchi L, Rongo R, Michelotti A, Martina R.J Oral Rehabil. 2015 Aug;42(8):624–42.

Treatment effects of removable functional appliances in patients with Class II malocclusion: a systematic review and meta-analysis. Koretsi V, Zymperdikas VF, Papageorgiou SN, Papadopoulos MA. Eur J Orthod. 2015 Aug;37(4):418–34.

Effects of cervical headgear appliance: a systematic review. Henriques FP, Janson G, Henriques JF, Pupulim DC. Dental Press J Orthod. 2015 Jul-Aug;20(4):76–81.

Meta-analysis on the mandibular dimensions effects of the MARA appliance in patients with Class II malocclusions. Al-Jewair TS. Angle Orthod. 2015 Jul;85(4):706–14.

Class II malocclusion treatment using high-pull headgear with a splint: a systematic review. Jacob HB, Buschang PH, dos Santos-Pinto A. Dental Press J Orthod. 2013 Mar 15;18(2):21. e1–7.

Meta-analysis of skeletal mandibular changes during Frankel appliance treatment. Perillo L, Cannavale R, Ferro F, Franchi L, Masucci C, Chiodini P, Baccetti T. Eur J Orthod. 2011 Feb;33(1):84–92.

Effectiveness of orthodontic treatment with functional appliances on mandibular growth in the short term. Marsico E, Gatto E, Burrascano M, Matarese G, Cordasco G. Am J Orthod Dentofacial Orthop. 2011 Jan;139(1):24–36.

Skeletal and dental changes in Class II division 1 malocclusions treated with splint-type Herbst appliances. A systematic review. Flores-Mir C, Ayeh A, Goswani A, Charkhandeh S. Angle Orthod. 2007 Mar;77(2):376–81.

A systematic review of cephalometric facial soft tissue changes with the Activator and Bionator appliances in Class II division 1 subjects. Flores-Mir C, Major PW. Eur J Orthod. 2006 Dec;28(6):586–93.

Mandibular changes produced by functional appliances in Class II malocclusion: a systematic review. Cozza P, Baccetti T, Franchi L, De Toffol L, McNamara JA Jr. Am J Orthod Dentofacial Orthop. 2006 May;129(5):599. e1–12.

Analysis of efficacy of functional appliances on mandibular growth. Chen JY, Will LA, Niederman R. Am J Orthod Dentofacial Orthop 2002;122(5):470–6.

Class III

Skeletal and dental effects of Class III orthopaedic treatment: a systematic review and meta-analysis. Rongo R, D'Antò V, Bucci R, Polito I, Martina R, Michelotti A. J Oral Rehabil. 2017 Jul;44(7):545–562.

The Effect of Chin-cup Therapy in Class III Malocclusion: A Systematic Review. Mousoulea S, Tsolakis I, Ferdianakis E, Tsolakis AI. Open Dent J. 2016 Dec 9;10:664–679.

Is alternate rapid maxillary expansion and constriction an effective protocol in the treatment of Class III malocclusion? A systematic review. Pithon MM, Santos NL, Santos CR, Baião FC, Pinheiro MC, Matos M Neto, Souza IA, Paula RP. Dental Press J Orthod. 2016 Nov-Dec;21(6):34–42.

Methodological quality and outcome of systematic reviews reporting on orthopaedic treatment for class III malocclusion: Overview of systematic reviews. Jamilian A, Cannavale R, Piancino MG, Eslami S, Perillo L. J Orthod. 2016 Jun;43(2):102–20.

Effectiveness of maxillary protraction using facemask with or without maxillary expansion: a systematic review and meta-analysis. Foersch M, Jacobs C, Wriedt S, Hechtner M, Wehrbein H. Clin Oral Investig. 2015 Jul;19(6):1181–92.

Clinical effectiveness of chin cup treatment for the management of Class III malocclusion in pre-pubertal patients: a systematic review and meta-analysis. Chatzoudi MI, Ioannidou-Marathiotou I, Papadopoulos MA. Prog Orthod. 2014 Dec 2;15:62.

Treatment effectiveness of Frankel function regulator on the Class III malocclusion: a systematic review and meta-analysis. Yang X, Li C, Bai D, Su N, Chen T, Xu Y, Han X. Am J Orthod Dentofacial Orthop. 2014 Aug;146(2):143–54.

Efficacy of orthopedic treatment with protraction facemask on skeletal Class III malocclusion: a systematic review and meta-analysis. Cordasco G, Matarese G, Rustico L, Fastuca S, Caprioglio A, Lindauer SJ, Nucera R. Orthod Craniofac Res. 2014 Aug;17(3):133–43.

Orthodontic treatment for prominent lower front teeth (Class III malocclusion) in children. Watkinson S, Harrison JE, Furness S, Worthington HV. Cochrane Database Syst Rev. 2013 Sep 30;(9):CD003451.

Orthopedic treatment outcomes in Class III malocclusion. A systematic review. Toffol LD, Pavoni C, Baccetti T, Franchi L, Cozza P. Angle Orthod. 2008 May;78(3):561–73.

Skeletal and dental effects of maxillary protraction in patients with angle class III malocclusion: A meta-analysis. Jager A, Braumann B, Kim C, Wahner S. J Orofac Orthop 2001;62(4):275–84.

The effectiveness of protraction face mask therapy: A meta-analysis. Kim JH, Viana MA, Graber TM, Omerza FF, BeGole EA. Am J Orthod Dentofacial Orthop 1999;115(6):675–85.

Obstructive sleep apnea

Effects of CPAP and Mandibular Advancement Devices on Health-Related Quality of Life in OSA: A Systematic Review and Meta-analysis. Kuhn E, Schwarz EI, Bratton DJ, Rossi VA, Kohler M. Chest. 2017 Apr;151(4):786–794.

Craniofacial and upper airway morphology in adult obstructive sleep apnea patients: A systematic review and meta-analysis of cephalometric studies. Neelapu BC, Kharbanda OP, Sardana HK, Balachandran R, Sardana V, Kapoor P, Gupta A, Vasamsetti S. Sleep Med Rev. 2017 Feb;31:79–90.

Oral appliances and functional orthopaedic appliances for obstructive sleep apnoea in children. Carvalho FR, Lentini-Oliveira DA, Prado LB, Prado GF, Carvalho LB. Cochrane Database Syst Rev. 2016 Oct 5;(10):CD005520.

The effectiveness of different mandibular advancement amounts in OSA patients: a systematic review and meta-regression analysis. Bartolucci ML, Bortolotti F, Raffaelli E, D'Antò V, Michelotti A, Alessandri Bonetti G. Sleep Breath. 2016 Sep;20(3):911–9.

Quality Assessment of Systematic Reviews on the Efficacy of Oral Appliance Therapy for Adult and Pediatric Sleep-Disordered Breathing.Al-Jewair TS, Gaffar BO, Flores-Mir C.J Clin Sleep Med. 2016 Aug 15;12(8):1175–83.

Meta-analysis of randomised controlled trials of oral mandibular advancement devices and continuous positive airway pressure for obstructive sleep apnoea-hypopnoea. Sharples LD, Clutterbuck-James AL, Glover MJ, Bennett MS, Chadwick R, Pittman MA, Quinnell TG. Sleep Med Rev. 2016 Jun;27:108–24.

Effectiveness of mandibular advancement appliances in treating obstructive sleep apnea syndrome: A systematic review. Serra-Torres S, Bellot-Arcís C, Montiel-Company JM, Marco-Algarra J, Almerich-Silla M. Laryngoscope. 2016 Feb;126(2):507–14.

Orthodontics treatments for managing obstructive sleep apnea syndrome in children: A systematic review and meta-analysis. Huynh NT, Desplats E, Almeida FR. Sleep Med Rev. 2016 Feb;25:84–94.

Maxillomandibular Advancement for Treatment of Obstructive Sleep Apnea: A Meta-analysis. Zaghi S, Holty JE, Certal V, Abdullatif J, Guilleminault C, Powell NB, Riley RW, Camacho M. JAMA Otolaryngol Head Neck Surg. 2016 Jan;142(1):58–66.

Myofunctional Therapy to Treat Obstructive Sleep Apnea: A Systematic Review and Meta-analysis. Camacho M, Certal V, Abdullatif J, Zaghi S, Ruoff CM, Capasso R, Kushida CA. Sleep. 2015 May 1;38(5):669–75.

Effect of oral appliances on blood pressure in obstructive sleep apnea: a systematic review and meta-analysis. Iftikhar IH, Hays ER, Iverson MA, Magalang UJ, Maas AK. J Clin Sleep Med. 2013 Feb 1;9(2):165–74.

A systematic review of the efficacy of oral appliance design in the management of obstructive sleep apnoea. Ahrens A, McGrath C, Hagg U. Eur J Orthod. 2011 Jun;33(3):318–24.

Subjective efficacy of oral appliance design features in the management of obstructive sleep apnea: a systematic review. Ahrens A, McGrath C, Hagg U. Am J Orthod Dentofacial Orthop. 2010 Nov;138(5):559–76.

Maxillomandibular advancement for the treatment of obstructive sleep apnea: a systematic review and meta-analysis. Holty JE, Guilleminault C. Sleep Med Rev. 2010 Oct;14(5):287–97.

Oral appliances and functional orthopaedic appliances for obstructive sleep apnoea in children. Carvalho FR, Lentini-Oliveira D, Machado MA, Prado GF, Prado LB, Saconato H. Cochrane Database Syst Rev. 2007 Apr 18;(2):CD005520.

Oral appliances for obstructive sleep apnoea. Lim J, Lasserson TJ, Fleetham J, Wright J. Cochrane Database Syst Rev. 2006 Jan 25;(1):CD004435.

Open bite

Systematic review for orthodontic and orthopedic treatments for anterior open bite in the mixed dentition. Pisani L, Bonaccorso L, Fastuca R, Spena R, Lombardo L, Caprioglio A. Prog Orthod. 2016 Dec;17(1):28.

Orthodontic and orthopaedic treatment for anterior open bite in children. Lentini-Oliveira DA, Carvalho FR, Rodrigues CG, Ye Q, Prado LB, Prado GF, Hu R. Cochrane Database Syst Rev. 2014 Sep 24;(9):CD005515.

Temporomandibular joint

Changes in temporomandibular joint morphology in class II patients treated with fixed mandibular repositioning and evaluated through 3D imaging: a systematic review. Al-Saleh MA, Alsufyani N, Flores-Mir C, Nebbe B, Major PW. Orthod Craniofac Res. 2015 Nov;18(4):185–201.

Effect of chin-cup treatment on the temporomandibular joint: a systematic review. Zurfluh MA, Kloukos D, Patcas R, Eliades T. Eur J Orthod. 2015 Jun;37(3):314–24.

Systematic review and meta-analysis of randomized controlled trials evaluating intraoral orthopedic appliances for temporomandibular disorders. Fricton J, Look JO, Wright E, Alencar FG Jr, Chen H, Lang M, Ouyang W, Velly AM. J Orofac Pain. 2010 Summer;24(3):237–54.

Effect of Herbst treatment on temporomandibular joint morphology: a systematic literature review. Popowich K, Nebbe B, Major PW. Am J Orthod Dentofacial Orthop 2003;123(4):388–94.

Genetics

Cleft lip and palate

Genome-wide meta-analyses of nonsyndromic orofacial clefts identify novel associations between FOXE1 and all orofacial clefts, and TP63 and cleft lip with or without cleft palate. Leslie EJ, Carlson JC, Shaffer JR, Butali A, Buxó CJ, Castilla EE, Christensen K, Deleyiannis FW, Leigh Field L, Hecht JT, Moreno L, Orioli IM, Padilla C, Vieira AR, Wehby GL, Feingold E, Weinberg SM, Murray JC, Beaty TH, Marazita ML. Hum Genet. 2017 Mar;136(3):275–286.

Association between polymorphism of TGFA Taq I and cleft lip and/or palate: A meta-analysis. Feng C, Zhang E, Duan W, Xu Z, Zhang Y, Lu L. BMC Oral Health. 2014 Jul 11;14:88.

Nonsyndromic oligodontia

Genetic Etiology in Nonsyndromic Mandibular Prognathism. Liu H, Wu C, Lin J, Shao J, Chen Q, Luo E. J Craniofac Surg. 2017 Jan;28(1):161–169.

Genetic background of nonsyndromic oligodontia: a systematic review and meta-analysis. Ruf S, Klimas D, Honemann M, Jabir S. J Orofac Orthop. 2013 Jul;74(4):295–308.

Root resorption

Association of genetic polymorphism and external apical root resorption. Aminoshariae A, Aminoshariae A, Valiathan M, Kulild JC. Angle Orthod. 2016 Nov;86(6):1042–1049.

Gingival recession

Indication and timing of soft tissue augmentation at maxillary and mandibular incisors in orthodontic patients. A systematic review. Kloukos D, Eliades T, Sculean A, Katsaros C. Eur J Orthod. 2014 Aug;36(4):442–9.

A systematic review of the association between appliance-induced labial movement of mandibular incisors and gingival recession Aziz T, Flores-Mir C. Aust Orthod J. 2011 May;27(1):33–9.

Orthodontic therapy and gingival recession: a systematic review. Joss-Vassalli I, Grebenstein C, Topouzelis N, Sculean A, Katsaros C. Orthod Craniofac Res. 2010 Aug;13(3):127–41.

Gingival display

Botulinum toxin for the treatment of excessive gingival display: a systematic review. Marwan W, Nasr MD, Samer F, Jabbour MD, Joseph A, Sidaoui MD, Roger N, Haber MD, Elio G, Kechichian MD. Aesthetic Surg J 2016;36(1):82–88.

Growth prediction

Methods to quantify soft tissue-based cranial growth and treatment outcomes in children: a systematic review. Brons S, van Beusichem ME, Bronkhorst EM, Draaisma JM, Berge SJ, Schols JG, Kuijpers-Jagtman AM. PLoS One. 2014 Feb 27;9(2):e89602.

The diagnostic performance of dental maturity for identification of the circumpubertal growth phases: a meta-analysis. Perinetti G, Westphalen GH, Biasotto M, Salgarello S, Contardo L. Prog Orthod. 2013 May 23;14:8.

Use of skeletal maturation based on hand-wrist radiographic analysis as a predictor of facial growth: a systematic review. Flores-Mir C, Nebbe B, Major PW. Angle Orthod 2004;74(1):118–24.

Habits

Interventions for the cessation of non-nutritive sucking habits in children. Borrie FR, Bearn DR, Innes NP, Iheozor-Ejiofor Z. Cochrane Database Syst Rev. 2015 Mar 31;(3):CD008694.

Headgear

Please see Class II.

Herbst appliance

Please see Functional and orthopedic appliances.

Imaging

Please see Diagnostic records.

Impaction

Please see Canine impaction and transmigration and Third molars.

Implant site development

Please see Extrusion.

Interdisciplinary orthodontics

Treatment options for congenitally missing lateral incisors. Kiliaridis S, Sidira M, Kirmanidou Y, Michalakis K. Eur J Oral Implantol 2016;9 Suppl 1:S5–24.

Prosthetic replacement vs space closure for maxillary lateral incisor agenesis: A systematic review. Silveira GS, de Almeida NV Pereira DM, Mattos CT, Mucha JN. Am J Orthod Dentofacial Orthop. 2016 Aug;150(2):228–37.

Orthodontic treatment of periodontal defects. Part II: A systematic review on human and animal studies. Rotundo R, Bassarelli T, Pace E, Iachetti G, Mervelt J, Pini Prato G. Prog Orthod. 2011;12(1):45–52.

Orthodontic treatment of periodontal defects. A systematic review. Rotundo R, Nieri M, Iachetti G, Mervelt J, Cairo F, Baccetti T, Franchi L, Prato GP. Prog Orthod. 2010;11(1):41–4.

The orthodontic-periodontic interrelationship in integrated treatment challenges: a systematic review. Gkantidis N, Christou P, Topouzelis N. J Oral Rehabil. 2010 May 1;37(5):377–90.

Implant site development by orthodontic extrusion. A systematic review. Korayem M, Flores-Mir C, Nassar U, Olfert K. Angle Orthod. 2008 Jul;78(4):752–60.

Occlusal interventions for periodontitis in adults. Weston P, Yaziz YA, Moles DR, Needleman I. Cochrane Database Syst Rev. 2008 Jul 16;(3):CD004968.

Orthodontic space closure versus implant placement in subjects with missing teeth. Thilander B. J Oral Rehabil. 2008 Jan;35 Suppl 1:64–71.

Interproximal reduction

Interproximal wear versus incisors extraction to solve anterior lower crowding: a systematic review. Almeida NV, Silveira GS, Pereira DM, Mattos CT, Mucha JN. Dental Press J Orthod. 2015 Jan-Feb;20(1):66–73.

Enamel roughness and incidence of caries after interproximal enamel reduction: a systematic review. Koretsi V, Chatzigianni A, Sidiropoulou S. Orthod Craniofac Res. 2014 Feb;17(1):1–13.

Intra-arch width

Intra-arch widths: a meta-analysis. Lombardo L, Setti S, Molinari C, Siciliani G. Int Orthod. 2013 Jun;11(2):177–92.
A meta-analysis of mandibular intercanine width in treatment and postretention. Burke SP, Silveira AM, Goldsmith LJ, Yancey JM, Van Stewart A, Scarfe WC. Angle Orthod 1998;68(1):53–60.

Intraoral scanners

Please see Diagnostic records.

Intrusion

True molar intrusion attained during orthodontic treatment: a systematic review. Ng J, Major PW, Flores-Mir C. Am J Orthod Dentofacial Orthop. 2006 Dec;130(6):709–14.
True incisor intrusion attained during orthodontic treatment: a systematic review and meta-analysis. Ng J, Major PW, Heo G, Flores-Mir C. Am J Orthod Dentofacial Orthop. 2005 Aug;128(2):212–9.

Invisalign

The treatment effects of Invisalign orthodontic aligners: a systematic review. Lagravere MO, Flores-Mir C. J Am Dent Assoc. 2005 Dec;136(12):1724–9.

Juvenile idiopathic arthritis

Orthodontic and dentofacial orthopedic management of juvenile idiopathic arthritis: a systematic review of the literature. von Bremen J, Ruf S. Orthod Craniofac Res. 2011 Aug;14(3):107–15.

Laceback ligatures

The effectiveness of laceback ligatures during initial orthodontic alignment: a systematic review and meta-analysis. Fleming PS, Johal A, Pandis N. Eur J Orthod. 2013 Aug;35(4):539–46.

Lateral incisors

Prosthetic replacement vs space closure for maxillary lateral incisor agenesis: A systematic review. Silveira GS, de Almeida NV, Pereira DM, Mattos CT, Mucha JN. Am J Orthod Dentofacial Orthop. 2016 Aug;150(2):228–37.
Treatment options for congenitally missing lateral incisors. Kiliaridis S, Sidira M, Kirmanidou Y, Michalakis K. Eur J Oral Implantol. 2016;9 Suppl 1:S5–24.

Prevalence of peg-shaped maxillary permanent lateral incisors: A meta-analysis. Hua F, He H, Ngan P, Bouzid W. Am J Orthod Dentofacial Orthop. 2013 Jul;144(1):97–109.

Lingual orthodontics

Please see Brackets.

Lip bumper

Please see Space maintenenece.

Low level laser therapy and pain

Please see Pain.

Low level laser therapy and tooth movement

Please see Accelerated tooth movement.

Maxillary expansion

Please see Crossbite (posterior).

Medications affecting tooth movement

Escaping the adverse impacts of NSAIDs on tooth movement during orthodontics: current evidence based on a meta-analysis. Fang J, Li Y, Zhang K, Zhao Z, Mei L. Medicine (Baltimore). 2016 Apr;95(16):e3256.
Effects of bisphosphonates in orthodontic therapy: systematic review. Rodolfino D, Saccucci M, Filippakos A, Gerxhani R, Lopez G, Felice F, D'Arcangelo C. J Biol Regul Homeost Agents. 2012 Apr-Jun;26(2 Suppl):29–33.
Influence of bisphosphonates in orthodontic therapy: Systematic review. Iglesias-Linares A, Yanez-Vico RM, Solano-Reina E, Torres-Lagares D, Gonzalez Moles MA. J Dent. 2010 Aug;38(8):603–11.

Mini-implants and mini-plates

Please see Anchorage.

Mixed dentition

Moyer's method of mixed dentition analysis: a meta-analysis. Buwembo W, Luboga S. Afr Health Sci 2004;4(1):63–6.

Molar distalization

Orthodontic treatment for distalising upper first molars in children and adolescents. Jambi S, Thiruvenkatachari B, O'Brien KD, Walsh T. Cochrane Database Syst Rev. 2013 Oct 23;(10):CD008375.

Efficiency of molar distalization associated with second and third molar eruption stage. Flores-Mir C, McGrath L, Heo G, Major PW. Angle Orthod. 2013 Jul;83(4):735–42.

Intraoral distalizer effects with conventional and skeletal anchorage: a meta-analysis. Grec RH, Janson G, Branco NC, Moura-Grec PG, Patel MP, Castanha Henriques JF. Am J Orthod Dentofacial Orthop. 2013 May;143(5):602–15.

Mouthguards

Dentofacial trauma and players attitude towards mouthguard use in field hockey: a systematic review and meta-analysis. Vucic S, Drost RW, Ongkosuwito EM, Wolvius EB. Br J Sports Med. 2016 Mar;50(5):298–304.

Myofunctional therapy

Effectiveness of orofacial myofunctional therapy in orthodontic patients: a systematic review. Homem MA, Vieira-Andrade RG, Falci SG, Ramos-Jorge ML, Marques LS. Dental Press J Orthod. 2014 Jul-Aug;19(4):94–9.

Nickel hypersensitivity

Nickel hypersensitivity and orthodontic treatment: a systematic review and meta-analysis. Golz L, Papageorgiou SN, Jager A. Contact Dermatitis. 2015 Jul;73(1):1–14.

Cytocompatibility of medical biomaterials containing nickel by osteoblasts: a systematic literature review. Mikulewicz M, Chojnacka K. Biol Trace Elem Res. 2011 Sep;142(3):865–89.

Allergic reactions and nickel-free braces: a systematic review. Pazzini CA, Marques LS, Pereira LJ, Correa-Faria P, Paiva SM. Braz Oral Res. 2011 Jan–Feb;25(1):85–90.

Prevalence of nickel hypersensitivity in orthodontic patients: a meta-analysis. Kolokitha OE, Kaklamanos EG, Papadopoulos MA. Am J Orthod Dentofacial Orthop. 2008 Dec;134(6):722.e1–722.e12; discussion 722–3.

Obstructive sleep apnea

Please also see Airway.

Airway morphology

Craniofacial and upper airway morphology in adult obstructive sleep apnea patients: A systematic review and meta-analysis of cephalometric studies. Neelapu BC, Kharbanda OP, Sardana HK, Balachandran R, Sardana V, Kapoor P, Gupta A, Vasamsetti S. Sleep Med Rev. 2017 Feb;31:79–90.

CBCT assessment of upper airway changes and treatment outcomes of obstructive sleep apnoea: a systematic review. Alsufyani NA, Al-Saleh MA, Major PW. Sleep Breath. 2013 Sep;17(3):911–23.

CPAP

Effects of CPAP and Mandibular Advancement Devices on Health-Related Quality of Life in OSA: A Systematic Review and Meta-analysis. Kuhn E, Schwarz EI, Bratton DJ, Rossi VA, Kohler M. Chest. 2017 Apr;151(4):786–794.

CPAP vs Mandibular Advancement Devices and Blood Pressure in Patients with Obstructive Sleep Apnea: A Systematic Review and Meta-analysis. Bratton DJ, Gaisl T, Wons AM, Kohler M. JAMA. 2015 Dec 1;314(21):2280–93.

Extraction

The effect of teeth extraction for orthodontic treatment on the upper airway: a systematic review. Hu Z, Yin X, Liao J, Zhou C, Yang Z, Zou S. Sleep Breath. 2015 May;19(2):441–51.

Oral appliances

Effects of CPAP and Mandibular Advancement Devices on Health-Related Quality of Life in OSA: A Systematic Review and Meta-analysis. Kuhn E, Schwarz EI, Bratton DJ, Rossi VA, Kohler M. Chest. 2017 Apr;151(4):786–794.

Oral appliances and functional orthopaedic appliances for obstructive sleep apnoea in children. Carvalho FR, Lentini-Oliveira DA, Prado LB, Prado GF, Carvalho LB. Cochrane Database Syst Rev. 2016 Oct 5;(10):CD005520.

Quality Assessment of Systematic Reviews on the Efficacy of Oral Appliance Therapy for Adult and Pediatric Sleep-Disordered Breathing.Al-Jewair TS, Gaffar BO, Flores-Mir C.J Clin Sleep Med. 2016 Aug 15;12(8):1175–83.

Meta-analysis of randomised controlled trials of oral mandibular advancement devices and continuous positive airway pressure for obstructive sleep apnoea-hypopnoea. Sharples LD, Clutterbuck-James AL, Glover MJ, Bennett MS, Chadwick R, Pittman MA, Quinnell TG. Sleep Med Rev. 2016 Jun;27:108–24.

Effectiveness of mandibular advancement appliances in treating obstructive sleep apnea syndrome: A systematic review. Serra-Torres S, Bellot-Arcís C, Montiel-Company JM, Marco-Algarra J, Almerich-Silla M. Laryngoscope. 2016 Feb;126(2):507–14.

Orthodontics treatments for managing obstructive sleep apnea syndrome in children: A systematic review and meta-analysis. Huynh NT, Desplats E, Almeida FR. Sleep Med Rev. 2016 Feb;25:84–94.

Maxillomandibular Advancement for Treatment of Obstructive Sleep Apnea: A Meta-analysis. Zaghi S, Holty JE, Certal V, Abdullatif J, Guilleminault C, Powell NB, Riley RW, Camacho M. JAMA Otolaryngol Head Neck Surg. 2016 Jan;142(1):58–66.

The effectiveness of different mandibular advancement amounts in OSA patients: a systematic review and meta-regression analysis. Bartolucci ML, Bortolotti F, Raffaelli E, D'Antò V, Michelotti A, Alessandri Bonetti G. Sleep Breath. 2016 Jan 15.

CPAP vs Mandibular Advancement Devices and Blood Pressure in Patients with Obstructive Sleep Apnea: A Systematic Review and Meta-analysis. Bratton DJ, Gaisl T, Wons AM, Kohler M. JAMA. 2015 Dec 1;314(21):2280–93

Myofunctional Therapy to Treat Obstructive Sleep Apnea: A Systematic Review and Meta-analysis. Camacho M, Certal V, Abdullatif J, Zaghi S, Ruoff CM, Capasso R, Kushida CA. Sleep. 2015 May 1;38(5):669–75.

Effect of oral appliances on blood pressure in obstructive sleep apnea: a systematic review and meta-analysis. Iftikhar IH, Hays ER, Iverson MA, Magalang UJ, Maas AK. J Clin Sleep Med. 2013 Feb 1;9(2):165–74.

A systematic review of the efficacy of oral appliance design in the management of obstructive sleep apnoea. Ahrens A, McGrath C, Hagg U. Eur J Orthod. 2011 Jun;33(3):318–24.

Subjective efficacy of oral appliance design features in the management of obstructive sleep apnea: a systematic review. Ahrens A, McGrath C, Hagg U. Am J Orthod Dentofacial Orthop. 2010 Nov;138(5):559–76.

Maxillomandibular advancement for the treatment of obstructive sleep apnea: a systematic review and meta-analysis. Holty JE, Guilleminault C. Sleep Med Rev. 2010 Oct;14(5):287–97.

Oral appliances and functional orthopaedic appliances for obstructive sleep apnoea in children. Carvalho FR, Lentini-Oliveira D, Machado MA, Prado GF, Prado LB, Saconato H. Cochrane Database Syst Rev. 2007 Apr 18;(2):CD005520.

Oral appliances for obstructive sleep apnoea. Lim J, Lasserson TJ, Fleetham J, Wright J. Cochrane Database Syst Rev. 2006 Jan 25;(1):CD004435.

Orthognathic surgery

Distraction osteogenesis as a treatment of obstructive sleep apnea syndrome: A systematic review. Tsui WK, Yang Y, Cheung LK, Leung YY. Medicine (Baltimore). 2016 Sep;95(36):e4674.

The effectiveness of different mandibular advancement amounts in OSA patients: a systematic review and meta-regression analysis. Bartolucci ML, Bortolotti F, Raffaelli E, D'Antò V, Michelotti A, Alessandri Bonetti G. Sleep Breath. 2016 Sep;20(3):911–9.

Improved apnea-hypopnea index and lowest oxygen saturation after maxillomandibular advancement with or without counterclockwise rotation in patients with obstructive sleep apnea: a meta-analysis. Knudsen TB, Laulund AS, Ingerslev J, HomÃ¸e P, Pinholt EM. J Oral Maxillofac Surg. 2015 Apr;73(4):719–26.

Effects of maxillomandibular advancement on the upper airway and surrounding structures in patients with obstructive sleep apnoea: a systematic review. Hsieh YJ, Liao YF. Br J Oral Maxillofac Surg. 2013 Dec;51(8):834–40.

Maxillomandibular advancement for treatment of obstructive sleep apnea syndrome: a systematic review. Pirklbauer K, Russmueller G, Stiebellehner L, Nell C, Sinko K, Millesi G, Klug C. J Oral Maxillofac Surg. 2011 Jun;69(6):e165–76.

Oligodontia

Please see Genetics.

Open bite

Treatment

Effectiveness of open bite correction when managing deleterious oral habits in growing children and adolescents: a systematic review and meta-analysis. Feres MF, Abreu LG, Insabralde NM, de Almeida MR, Flores-Mir C. Eur J Orthod. 2017 Feb;39(1):31–42.

Systematic review for orthodontic and orthopedic treatments for anterior open bite in the mixed dentition. Pisani L, Bonaccorso L, Fastuca R, Spena R, Lombardo L, Caprioglio A. Prog Orthod. 2016 Dec;17(1):28.

Effectiveness of the open bite treatment in growing children and adolescents. A systematic review. Feres MF, Abreu LG, Insabralde NM, Almeida MR, Flores-Mir C. Eur J Orthod. 2016 Jun;38(3):237–50.

Effect of molar intrusion with temporary anchorage devices in patients with anterior open bite: a systematic review. Alsafadi AS, Alabdullah MM, Saltaji H, Abdo A, Youssef M. Prog Orthod. 2016;17:9.

Orthodontic and orthopaedic treatment for anterior open bite in children. Lentini-Oliveira DA, Carvalho FR, Rodrigues CG, Ye Q, Prado LB, Prado GF, Hu R. Cochrane Database Syst Rev. 2014 Sep 24;(9):CD005515.

Effectiveness of orofacial myofunctional therapy in orthodontic patients: a systematic review. Homem MA, Vieira-Andrade RG, Falci SG, Ramos-Jorge ML, Marques LS. Dental Press J Orthod. 2014 Jul-Aug;19(4):94–9.

Early orthodontic treatment of skeletal open-bite malocclusion: a systematic review. Cozza P, Mucedero M, Baccetti T, Franchi L. Angle Orthod. 2005 Sep;75(5):707–13.

Stability

Combined orthodontic and orthognathic surgical treatment for the correction of skeletal anterior open-bite malocclusion: a systematic review on vertical stability. Solano-Hernandez B, Antonarakis GS, Scolozzi P, Kiliaridis S. J Oral Maxillofac Surg. 2013 Jan;71(1):98–109.

Stability of treatment for anterior open-bite malocclusion: a meta-analysis. Greenlee GM, Huang GJ, Chen SS, Chen J, Koepsell T, Hujoel P. Am J Orthod Dentofacial Orthop. 2011 Feb;139(2):154–69.

Oral health promotion

Please also see Antimicrobials.

Efficacy of professional hygiene and prophylaxis on preventing plaque increase in orthodontic patients with multibracket appliances: a systematic review. Migliorati M, Isaia L, Cassaro A, Rivetti A, Silvestrini-Biavati F, Gastaldo L, Piccardo I, Dalessandri D, Silvestrini-Biavati A. Eur J Orthod. 2015 Jun;37(3):297–307.

The influence of orthodontic fixed appliances on the oral microbiota: a systematic review. Freitas AO, Marquezan M, Nojima Mda C, Alviano DS, Maia LC. Dental Press J Orthod. 2014 Mar-Apr;19(2):46–55.

Caries preventive effects of xylitol-based candies and lozenges: a systematic review. Antonio AG, Pierro VS, Maia LC. J Public Health Dent. 2011 Spring;71(2):117–24.

Does oral health promotion influence the oral hygiene and gingival health of patients undergoing fixed appliance orthodontic treatment? A systematic literature review. Gray D, McIntyre G. J Orthod. 2008 Dec;35(4):262–9.

Meta-analysis on the effectiveness of powered toothbrushes for orthodontic patients. Kaklamanos EG, Kalfas S. Am J Orthod Dentofacial Orthop. 2008 Feb;133(2):187.e1–14.

Caries-Inhibiting Effect of Preventive Measures during Orthodontic Treatment with Fixed Appliances. A Systematic Review. Derks A, Katsaros C, Frencken JE, Van't Hof MA, Kuijpers-Jagtman AM. Caries Res 2004;38(5):413–20

Orthognathic surgery

Class II treatment

Effects of mandibular advancement surgery on the temporomandibular joint and muscular and articular adaptive changes--a systematic review. Bermell-Baviera A, Bellot-Arcis C, Montiel-Company JM, Almerich-Silla JM. Int J Oral Maxillofac Surg. 2016 May;45(5):545–52.

Class III treatment

Relation between soft tissue and skeletal changes after mandibular setback surgery: A systematic review and meta-analysis. Kaklamanos EG, Kolokitha OE. J Craniomaxillofac Surg. 2016 Apr;44(4):427–35.

Soft tissue profile changes after bilateral sagittal split osteotomy for mandibular setback: A systematic review. Joss CU, Joss-Vassalli IM, Berge SJ, Kuijpers-Jagtman AM. J Oral Maxillofac Surg. 2010 Nov;68(11): 2792–801

Miscellaneous

Mandible-first sequence in bimaxillary orthognathic surgery: a systematic review. Borba AM, Borges AH, Cé PS, Venturi BA, Naclério-Homem MG, Miloro M. Int J Oral Maxillofac Surg. 2016 Apr;45(4):472–5.

Accuracy of computer programs in predicting orthognathic surgery soft tissue response. Kaipatur NR, Flores-Mir C. J Oral Maxillofac Surg. 2009 Apr;67(4):751–9.

Obstructive sleep apnea

Distraction osteogenesis as a treatment of obstructive sleep apnea syndrome: A systematic review. Tsui WK, Yang Y, Cheung LK, Leung YY. Medicine (Baltimore). 2016 Sep;95(36):e4674.

The effectiveness of different mandibular advancement amounts in OSA patients: a systematic review and meta-regression analysis. Bartolucci ML, Bortolotti F, Raffaelli E, D'Antò V, Michelotti A, Alessandri Bonetti G. Sleep Breath. 2016 Sep;20(3):911–9.

Improved apnea-hypopnea index and lowest oxygen saturation after maxillomandibular advancement with or without counterclockwise rotation in patients with obstructive sleep apnea: a meta-analysis. Knudsen TB, Laulund AS, Ingerslev J, Homäe P, Pinholt EM. J Oral Maxillofac Surg. 2015 Apr;73(4):719–26.

Effects of maxillomandibular advancement on the upper airway and surrounding structures in patients with obstructive sleep apnoea: a systematic review. Hsieh YJ, Liao YF. Br J Oral Maxillofac Surg. 2013 Dec;51(8):834–40.

Maxillomandibular advancement for treatment of obstructive sleep apnea syndrome: a systematic review. Pirklbauer K, Russmueller G, Stiebellehner L, Nell C, Sinko K, Millesi G, Klug C. J Oral Maxillofac Surg. 2011 Jun;69(6):e165–76.

Stability

Is Counterclockwise Rotation of the Maxillomandibular Complex Stable Compared with Clockwise Rotation in the Correction of Dentofacial Deformities? A Systematic Review and Meta-Analysis. Al-Moraissi EA, Wolford LM. J Oral Maxillofac Surg. 2016 Oct;74(10):2066.e1–2066.e12.

Are bicortical screw and plate osteosynthesis techniques equal in providing skeletal stability with the bilateral sagittal split osteotomy when used for mandibular advancement surgery? A systematic review and meta-analysis. Al-Moraissi EA, Al-Hendi EA. Int J Oral Maxillofac Surg. 2016 Oct;45(10):1195–200.

Stability of Le Fort I maxillary inferior repositioning surgery with rigid internal fixation: a systematic review. Convens JM, Kiekens RM, Kuijpers-Jagtman AM, Fudalej PS. Int J Oral Maxillofac Surg. 2015 May;44(5):609–14.

Combined orthodontic and orthognathic surgical treatment for the correction of skeletal anterior open-bite malocclusion: a systematic review on vertical stability. Solano-Hernández B, Antonarakis GS, Scolozzi P, Kiliaridis S. J Oral Maxillofac Surg. 2013 Jan;71(1):98–109.

Skeletal stability and complications of bilateral sagittal split osteotomies and mandibular distraction osteogenesis: an evidence-based review. Ow A, Cheung LK. J Oral Maxillofac Surg. 2009 Nov;67(11):2344–53.

Stability after bilateral sagittal split osteotomy advancement surgery with rigid internal fixation: a systematic review. Joss CU, Vassalli, IM. J Oral Maxillofac Surg. 2009 Feb;67(2):301–13.

Stability factors after double-jaw surgery in Class III malocclusion. A systematic review. Mucedero M, Coviello A, Baccetti T, Franchi L, Cozza P. Angle Orthod. 2008 Nov;78(6):1141–52.

Surgery first approach

Does the Surgery-First Approach Produce Better Outcomes in Orthognathic Surgery? A Systematic Review and Meta-Analysis. Yang L, Xiao YD, Liang YJ, Wang X, Li JY, Liao GQ. J Oral Maxillofac Surg. 2017 Nov;75(11):2422–2429.

Surgery first in orthognathic surgery: A systematic review of the literature. Peiro-Guijarro MA, Guijarro-Martínez R, Hernández-Alfaro F. Am J Orthod Dentofacial Orthop. 2016 Apr;149(4):448–62.

Systematic review of the surgery-first approach in orthognathic surgery. Huang CS, Hsu SS, Chen YR. Biomed J. 2014 Jul-Aug;37(4):184–90.

Temporomandibular joint

Does orthognathic surgery cause or cure temporomandibular disorders? a systematic review and meta-analysis. Al-Moraissi EA, Wolford LM, Perez D, Laskin DM, Ellis E 3rd. J Oral Maxillofac Surg. 2017 Sep;75(9):1835–1847.

The effect of orthognathic surgery on the temporomandibular joint and oral function: a systematic review. Te Veldhuis EC, Te Veldhuis AH, Bramer WM, Wolvius EB, Koudstaal MJ. Int J Oral Maxillofac Surg. 2017 May;46(5):554–563.

Does temporomandibular joint pathology with or without surgical management affect the stability of counterclockwise rotation of the maxillomandibular complex in orthognathic surgery? A systematic review and meta-analysis. Al-Moraissi EA, Wolford LM. J Oral Maxillofac Surg. 2017 Apr;75(4):805–821.

Orthognathic treatment of dentofacial disharmonies: its impact on temporomandibular disorders, quality of life, and psychosocial wellness. Song YL, Yap AU. Cranio. 2017 Jan;35(1):52–57.

Condylar resorption in orthognathic patients after mandibular bilateral sagittal split osteotomy: a systematic review. Mousoulea S, Kloukos D, Sampaziotis D, Vogiatzi T, Eliades T. Eur J Orthod. 2016 Jun;22:294–309.

Effects of mandibular advancement surgery on the temporomandibular joint and muscular and articular adaptive changes--a systematic review. Bermell-Baviera A, Bellot-Arcís C, Montiel-Company JM, Almerich-Silla JM. Int J Oral Maxillofac Surg. 2016 May;45(5):545–52.

TMJ response to mandibular advancement surgery: an overview of risk factors. Valladares-Neto J, Cevidanes LH, Rocha WC, Almeida Gde A, Paiva JB, Rino-Neto J. J Appl Oral Sci. 2014 Jan–Feb;22(1):2–14.

Orthognathic treatment and temporomandibular disorders: a systematic review. Part 2. Signs and symptoms and meta-analyses. Al-Riyami S, Cunningham SJ, Moles DR. Am J Orthod Dentofacial Orthop. 2009 Nov;136(5):626.e1–16.

Orthognathic treatment and temporomandibular disorders: A systematic review. Part 1. A new quality-assessment technique and analysis of study characteristics and classifications. Al-Riyami S, Cunningham SJ, Moles DR. Am J Orthod Dentofacial Orthop. 2009 Nov;136(5):624.e1–15.

Temporomandibular joint morphology changes with mandibular advancement surgery and rigid internal fixation: a systematic. literature review. Kersey ML, Nebbe B, Major PW. Angle Orthod 2003;73(1):79–85.

Osteoarthritis

Interventions for the management of temporomandibular joint osteoarthritis. de Souza RF, Lovato da Silva CH, Nasser M, Fedorowicz Z, Al-Muharraqi MA. Cochrane Database Syst Rev. 2012 Apr 18;(4):CD007261.

Overlay retainer

Please see Retention and relapse.

Pain

Adverse effects

Pain and tissue damage in response to orthodontic tooth movement: are they correlated? Cuoghi OA, Topolski F, de Faria LP, de Mendonça MR. J Contemp Dent Pract. 2016 Sep 1;17(9):713–720.

Adverse effects of lingual and buccal orthodontic techniques: A systematic review and meta-analysis. Ata-Ali F, Ata-Ali J, Ferrer-Molina M, Cobo T, De Carlos F, Cobo J. Am J Orthod Dentofacial Orthop. 2016 Jun;149(6):820–9.

Comparison of interventions

Non-pharmacological interventions for alleviating pain during orthodontic treatment. Fleming PS, Strydom H, Katsaros C, MacDonald L, Curatolo M, Fudalej P, Pandis N. Cochrane Database Syst Rev. 2016 Dec 23;(12):CD010263.

Comparative effectiveness of pharmacologic and nonpharmacologic interventions for orthodontic pain relief at peak pain intensity: A Bayesian network meta-analysis. Sandhu SS, Cheema MS, Khehra HS. Am J Orthod Dentofacial Orthop. 2016 Jul;150(1):13–32.

Interventions for pain during fixed orthodontic appliance therapy. A systematic review. Xiaoting L, Yin T, Yangxi C. Angle Orthod. 2010 Sep;80(5):925–32.

Low level laser therapy

Low-level laser therapy for orthodontic pain: a systematic review. Li FJ, Zhang JY, Zeng XT, Guo Y. Lasers Med Sci. 2015 Aug;30(6):1789–803.

Systematic literature review: influence of low-level laser on orthodontic movement and pain control in humans. Sousa MV, Pinzan A, Consolaro A, Henriques JF, de Freitas MR. Photomed Laser Surg. 2014 Nov;32(11):592–9.

Efficacy of low-level laser therapy in the management of orthodontic pain: a systematic review and meta-analysis. He WL, Li CJ, Liu ZP, Sun JF, Hu ZA, Yin X, Zou SJ. Lasers Med Sci. 2013 Nov;28(6):1581–9.

Pharmacological intervention

Preoperative analgesics for additional pain relief in children and adolescents having dental treatment. Ashley PF, Parekh S, Moles DR, Anand P, MacDonald LC. Cochrane Database Syst Rev. 2016 Aug 8;(8):CD008392.

Escaping the Adverse Impacts of NSAIDs on Tooth Movement During Orthodontics: Current Evidence Based on a Meta-Analysis. Fang J, Li Y, Zhang K, Zhao Z, Mei L. Medicine (Baltimore). 2016 Apr;95(16):e3256.

Pharmacological management of pain during orthodontic treatment: a meta-analysis. Angelopoulou MV, Vlachou V, Halazonetis DJ. Orthod Craniofac Res. 2012 May;15(2):71–83.

Peg lateral incisors

Please see Epidemiology.

Patient-centered outcomes

Patient satisfaction and expectations

Patient satisfaction after orthodontic treatment combined with orthognathic surgery: A systematic review. Pacheco-Pereira C, Abreu LG, Dick BD, De Luca Canto G, Paiva SM, Flores-Mir C. Angle Orthod. 2016 May;86(3):495–508.

What are patients' expectations of orthodontic treatment: a systematic review. Yao J, Li DD, Yang YQ, McGrath CP, Mattheos N. BMC Oral Health. 2016 Feb 17;16:19.

Factors associated with patient and parent satisfaction after orthodontic treatment: a systematic review. Pacheco-Pereira C, Pereira JR, Dick BD, Perez A, Flores-Mir C. Am J Orthod Dentofacial Orthop. 2015 Oct;148(4):652–9.

Do orthodontic research outcomes reflect patient values? A systematic review of randomized controlled trials involving children. Tsichlaki A, O'Brien K. Am J Orthod Dentofacial Orthop. 2014 Sep;146(3):279–85.

Subjective and objective perception of orthodontic treatment need: a systematic review. Livas C, Delli K. Eur J Orthod. 2013 Jun;35(3):347–53.

Patients' perceptions of orthognathic treatment, well-being, and psychological or psychiatric status: a systematic review. Alanko OM, Svedstrom-Oristo AL, Tuomisto MT. Acta Odontol Scand. 2010 Sep;68(5):249–60.

Long-term stability of orthodontic treatment and patient satisfaction. A systematic review. Bondemark L, Holm AK, Hansen K, Axelsson S, Mohlin B, Brattstrom V, Paulin G, Pietila T. Angle Orthodon 2007;77:181–191.

Psychological impact

The psychosocial impact of orthognathic surgery: a systematic review. Hunt OT, Johnston CD, Hepper PG, Burden DJ. Am J Orthod Dentofacial Orthop 2001;120(5):490–7.

Quality of life

Does orthodontic treatment before the age of 18 years improve oral health-related quality of life? A systematic review and meta-analysis. Javidi H, Vettore M, Benson PE. Am J Orthod Dentofacial Orthop. 2017 Apr;151(4):644–655.

Orthognathic treatment of dentofacial disharmonies: its impact on temporomandibular disorders, quality of life, and psychosocial wellness. Song YL Bds Mds M Ortho Rcs, Yap AU Bds MSc PhD. Cranio. 2017 Jan;35(1):52–57.

The impact of malocclusions on oral health-related quality of life in children-a systematic review and meta-analysis. Kragt L, Dhamo B, Wolvius EB, Ongkosuwito EM. Clin Oral Investig. 2016 Nov;20(8):1881–1894.

Malocclusion, orthodontic treatment, and the Oral Health Impact Profile (OHIP-14): Systematic review and meta-analysis. Andiappan M, Gao W, Bernabe E, Kandala NB, Donaldson AN. Angle Orthod. 2015 May;85(3):493–500.

The impact of orthodontic treatment on the quality of life a systematic review. Zhou Y, Wang Y, Wang X, Voliere G, Hu R. BMC Oral Health. 2014 Jun 10;14:66.

Research methods

Expert panels as a reference standard in orthodontic research: An assessment of published methods and reporting. Lempesi E, Toulia E, Pandis N. Am J Orthod Dentofacial Orthop. 2017 Apr;151(4):656–668.

Bias from historical control groups used in orthodontic research: a meta-epidemiological study. Papageorgiou SN, Koretsi V, Jager A. Eur J Orthod. 2017 Feb;39(1):98–105.

Health economic evaluations in orthodontics: a systematic review. Sollenius O, Petrén S, Björnsson L, Norlund A, Bondemark L. Eur J Orthod. 2016 Jun;38(3):259–65.

Demographic characteristics of systematic reviews, meta-analyses, and randomized controlled trials in orthodontic journals with impact factor. Kanavakis G, Dombroski MM, Malouf DP, Athanasiou AE. Eur J Orthod. 2016 Feb;38(1):57–65.

Statistical analysis in orthodontic journals: are we ignoring confounding? Spanou A, Koletsi D, Fleming PS, Polychronopoulou A, Pandis N. Eur J Orthod. 2016 Feb;38(1):32–38.

Cochrane systematic reviews in orthodontics. Deliere M, Yan-Vergnes W, Hamel O, Marchal-Sixou C, Vergnes JN. Int Orthod. 2010 Sep;8(3):278–92.

A critical evaluation of meta-analyses in orthodontics. Papadopoulos MA, Gkiaouris I. Am J Orthod Dentofacial Orthop. 2007 May;131(5):589–99

Periodontal health

Brackets

The effect of bracket ligation on the periodontal status of adolescents undergoing orthodontic treatment. A systematic review and meta-analysis. Arnold S, Koletsi D, Patcas R, Eliades T. J Dent. 2016 Nov;54:13–24.

Adverse effects of lingual and buccal orthodontic techniques: A systematic review and meta-analysis. Ata-Ali F, Ata-Ali J, Ferrer-Molina M, Cobo T, De Carlos F, Cobo J. Am J Orthod Dentofacial Orthop. 2016 Jun;149(6):820–9.

Clear aligners

Periodontal health during clear aligners treatment: a systematic review. Rossini G, Parrini S, Castroflorio T, Deregibus A, Debernardi CL. Eur J Orthod. 2015 Oct;37(5):539–43.

Gingival recession

Indication and timing of soft tissue augmentation at maxillary and mandibular incisors in orthodontic patients. A systematic review. Kloukos D, Eliades T, Sculean A, Katsaros C. Eur J Orthod. 2014 Aug;36(4):442–9.

A systematic review of the association between appliance-induced labial movement of mandibular incisors and gingival recession. Aziz T, Flores-Mir C. Aust Orthod J. 2011 May;27(1):33–9.

Orthodontic therapy and gingival recession: a systematic review. Joss-Vassalli I, Grebenstein C, Topouzelis N, Sculean A, Katsaros C. Orthod Craniofac Res. 2010 Aug;13(3):127–41.

Orthodontic therapy

The microbial changes in subgingival plaques of orthodontic patients: a systematic review and meta-analysis of clinical trials. Guo R, Lin Y, Zheng Y, Li W. BMC Oral Health. 2017 Jun 2;17(1):90.

Pain and Tissue Damage in Response to Orthodontic Tooth Movement: Are They Correlated? Cuoghi OA, Topolski F, de Faria LP, de Mendonça MR. J Contemp Dent Pract. 2016 Sep 1;17(9):713–720.

The effects of orthodontic therapy on periodontal health: a systematic review of controlled evidence. Bollen AM, Cunha-Cruz J, Bakko DW, Huang GJ, Hujoel PP. J Am Dent Assoc. 2008 Apr;139(4):413–22.

Effects of malocclusions and orthodontics on periodontal health: evidence from a systematic review. Bollen, AM. J Dent Educ. 2008 Aug;72(8):912–8.

The relationships between malocclusion, fixed orthodontic appliances and periodontal disease. A review of the literature van Gastel J, Quirynen M, Teughels W, Carels C. Aust Orthod J. 2007 Nov;23(2):121–9.

Gingival invagination--a systematic review. Golz L, Reichert C, Jager A. J Orofac Orthop. 2011 Nov;72(6):409–20.

Retainers

Gingival condition associated with two types of orthodontic fixed retainers: a meta-analysis. Buzatta LN, Shimizu RH, Shimizu IA, Pachêco-Pereira C, Flores-Mir C, Taba M Jr, Porporatti AL, De Luca Canto G. Eur J Orthod. 2017 Aug 1;39(4):446–452.

Surgical- orthodontic treatment of impacted canines

Periodontal status after surgical-orthodontic treatment of labially impacted canines with different surgical techniques: A systematic review. Incerti-Parenti S, Checchi V, Ippolito DR, Gracco A, Alessandri-Bonetti G. Am J Orthod Dentofacial Orthop. 2016 Apr;149(4):463–72.

Pharmacological agents

Please see Accelerated tooth movement.

Piezocision

Please see Accelerated tooth movement.

Posterior crossbite

Please see Crossbites (posterior).

Powered toothbrush

Meta-analysis on the effectiveness of powered toothbrushes for orthodontic patients. Kaklamanos EG, Kalfas S. Am J Orthod Dentofacial Orthop. 2008 Feb;133(2):187.e1–14.

Premature loss of deciduous teeth

Dental arch space changes following premature loss of primary first molars: a systematic review. Tunison W, Flores-Mir C, ElBadrawy H, Nassar U, El-Bialy T. Pediatr Dent. 2008 Jul-Aug;30(4):297–302.

Profile

Please see Soft tissue profile.

Pulpal health

Influence of orthodontic forces on human dental pulp: a systematic review. Javed F, Al-Kheraif AA, Romanos EB, Romanos GE. Arch Oral Biol. 2015 Feb;60(2):347–56.
Pulpal reactions to orthodontic force application in humans: a systematic review. von Bohl M, Ren Y, Fudalej PS, Kuijpers-Jagtman AM. J Endod. 2012 Nov;38(11):1463–9.

Quality of life

Please see Patient-centered outcomes.

Recession

Please see Gingival recession and Periodontal health.

Retention and relapse

Low laser therapy

Effect of Low-Level Laser Therapy on Relapse of Rotated Teeth: A Systematic Review of Human and Animal Study. Meng M, Yang M, Lv C, Yang Q, Yang Z, Chen S. Photomed Laser Surg. 2017 Jan;35(1):3–11.

Efficacy of low-level laser therapy in accelerating tooth movement, preventing relapse and managing acute pain during orthodontic treatment in humans: a systematic review. Sonesson M, De Geer E, Subraian J, Petrén S. BMC Oral Health. 2016 Jul 7;17(1):11.

Periodontal health

Gingival condition associated with two types of orthodontic fixed retainers: a meta-analysis. Buzatta LN, Shimizu RH, Shimizu IA, Pacheco-Pereira C, Flores-Mir C, Taba M Jr, Porporatti AL, De Luca Canto G. Eur J Orthod. 2017 Aug 1;39(4):446–452.

Retention procedures

Retention procedures for stabilising tooth position after treatment with orthodontic braces. Littlewood SJ, Millett DT, Doubleday B, Bearn DR, Worthington HV. Cochrane Database Syst Rev. 2016 Jan 29;(1):CD002283.

Interventions for managing relapse of the lower front teeth after orthodontic treatment. Yu Y, Sun J, Lai W, Wu T, Koshy S, Shi Z. Cochrane Database Syst Rev. 2013 Sep 6;(9):CD008734.

Orthodontic retention: A systematic review. Littlewood SJ, Millett DT, Doubleday B, Bearn DR, Worthington HV. J Orthod. 2006 Sep;33(3):205–212.

Success and failures

Failure of fixed orthodontic retainers: A systematic review. Iliadi A, Kloukos D, Gkantidis N, Katsaros C, Pandis N. J Dent. 2015 Aug;43(8):876–96.

Surgery

Is Counterclockwise Rotation of the Maxillomandibular Complex Stable Compared with Clockwise Rotation in the Correction of Dentofacial Deformities? A Systematic Review and Meta-Analysis. Al-Moraissi EA, Wolford LM. J Oral Maxillofac Surg. 2016 Oct;74(10):2066.e1–2066.e12.

Are bicortical screw and plate osteosynthesis techniques equal in providing skeletal stability with the bilateral sagittal split osteotomy when used for mandibular advancement surgery? A systematic review and meta-analysis. Al-Moraissi EA, Al-Hendi EA. Int J Oral Maxillofac Surg. 2016 Oct;45(10):1195–200.

Vacuum formed retainers

Performance of clear vacuum-formed thermoplastic retainers depending on retention protocol: a systematic review. Kaklamanos EG, Kourakou M, Kloukos D, Doulis I, Kavvadia S. Odontology. 2017 Apr;105(2):237–247.

Comparison of vacuum-formed and Hawley retainers: a systematic review. Mai W, He J, Meng H, Jiang Y, Huang C, Li M, Yuan K, Kang N. Am J Orthod Dentofacial Orthop. 2014 Jun;145(6):720–7.

Remineralizing agents

Please see Caries and White spot lesions.

Root damage/repair

Root repair after contact with mini-implants: systematic review of the literature. Alves M Jr, Baratieri C, Mattos CT, Araujo MT, Maia LC. Eur J Orthod. 2013 Aug;35(4):491–9.

Root damage associated with intermaxillary screws: a systematic review. Alves M Jr, Baratieri C, Araujo MT, Souza MM, Maia LC. Int J Oral Maxillofac Surg. 2012 Nov;41(11):1445–50.

Root resorption

Class II

Radiologically determined orthodontically induced external apical root resorption in incisors after non-surgical orthodontic treatment of class II division 1 malocclusion: a systematic review. Tieu LD, Saltaji H, Normando D, Flores-Mir C. Prog Orthod. 2014 Jul 23;15:48.

Cytokines and receptor levels

Effect of orthodontic forces on cytokine and receptor levels in gingival crevicular fluid: a systematic review. Kapoor P, Kharbanda OP, Monga N, Miglani R, Kapila S. Prog Orthod. 2014 Dec 9;15:65.

Interleukin-1β +3954 polymorphisms and risk of external apical root resorption in orthodontic treatment: a meta-analysis. Wu FL, Wang LY, Huang YQ, Guo WB, Liu CD, Li SG. Genet Mol Res. 2013 Oct 18;12(4):4678–86.

Endodontically treated teeth

Radiographic comparison of the extent of orthodontically induced external apical root resorption in vital and root-filled teeth: a systematic review. Walker SL, Tieu LD, Flores-Mir C. Eur J Orthod. 2013 Dec;35(6):796–802.

Root resorption of endodontically treated teeth following orthodontic treatment: a meta-analysis Ioannidou-Marathiotou I, Zafeiriadis AA, Papadopoulos MA. Clin Oral Investig. 2013 Sep;17(7):1733–44.

Expansion

Radiographic assessment of external root resorption associated with jackscrew-based maxillary expansion therapies: a systematic review. Forst D, Nijjar S, Khaled Y, Lagravere M, Flores-Mir C. Eur J Orthod. 2014 Oct;36(5):576–85.

Force level

Association of orthodontic force system and root resorption: A systematic review. Roscoe MG, Meira JB, Cattaneo PM. Am J Orthod Dentofacial Orthop. 2015 May;147(5):610–26.

Genetics

Association of genetic polymorphism and external apical root resorption. Aminoshariae A, Aminoshariae A, Valiathan M, Kulild JC. Angle Orthod. 2016 Nov;86(6):1042–1049.

Risk factors

Root resorption associated with orthodontic tooth movement: a systematic review. Weltman B, Vig KW, Fields HW, Shanker S, Kaizar EE. Am J Orthod Dentofacial Orthop. 2010 Apr;137(4):462–76.

Root resorption and orthodontic treatment. Review of the literature. Pizzo G, Licata ME, Guiglia R, Giuliana G. Minerva Stomatol. 2007 Jan-Feb;56(1-2):31–44.

Self ligating brackets

Root resorption during orthodontic treatment with self-ligating or conventional brackets: a systematic review and meta-analysis. Yi J, Li M, Li Y, Li X, Zhao Z. BMC Oral Health. 2016 Nov 21;16(1):125.

Scanners, intraoral

Please see Diagnostic records.

Self-ligating brackets

Please see Brackets.

Smile esthetics

Laypeople's perceptions of frontal smile esthetics: A systematic review. Parrini S, Rossini G, Castroflorio T, Fortini A, Deregibus A, Debernardi C. Am J Orthod Dentofacial Orthop. 2016 Nov;150(5):740–750.

Influence of orthodontic treatment, midline position, buccal corridor and smile arc on smile attractiveness. Janson G, Branco NC, Fernandes TM, Sathler R, Garib D, Lauris A. Angle Orthod. 2011 Jan;81(1):153–61.

Soft tissue profile

Esthetic perception of changes in facial profile resulting from orthodontic treatment with extraction of premolars: A systematic review. Iared W, Koga da Silva EM, Iared W, Rufino Macedo C. J Am Dent Assoc. 2017 Jan;148(1):9–16.

Soft-tissue changes in Class II malocclusion patients treated with extractions: a systematic review. Janson G, Mendes LM, Junqueira CH, Garib DG. Eur J Orthod. 2016 Dec;38(6):631–637.

Relation between soft tissue and skeletal changes after mandibular setback surgery: A systematic review and meta-analysis. Kaklamanos EG, Kolokitha OE. J Craniomaxillofac Surg. 2016 Apr;44(4):427–35.

Soft tissue profile changes after bilateral sagittal split osteotomy for mandibular setback: a systematic review. Joss CU, Joss-Vassalli IM, Berge SJ, Kuijpers-Jagtman AM. J Oral Maxillofac Surg. 2010 Nov;68(11): 2792–801.

Soft tissue changes following the extraction of premolars in nongrowing patients with bimaxillary protrusion. A systematic review. Leonardi R, Annunziata A, Licciardello V, Barbato E. Angle Orthod. 2010 Jan;80(1):211–6.

A systematic review of cephalometric facial soft tissue changes with the Activator and Bionator appliances in Class II division 1 subjects. Flores-Mir C, Major PW. Eur J Orthod. 2006 Dec;28(6):586–93.

Cephalometric facial soft tissue changes with the twin block appliance in Class II division 1 malocclusion patients. A systematic review. Flores-Mir C, Major PW. Angle Orthod. 2006 Sep;76(5):876–81.

Soft tissue changes with fixed functional appliances in Class II division 1. Flores-Mir C, Major MP, Major PW. Angle Orthod. 2006 Jul;76(4):712–20.

Space maintenance

Effects of lingual arch used as space maintainer on mandibular arch dimension: a systematic review. Viglianisi, A. Am J Orthod Dentofacial Orthop. 2010 Oct;138(4):382.e1–4; discussion 382–3.

Effect of lip bumpers on mandibular arch dimensions. Hashish DI, Mostafa, YA. Am J Orthod Dentofacial Orthop. 2009 Jan;135(1):106–9.

Guidelines on the use of space maintainers following premature loss of primary teeth. Brothwell, DJ. J Can Dent Assoc. 1997 Nov;63(10):753, 757–60, 764–6.

Speech

Speech and orthodontic appliances: a systematic literature review. Chen J, Wan J, You L. Eur J Orthod. doi: 10.1093/ejo/cjx023. [Epub ahead of print].

Adverse effects of lingual and buccal orthodontic techniques: A systematic review and meta-analysis. Ata-Ali F, Ata-Ali J, Ferrer-Molina M, Cobo T, De Carlos F, Cobo J. Am J Orthod Dentofacial Orthop. 2016 Jun;149(6):820–9.

The effects of orthognathic surgery on speech: a review. Hassan T, Naini FB, Gill DS. J Oral Maxillofac Surg. 2007 Dec;65(12):2536–43.

Stability

Class II

Predictive factors of sagittal stability after treatment of Class II malocclusions. Maniewicz Wins S, Antonarakis GS, Kiliaridis S. Angle Orthod. 2016 Nov;86(6):1033–1041.

Stability of Class II fixed functional appliance therapy-a systematic review and meta-analysis. Bock NC, von Bremen J, Ruf S. Eur J Orthod. 2016 Apr;38(2):129–39.

Class III

Stability factors after double-jaw surgery in Class III malocclusion. A systematic review. Mucedero M, Coviello A, Baccetti T, Franchi L, Cozza P. Angle Orthod. 2008 Nov;78(6):1141–52.

Deepbite

Stability of deep-bite correction: A systematic review. Huang GJ, Bates SB, Ehlert AA, Whiting DP, Chen SS, Bollen AM. J World Fed Orthod. 2012 Sep 1;1(3):e89–e86.

Methodology to evaluate stability

Methodologies for evaluating long-term stability of dental relationships after orthodontic treatment. BeGole EA, Sadowsky C. Semin Orthod 1999;5(3):142–50.

Openbite

Combined orthodontic and orthognathic surgical treatment for the correction of skeletal anterior open-bite malocclusion: a systematic review on vertical stability. Solano-Hernández B, Antonarakis GS, Scolozzi P, Kiliaridis S. J Oral Maxillofac Surg. 2013 Jan;71(1):98–109.

Stability of treatment for anterior open-bite malocclusion: a meta-analysis. Greenlee GM, Huang GJ, Chen SS, Chen J, Koepsell T, Hujoel P. Am J Orthod Dentofacial Orthop. 2011 Feb;139(2):154–69.

Orthognathic surgery

Is Counterclockwise Rotation of the Maxillomandibular Complex Stable Compared with Clockwise Rotation in the Correction of Dentofacial Deformities? A Systematic Review and Meta-Analysis. Al-Moraissi EA, Wolford LM. J Oral Maxillofac Surg. 2016 Oct;74(10):2066.e1–2066.e12.

Are bicortical screw and plate osteosynthesis techniques equal in providing skeletal stability with the bilateral sagittal split osteotomy when used for mandibular advancement surgery? A systematic review and meta-analysis. Al-Moraissi EA, Al-Hendi EA. Int J Oral Maxillofac Surg. 2016 Oct;45(10):1195–200.

Stability of Le Fort I maxillary inferior repositioning surgery with rigid internal fixation: a systematic review. Convens JM, Kiekens RM, Kuijpers-Jagtman AM, Fudalej PS. Int J Oral Maxillofac Surg. 2015 May;44(5):609–14.

Stability after bilateral sagittal split osteotomy advancement surgery with rigid internal fixation: a systematic review. Joss CU, Vassalli IM. J Oral Maxillofac Surg. 2009 Feb;67(2):301–13.

Skeletal stability and complications of bilateral sagittal split osteotomies and mandibular distraction osteogenesis: an evidence-based review. Ow A, Cheung LK. J Oral Maxillofac Surg. 2009 Nov;67(11):2344–53.

Stability factors after double-jaw surgery in Class III malocclusion. A systematic review. Mucedero M, Coviello A, Baccetti T, Franchi L, Cozza, P. Angle Orthod. 2008 Nov;78(6):1141–52.

Surgically assisted maxillary expansion

Please see Crossbites (posterior).

Surgery first approach

Please see Orthognathic surgery.

Temporary anchorage devices (TADs)

Please see Anchorage.

Temporomandibular joint

Juvenile idiopathic arthritis

Orthodontic and dentofacial orthopedic management of juvenile idiopathic arthritis: A systematic review of the literature. von Bremen J, Ruf S. Orthod Craniofac Res. 2011 Aug;14(3):107–15.

Occlusion

Temporomandibular disorders and dental occlusion. A systematic review of association studies: end of an era? Manfredini D, Lombardo L, Siciliani G. J Oral Rehabil. 2017 Nov;44(11):908–923.

Posterior crossbite and temporomandibular disorders (TMDs): need for orthodontic treatment? Thilander B, Bjerklin K. Eur J Orthod. 2012 Dec;34(6):667–73.

Orthodontics for treating temporomandibular joint (TMJ) disorders. Luther F, Layton S, McDonald F. Cochrane Database Syst Rev. 2010 Jul 7;(7):CD006541.

Occlusal adjustment for treating and preventing temporomandibular joint disorders. Koh H, Robinson PG. Cochrane Database Syst Rev 2003(1):CD003812.

Orthodontics and temporomandibular disorder: a meta-analysis. Kim MR, Graber TM, Viana MA. Am J Orthod Dentofacial Orthop 2002;121(5):438–46.

Occlusal treatments in temporomandibular disorders: a qualitative systematic review of randomized controlled trials. Forssell H, Kalso E, Koskela P, Vehmanen R, Puukka P, Alanen P. Pain 1999;83(3):549–60.

Oral appliances

Changes in temporomandibular joint morphology in class II patients treated with fixed mandibular repositioning and evaluated through 3D imaging: a systematic review. Al-Saleh MA, Alsufyani N, Flores-Mir C, Nebbe B, Major PW. Orthod Craniofac Res. 2015 Nov;18(4):185–201.

Effect of chin-cup treatment on the temporomandibular joint: a systematic review. Zurfluh MA, Kloukos D, Patcas R, Eliades T. Eur J Orthod. 2015 Jun;37(3):314–24.

The effectiveness of splint therapy in patients with temporomandibular disorders: a systematic review and meta-analysis. Ebrahim S, Montoya L, Busse JW, Carrasco-Labra A, Guyatt GH; Medically Unexplained Syndromes Research Group. J Am Dent Assoc. 2012 Aug;143(8):847–57.

Systematic review and meta-analysis of randomized controlled trials evaluating intraoral orthopedic appliances for temporomandibular disorders. Fricton J, Look JO, Wright E, Alencar FG Jr, Chen H, Lang M, Ouyang W, Velly AM. J Orofac Pain. 2010 Summer;24(3):237–54.

Stabilization splint therapy for the treatment of temporomandibular myofascial pain: a systematic review. Al-Ani Z, Gray RJ, Davies SJ, Sloan P, Glenny AM. J Dent Educ. 2005 Nov;69(11):1242–50.

Efficacy of stabilization splints for the management of patients with masticatory muscle pain: a qualitative systematic review Turp JC, Komine F, Hugger A. Clin Oral Investig. 2004 Dec;8(4):179–95.

Effect of Herbst treatment on temporomandibular joint morphology: a systematic literature review. Popowich K, Nebbe B, Major PW. Am J Orthod Dentofacial Orthop 2003;123(4):388–94.

Orthognathic surgery

The effect of orthognathic surgery on the temporomandibular joint and oral function: a systematic review. Te Veldhuis EC, Te Veldhuis AH, Bramer WM, Wolvius EB, Koudstaal MJ. Int J Oral Maxillofac Surg. 2017 May;46(5):554–563.

Does temporomandibular joint pathology with or without surgical management affect the stability of counterclockwise rotation of the maxillomandibular complex in orthognathic surgery? A Systematic Review and Meta-Analysis. Al-Moraissi EA, Wolford LM. J Oral Maxillofac Surg. 2017 Apr;75(4):805–821.

Does orthognathic surgery cause or cure temporomandibular disorders? A systematic review and meta-analysis. Al-Moraissi EA, Wolford LM, Perez D, Laskin DM, Ellis E 3rd. J Oral Maxillofac Surg. 2017 Sep;75(9):1835–1847.

Orthognathic treatment of dentofacial disharmonies: its impact on temporomandibular disorders, quality of life, and psychosocial wellness. Song YL, Yap AU. Cranio. 2017 Jan;35(1):52–57.

Condylar resorption in orthognathic patients after mandibular bilateral sagittal split osteotomy: a systematic review. Mousoulea S, Kloukos D, Sampaziotis D, Vogiatzi T, Eliades T. Eur J Orthod. 2016 Jun 22:294–309.

Effects of mandibular advancement surgery on the temporomandibular joint and muscular and articular adaptive changes--a systematic review. Bermell-Baviera A, Bellot-Arcís C, Montiel-Company JM, Almerich-Silla JM. Int J Oral Maxillofac Surg. 2016 May;45(5):545–52.

TMJ response to mandibular advancement surgery: an overview of risk factors. Valladares-Neto J, Cevidanes LH, Rocha WC, Almeida Gde A, Paiva JB, Rino-Neto J. J Appl Oral Sci. 2014 Jan-Feb;22(1):2–14.

Orthognathic treatment and temporomandibular disorders: a systematic review. Part 2. Signs and symptoms and meta-analyses. Al-Riyami S, Cunningham SJ, Moles DR. Am J Orthod Dentofacial Orthop. 2009 Nov;136(5):626.e1–16.

Orthognathic treatment and temporomandibular disorders: A systematic review. Part 1. A new quality-assessment technique and analysis of study characteristics and classifications. Al-Riyami S, Cunningham SJ, Moles DR. Am J Orthod Dentofacial Orthop. 2009 Nov;136(5):624.e1–15.

Temporomandibular joint morphology changes with mandibular advancement surgery and rigid internal fixation: a systematic. literature review. Kersey ML, Nebbe B, Major PW. Angle Orthod 2003;73(1):79–85.

Osteoarthritis

Interventions for the management of temporomandibular joint osteoarthritis. de Souza RF, Lovato da Silva CH, Nasser M, Fedorowicz Z, Al-Muharraqi MA. Cochrane Database Syst Rev. 2012 Apr 18;(4):CD007261.

Third molars

Does orthodontic extraction treatment improve the angular position of third molars? A systematic review. Livas C, Delli K. J Oral Maxillofac Surg. 2017 Mar;75(3):475–483.

Orthodontic extraction of high-risk impacted mandibular third molars in close proximity to the mandibular canal: a systematic review. Kalantar Motamedi MR, Heidarpour M, Siadat S, Kalantar Motamedi A, Bahreman AA. J Oral Maxillofac Surg. 2015 Sep;73(9):1672–85.

The role of mandibular third molars on lower anterior teeth crowding and relapse after orthodontic treatment: a systematic review. Zawawi KH, Melis M. ScientificWorldJournal. 2014;2014:615429.

Is there justification for prophylactic extraction of third molars? A systematic review. Costa MG, Pazzini CA, Pantuzo MC, Jorge ML, Marques LS. Braz Oral Res. 2013 Mar-Apr;27(2):183–8.

Coronectomy vs. total removal for third molar extraction: a systematic review. Long H, Zhou Y, Liao L, Pyakurel U, Wang Y, Lai W. J Dent Res. 2012 Jul;91(7):659–65.

Surgical removal versus retention for the management of asymptomatic impacted wisdom teeth. Cochrane Database Syst Rev. 2012 Jun 13;(6):CD003879.

How predictable is the position of third molars over time? Phillips C, White RP Jr. J Oral Maxillofac Surg. 2012 Sep;70:S11–4.

The effectiveness and cost-effectiveness of prophylactic removal of wisdom teeth. Song F, O'Meara S, Wilson P, Golder S, Kleijnen J. Health Technol Assess 2000;4(15):1–55.

Transposition of teeth

Prevalence of tooth transposition. A meta-analysis. Papadopoulos MA, Chatzoudi M, Kaklamanos EG. Angle Orthod. 2010 Mar;80(2):275–85.

Assessment of characteristic features and dental anomalies accompanying tooth transposition: a meta-analysis. Papadopoulos MA, Chatzoudi M, Karagiannis V. Am J Orthod Dentofacial Orthop. 2009 Sep;136(3):308.e1–10.

Trauma

Please see Dental trauma.

Treatment time

Please also see Accelerated tooth movement.

Effectiveness of biologic methods of inhibiting orthodontic tooth movement in animal studies. Cadenas-Perula M, Yañez-Vico RM, Solano-Reina E, Iglesias-Linares A. Am J Orthod Dentofacial Orthop. 2016 Jul;150(1):33–48.

Escaping the adverse impacts of NSAIDs on tooth movement during orthodontics: current evidence based on a meta-analysis. Fang J, Li Y, Zhang K, Zhao Z, Mei L. Medicine (Baltimore). 2016 Apr;95(16):e3256.

How long does treatment with fixed orthodontic appliances last? A systematic review. Tsichlaki A, Chin SY, Pandis N, Fleming PS. Am J Orthod Dentofacial Orthop. 2016 Mar;149(3):308–18.

A systematic review of force decay in orthodontic elastomeric power chains. Halimi A, Benyahia H, Doukkali A, Azeroual MF, Zaoui F. Int Orthod. 2012 Sep;10(3):223–40.

Effects of bisphosphonates in orthodontic therapy: systematic review. Rodolfino D, Saccucci M, Filippakos A, Gerxhani R, Lopez G, Felice F, D'Arcangelo C. J Biol Regul Homeost Agents. 2012 Apr-Jun;26(2 Suppl):29–33.

Influence of bisphosphonates in orthodontic therapy: Systematic review. Iglesias-Linares A, Yanez-Vico RM, Solano-Reina E, Torres-Lagares D, Gonzalez Moles MA. J Dent. 2010 Aug;38(8):603–11.

Hyalinization during orthodontic tooth movement: a systematic review on tissue reactions. von Bhl M, Kuijpers-Jagtman AM. Eur J Orthod. 2009 Feb;31(1):30–6.

Factors influencing efficiency of sliding mechanics to close extraction space: a systematic review. Barlow M, Kula K. Orthod Craniofac Res. 2008 May;11(2):65–73.

Factors affecting the duration of orthodontic treatment: a systematic review. Mavreas D, Athanasiou AE. Eur J Orthod. 2008 Aug;30(4):386–95.

Vacuum formed thermoplastic retainers

Please see Retention and relapse.

White spot lesions

Please also see Caries.

Interventions for orthodontically induced white spot lesions: a systematic review and meta-analysis. Hochli D, Hersberger-Zurfluh M, Papageorgiou SN, Eliades T. Eur J Orthod. 2017 Apr 1;39(2):122–133.

Management of post-orthodontic white spot lesions: an updated systematic review. Sonesson M, Bergstrand F, Gizani S, Twetman S. Eur J Orthod. 2017 Apr 1;39(2):116–121.

Therapies for white spot lesions-a systematic review. Paula AB, Fernandes AR, Coelho AS, Marto CM, Ferreira MM, Caramelo F, do Vale F, Carrilho E.J Evid Based Dent Pract. 2017 Mar;17(1):23–38.

Prevention and treatment of white spot lesions during and after treatment with fixed orthodontic appliances: a systematic literature review. Lopatiene K, Borisovaite M, Lapenaite E. J Oral Maxillofac Res. 2016 Jun 30;7(2):e1.

Fluoride-releasing materials to prevent white spot lesions around orthodontic brackets: a systematic review. Nascimento PL, Fernandes MT, Figueiredo FE, Faria-E-Silva AL. Braz Dent J. 2016 Jan-Feb;27(1):101–7.

Influence of orthodontic treatment with fixed appliances on enamel color: a systematic review. Chen Q, Zheng X, Chen W, Ni Z, Zhou Y.BMC Oral Health. 2015 Mar 10;15:31.

Long-term remineralizing effect of casein phosphopeptide-amorphous calcium phosphate (CPP-ACP) on early caries lesions in vivo: a systematic review. Li J, Xie X, Wang Y, Yin W, Antoun JS, Farella M, Mei L. J Dent. 2014 Jul;42(7):769–77.

Fluorides for the prevention of early tooth decay (demineralised white lesions) during fixed brace treatment. Benson PE, Parkin N, Dyer F, Millett DT, Furness S, Germain P. Cochrane Database Syst Rev. 2013 Dec 12;(12):CD003809.

Bisphenol-A and residual monomer leaching from orthodontic adhesive resins and polycarbonate brackets: a systematic review Kloukos D, Pandis N, Eliades T. Am J Orthod Dentofacial Orthop. 2013 Apr;143(4 Suppl):S104–12. e1–2.

Effect of remineralizing agents on white spot lesions after orthodontic treatment: a systematic review. Chen H, Liu X, Dai J, Jiang Z, Guo T, Ding Y. Am J Orthod Dentofacial Orthop. 2013 Mar;143(3):376–382.

Fluoride-containing orthodontic adhesives and decalcification in patients with fixed appliances: a systematic review. Rogers S, Chadwick B, Treasure E. Am J Orthod Dentofacial Orthop. 2010 Oct;138(4):390.e1–8.

The effect of topical fluorides on decalcification in patients with fixed orthodontic appliances: a systematic review. Chadwick BL, Roy J, Knox J, Treasure ET. Am J Orthod Dentofacial Orthop. 2005 Nov;128(5):601–6.

Fluorides, orthodontics and demineralization: a systematic review - More recent review. Benson PE, Shah AA, Millett DT, Dyer F, Parkin N, Vine RS. J Orthod. 2005 Jun;32(2):102–14.

Caries-inhibiting effect of preventive measures during orthodontic treatment with fixed appliances. a systematic review Derks A, Katsaros C, Frencken JE, Van't Hof MA, Kuijpers-Jagtman AM. Caries Res 2004;38(5):413–20.

Index

Page numbers in *italics* refer to figures.
Page numbers in **bold** refer to tables.
The suffix "r" indicates that page or page range has literature references only.

Evidence-Based Orthodontics, Second Edition. Edited by Greg J. Huang, Stephen Richmond and Katherine W. L. Vig.
© 2018 John Wiley & Sons, Inc. Published 2018 by John Wiley & Sons, Inc.